A Dictionary *of* Epidemiology

A Dictionary *of* Epidemiology

Fifth Edition

Edited for the
International Epidemiological Association
by
Miquel Porta
Professor of Preventive Medicine & Public Health
School of Medicine, Universitat Autònoma de Barcelona
Senior Scientist, Institut Municipal d'Investigació Mèdica
Barcelona, Spain
Adjunct Professor of Epidemiology, School of Public Health
University of North Carolina at Chapel Hill

Associate Editors
Sander Greenland
John M. Last

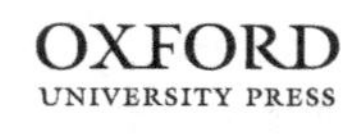

2008

OXFORD
UNIVERSITY PRESS

Oxford University Press, Inc., publishes works that further
Oxford University's objective excellence
in research, scholarship, and education

Oxford New York
Auckland Cape Town Dar es Salaam Hong Kong Karachi
Kuala Lumpur Madrid Melbourne Mexico City Nairobi
Shanghai Taipei Toronto

With offices in
Argentina Austria Brazil Chile Czech Republic France Greece
Guatemala Hungary Italy Japan Poland Portugal Singapore
South Korea Switzerland Thailand Turkey Ukraine Vietnam

Published by Oxford University Press, Inc.
198 Madison Avenue, New York, New York 10016
www.oup-usa.org

This edition was prepared with support from
Esteve Foundation (Barcelona, Catalonia, Spain)
(http://www.esteve.org)

Library of Congress Cataloging-in-Publication Data
A dictionary of epidemiology /
edited for the International Epidemiological Association
by Miquel Porta;
associate editors, John M. Last . . . [et al.].—5th ed.
p. cm. Includes bibliographical references and index.
ISBN 978-0-19-531449-6 ISBN 978-0-19-531450-2 (pbk.)
1. Epidemiology—Dictionaries.
I. Porta, Miquel–
II. International Epidemiological Association.
RA651.D553 2000
614.4′03—dc21 00-037504

8 9

Printed in the United States of America
on acid-free paper

Foreword

To write a dictionary in any scientific discipline is a risky endeavor, because scientists often disagree. The nature of science is not to reach consensus but to advance our knowledge by bringing conflicting ideas to critical examinations. That is true also for how we define the concepts we use. No dictionary will ever be able to satisfy all, nor should it try to.

The aim of the International Epidemiological Association (IEA) in cosponsoring this dictionary in its more than 20 years' history has been to facilitate communication among epidemiologists—to develop a "common language" to the extent that this is possible. We need a common language when we write papers, teach, and communicate findings to the public.

This "common language" changes over time, as anybody can see by reading the successive editions of this dictionary. The language changes because our understanding of the concepts changes over time and new research options bring forward new concepts.

From the IEA, we want to thank John Last for his tremendous achievements as editor of the dictionary, and we are happy to welcome Miquel Porta as the new editor. Miquel has provided the smooth transition we were looking for, and we are pleased to see that he continues the tradition of collaborating with leading epidemiologists worldwide to get the best possible result.

Jørn Olsen, Neil Pearce, and Chitr Sitthi-Amorn
Current, coming, and past presidents,
International Epidemiological Association
www.ieaweb.org

Foreword to the Fourth Edition, 2001

IF I HAD TO LIMIT MY PROFESSIONAL BOOKCASE TO A SINGLE VOLUME, I WOULD choose this dictionary. With many new entries, updates, and other refinements in the fourth edition, the dictionary has grown from the original slim pocket book into a mature and substantial volume. John Last and his collaborators must be congratulated for their extraordinary devotion and productivity over the past 20 years, from which epidemiologists around the world have benefited.

The dictionary's authority stems from its international recognition. It is an immediate source for students and practitioners to verify their understanding of the increasing number of technical words in epidemiologic practice. It clarifies concepts that may not have been understood in class, fills many gaps in anyone's education, and jogs the memory of near-forgotten terms. It has no equal in the field of epidemiology.

The International Epidemiological Association is proud to have had such a long-standing association with the dictionary. We all hope this relationship will continue indefinitely in the future, even though John Last, being mortal, will not. He has set a high standard for his successors. We are grateful that he has prepared the way so well to ensure that the dictionary remains of contemporary relevance in the coming decades.

Charles du V. Florey
President, 1999–2002
International Epidemiological Association
www.ieaweb.org

Preface

THERE WAS VIRTUALLY NO GOOGLE, AND NO WIKIPEDIA THEN, SEEMINGLY CENTURIES ago, when the previous edition of this dictionary came out in 2001. And of the respected dictionaries, very little was "posted on the Internet." Hard to believe. How did we manage, how could we ever have worked? But we did, we surely did: with open minds, critical sense, intellectual rigor. . . . No *google* or *wiki* or information technology (IT) whatsoever will change that. The need to do the epidemiological work with "that."

Now we have thousands of webs and wikis with millions of papers, definitions, and discussions regarding terms at our very fingertips. Many are truly authoritative. You'll find them – some, selected – duly referenced at the end of this book. Yes, we googled and used the Wikipedia, "surfed" and "visited" many remote, beautiful places. To surf, to post . . . whew, these terms will soon be obsolete, won't they?

We continue to seek and to find *meaning:* in PubMed/Medline, in online textbooks and websites. Foremost, within the main dictionaries,[1–3] which we read often while writing this new edition, and which I hope you will always use in case of doubt or simply to enrich the definitions that we offer here (See pages 265 and 273–289). At—and through—"places" such as HighWire, ScienceDirect, Scopus, SciELO, ProQuest, Synergy, ISI Web of knowledge, Google, Yahoo, Live Search . . . what yesterday was an unthinkable utopia has become an "achievable utopia," in many places actually achieved daily: the infinite library, and with it the unlimited dictionary too. I wish Borges were alive to enjoy it, if not actually to see it, since he was blind.

So what sense does it make, to craft a dictionary? Simple: in a radically new way, the "IEA dictionary," "Last's dictionary" can be as relevant—or more so—as it has been before. Because we have again, as always, critically listened and read, thought, discussed, and *selected* terms, meanings and definitions. With "that": open minds, critical sense, common sense, intellectual rigor, creativity, flexibility, craftsmanship. . . . And because nowadays, with more "noise" than ever in history, sifting, decanting—selection with "that"—is more valuable than ever before.

You will judge, but writing this dictionary confirmed to me that it was perfectly feasible to achieve a normative purpose and an informative one. With help of the highest possible academic level from many colleagues (duly acknowledged later), I tried to integrate two approaches to dictionary making: expert-opinion-based prescription (to aid production) and corpus-based description (to aid decoding).[395] Meanings of scientific terms need to be proposed —and may occasionally be imposed—on the basis of expert advice; yet experts and specialists can also keep an ear for actual usage, from which meanings must also be extracted. When we were choosing terms and meanings, we not only kept epidemiological theory and general logic in mind, but usage as well, and often attested explicitly the different uses of polysemic terms. The word "dictionary" is itself notoriously polysemic.[395] This book shows how comfortable the coexistence of diverse meanings of "dictionary" can be. More importantly, it also shows a healthy "micropolysemic" variation[395] in the terms and definitions. This edition also reflects, I believe, how plural—professionally, scientifically, culturally, and ideologically—epidemiologists are. John Last's outstanding first four editions were themselves the result of a highly comprehensive and inclusive process of selection of terms and definitions: some 20 years of fantastic collaborative work by several hundred contributors since the early 1980s. The five editions are an extraordinary "record" —a "DVD," if you wish, or an "mp4"— of the evolution of epidemiology during the last quarter century. I think they are also excellent materials for a sociology of epidemiology.

Therefore, as we continued the process and revised the last edition, we kept well in mind many types of reader, most with unimaginable resources, smart, "IT-wise." Although you are cordially invited to pull the many strings that this book holds by simply reading and turning its pages with your fingers (odd and familiar as this may at once seem), we assumed that these pages were just a stop on your journey: perhaps you just came here from Oxford Reference Online and will next be at The Cochrane Library. Who could know? You know.

Not only can you always expand and progress on what you find here, we know you can always assess, contrast, verify. Quite a responsibility for an editor of a dictionary. This duty is not new, but it surely works on a different scale nowadays. It is now so easy to find that we were wrong, narrow-minded, off beam, too punctilious . . .

In the meantime, the ancestral book and our beloved library have not died. Neither did the paper journal. News of the death of academic journals—loudly proclaimed in the early years of this, the long awaited twenty-first century—were premature. We therefore may hope that this book will again find a place in your mind and be close to your heart. It's light in weight, its pages will welcome your handwriting, it can be comfortably read out there in the sunlight—batteries are not needed.

* * *

My call for contributions to this 5th edition was widely disseminated beginning early in 2006—prominently, in the International Journal of Epidemiology and the Newsletter of the International Epidemiological Association (IEA), the worldwide scientific organization of epidemiologists that has nurtured all editions. The call was operationally answered by 224 professionals who registered in the wiki that we had set up with Oxford University Press. When invited to choose the sentence that best described their professional relationship with epidemiology, 67% of respondents selected "I have some to extensive training in epidemiology and currently work or have professional experience as an epidemiologist [you may also have professional experience in other fields]," 27% answered "While my main job is not as an epidemiologist, I often use epidemiologic knowledge, methods or reasoning in my work," 2% selected "I have little to no training in epidemiology and I seldom or never use it in my work [your contribution is nevertheless welcomed]," and 4% "Other." These data provide a factual background for the next paragraphs.

Is this dictionary an attempt to *demarcate* epidemiology neatly? I don't think so. Or I'd rather think it is not, to the extent that a dictionary can—or needs to—avoid demarcating a discipline.[4] Yet like many other scientists, every now and then epidemiologists engage in boundary-making endeavors and disciplinary demarcation. And then, as usual in other disciplines, epidemiologists assert or reclaim contested epistemic authority and may claim jurisdiction over areas of public health, medicine, statistics, or science. These efforts evolved in the course of the twentieth century while epidemiology developed as a very diverse, eclectic—and foremost, *integrative*—field of practice and academic discipline.[4–12] And so will they evolve as the societies of the twenty-first century continue developing. There is nothing wrong with that, it is the *natural* thing.

Is this dictionary an epistemic space? Well, of course it is, in the broadest sense: a space of knowledge. Does it belong to an epistemic community or to more than one? Both answers are true. It belongs to one very diverse community of knowledge—epidemiologists around the globe. And to a lesser but no less important extent, the dictionary pertains also to the many communities of knowledge that interact and cooperate with epidemiology, or with which epidemiology cooperates, or that simply use epidemiological reasoning, knowledge, methods, or techniques.

No matter how many mistakes we may have made (eventually, they are all my responsibility), I would like to think that in making this new edition we again practiced a high level of scientific and intellectual rigor in two opposite and complementary directions: (1) in selecting and defining terms that are at the ontological, epistemological, and methodological core of epidemiology, and (2) in selecting and defining terms that are near or within disciplines with which epidemiology maintains vital interactions—vital for epidemiology, the other disciplines, science, and society.

These I take to be facts: today research methods with strong epidemiological roots and properties are fruitfully applied "within" and "outside" epidemiology. A positive blurring of the boundaries of epidemiological research methods occurred in the last decades of the last century; e.g., the integration of population thinking and group comparison into clinical and public health research.[10] The expansion of this influence toward other research areas remains a significant—and in my view highly attractive—challenge for many scientists. Such an expansion of influence will not be identical to what occurred via clinical epidemiology and, later, evidence-based medicine and, today, evidence-based health care. The nature of the hypotheses at stake is often quite different in clinical medicine than in, say, molecular biology or proteomics. Largely because of this ontological fact, because biotechnologies generate and drive different types and amounts of information and research, and for other reasons, today epidemiological thinking continues to create new approaches, research designs, strategies of analysis, and ways to assess causality for such biological disciplines. Thus the influence of epidemiology continues. The potential to improve the health of citizens is there. In fact, the rationale for task (2) mentioned above also includes the relevance of epidemiological methods for research on the public health problems that are best tackled by blending the reasoning and the tools of epidemiology and of some of the social sciences. Therefore, this new edition aims at being useful not only to classic epidemiological and clinical research, but would also like to continue favoring the integration of epidemiology into "microbiological" and "macrosocial" health research and practice. I am confident and content that much of this is already happening, and thus feel this book is rather in harmony with most of the contemporary scientific world: wide open and interconnected—much more creative, relevant, efficient, and interesting because of the porousness and plasticity of the disciplines than because of the putative higher mission or language of their leaders and disciples.

In short, if you live in a foreign land and have come to visit this book from "outside" epidemiology, be welcome. If you are an epidemiologist on the eve of a "trip" to a foreign discipline, please take this book with you. And, again, if you mostly work "inside" epidemiology, please keep it at hand: this is your territory—yet I hope you will here discover new landscapes of unsuspected beauty.

Miquel Porta
January 2008
Barcelona

Preface to the Fourth Edition, 2001

DICTIONARY-MAKING, LIKE PAINTING THE SYDNEY HARBOUR BRIDGE, NEVER ENDS. As soon as an edition goes into production, I open a file for amendments to be made in the next one. Formal preparation of this edition began in April 1999, when I distributed by e-mail and airmail a list of proposed items to about 80 correspondents around the world. I sent an expanded list to more than 100 correspondents in June 1999, and in August 1999 I sent more items and questions to about 130 correspondents. Finally, in January 2000, I asked a small group—Janet Byron Anderson, Iain Chalmers, Gary Friedman, Sander Greenland, Susan Harris, Ian McDowell, Miquel Porta, Bob Spasoff, Mervyn Susser, Michel Thuriaux, and Don Wigle—to review the new and revised old entries. The entire process is as open and iterative as practical realities allow. The wording of many definitions has been refined in light of repeated discussions with many participants. This edition contains the fruits of these labors—amounting to more than 150 new items and about as many revisions of existing entries. There are more citations and statements about the provenance of terminology than in previous editions and several new illustrations. A few items previously included and several illustrations have been dropped. There are some notes for users. The acronyms have been integrated into the text.

As in previous editions, flexibility in the use of technical terms is implied, although preferred usage is suggested by placement of detailed entries. The guiding principle has been to create a dictionary that is authoritative but not authoritarian. The improvements in this revision reflect the help of all those named here and others not named. All the shortcomings are mine.

John M. Last
Ottawa, May 2000

Acknowledgments

It is a pleasure and a privilege to thank each and all individuals throughout the world who volunteered to contribute terms, definitions, or other ideas for this dictionary: never before had I enjoyed such a large, diverse, and creative group of coauthors. Thanks! I trust you will understand that I could not always make all your scientific, linguistic, and lexicographic dreams come true. And I very much hope you will have fun skimming through the pages that follow.

It is equally a joy and an honor to thank all members of the International Epidemiological Association (IEA), and in their name, especially, past, current or coming presidents Rodolfo Saracci, Charles du V. Florey, Chitr Sitthi-Amorn, Jørn Olsen, and Neil Pearce for their intellectual stimulus, personal encouragement, and institutional support in editing this book.

I feel extremely fortunate that Sander Greenland and John Last accepted my personal invitation to work as associate editors and that they offered extremely valuable contributions; I am sure that readers—some, perhaps unknowingly—will be equally fortunate: a lot in this volume is due to John and Sander. It is also my great pleasure to give special thanks to Miguel A. Hernán and Vasily Vlassov for their extremely thoughtful, insightful, and practical contributions, many made speedily and when it seemed impossible to achieve clarity for particularly complex or unusual terms. For what I have made of the advice of all contributors, and for any errors, I alone am responsible.

Warm thanks are also due to the linguistic and lexicographic consultants, Janet Byron Anderson (fourth edition), Lluís Quintana, Albert Rico and David J. MacFarlane (fifth edition). Skilled editorial assistance was kindly and efficiently provided by Joan Pau Millet, Eva Morales, Tomas Lopez and Silvia Geeraerd.

This edition was prepared with support from an unrestricted grant from the Esteve Foundation (Barcelona, Catalonia, Spain), a nonprofit, internationally focused institution with the primary goal of fostering progress in pharmacotherapy. Some operational costs were absorbed in our budget at the Institut Municipal d'Investigació Mèdica (IMIM) and at the Universitat Autònoma de Barcelona, for which I am also grateful.

Like many other human beings for centuries, I continue to treasure my love—both emotional and practical—for books, and have come to experience a somewhat peculiar bliss in reading prophecies on the death of the book. I am, therefore, so glad to acknowledge everyone at Oxford University Press, who with their outstanding editorial competence and wisdom also *made* this book. I dedicate it to the youngest generation of health scientists and advocates; and to Anna, Júlia, and Joan.

M. P.

About This Dictionary

(Advice on how best to use it)

Alphabetical Listing

The alphabetical listing is a guide to the placement of entries and follows a letter-by-letter sequence of headwords without regard to word spacing, hyphens, or apostrophes. For example:

Case classification
Case-control study
Case finding
Case-only study
Case-specular design
Case-time-control design

Headwords

Headwords are in bold small capitals. If there are several varieties of a concept, such as *bias*, all are listed alphabetically under the headword **BIAS**; but when customary epidemiological usage places an adjective before the headword, the alphabetical listing is usually a cross-reference to the entry where the definition is to be found. Thus **BIAS, CONFOUNDING** leads the user to the definition under **CONFOUNDING BIAS**. However, terms on the periphery of epidemiology are mostly located together under the pertinent headword. For example, most of those associated with *costs* appear under **COST**.

Compound Phrases

Epidemiology has many compound phrases, not all of which have an obvious headword. Thus *rare disease assumption* is found under **RARE**, not under disease.

Citations

In this edition all citations of articles and books have been moved to the back of the book (See pages 273–289). This allowed us to avoid repetition—some books and articles are cited several times. Most citations are just meant to help the reader follow-up on the definition; they just aim to *evoke* or *suggest* further avenues of thought. They cannot be and are not exhaustive. None is meant to endorse the definition or the comment. No citation is meant either to imply that an article or book is the original or most authoritative source on the issue. Many cited books will provide additional help on additional terms, that is, in definitions where they are not cited; this is particularly the case for definitions of terms on epidemiological methods.

Acronyms

There is no generally agreed way to pronounce or print acronyms, but some usages are commonly agreed. Thus, for instance, WHO is always spelled out in pronunciation ("W-H-O"), never pronounced "Hoo." By contrast, AIDS is always pronounced "Aids" and never spelled out. Acronyms can be made up of the initial letters of the words on which they are based, such as NIOSH (National Institute for Occupational Safety and Health, pronounced Ny-osh), or on parts of words or abbreviations, such as QUANGO (quasi-autonomous nongovernmental organization). Acronyms can survive after the organization they signify has changed names. UNICEF originally stood for United Nations International Children's Emergency Fund. This UN agency is now called the United Nations Children's Fund, but the acronym is unchanged. Generally, all the letters of an acronym are upper case, even when not all the letters are initial letters of individual words, so ANOVA, analysis of variance, is spelled as here, not AnOVa, although Anova is sometimes seen.

Cross-References

Most cross-references identified in the text of the definitions are in nonbold small capitals. Other important words and phrases mentioned in a definition are sometimes italicized to draw attention to their special significance in relation to that particular term and to signify the absence of a cross-reference. Cross-references are again just meant to *suggest*—to invite the reader to take a look elsewhere in the book. They are not exhaustive; a term may appear in another part of the book and yet not be marked in nonbold small capitals (one common reason for that is to avoid a baroque or visually confusing sentence).

Definitions and Discussions

A brief definition generally appears at the beginning of each entry. This usually follows dictionary conventions and is a statement of the meaning rather than an explanation. However, there are many discussions and, occasionally, illustrative examples and remarks on the provenance of terms. Admonitions and cautionary notes about use and abuse of terms have been kept to a minimum.

Evolving Language and Changing Usage

English and its technical varieties are evolving and changing, as do virtually all societies worldwide—and foremost the Internet and the virtual society. We aimed at sensibly respecting all sensitivities, and we found no major difficulties in doing so while at the same time ensuring precision and avoiding ambiguity in scientific communication.

Epidemiology is expanding and budding off subspecialties, each of which has its own vocabulary, terms, and meanings, adapting old words and phrases to new uses, creating its own neologisms. Epidemiology regularly absorbs, transforms, and embodies terms from other fields: as a living organism, it actively metabolizes language. We have tried to capture and present the *essential* terminology of clinical, environmental, genetic, social, and molecular epidemiology as well as core terms from pediatric epidemiology, pharmaco-epidemiology, and some other subspecialties of epidemiology. Of course, we did not wish to lengthen the book too much. Thus, the reader will sometimes need to go to the specialty books in seeking definitions of highly specialized terms. Finally, some common everyday words are defined and discussed because they often occur in epidemiological articles with a distinct meaning, they are particularly relevant to conduct health research, or because their sense is not always clear in these contexts to people whose first language is not English. Words and phrases from disciplines that overlap or interact with epidemiology are defined here for the same reasons.

We have tried to be highly rigorous, systematic, thorough, and to a reasonable extent, explicit and transparent; yet when necessary, these goals gave precedence to the primary objective: that the dictionary should be practical and plural, and that it should encourage critical and creative thinking.

M. P. and J. M. L.

Contributors to the Fourth and Fifth Editions

IBRAHIM ABDELNOUR
Damascus, Syria
THEO ABELIN
Berne, Switzerland
JOE ABRAMSON
Jerusalem, Israel
ANDERS AHLBOM
Stockholm, Sweden
MOHAMED FAROUK ALLAM
Córdoba, Spain
ÁLVARO ALONSO
Minneapolis, Minnesota, USA
DOUGLAS ALTMAN
London, England, UK
JANET BYRON ANDERSON
Rocky River, Ohio, USA
KUNIO AOKI
Nagoya, Japan
HAROUTUNE ARMENIAN
Baltimore, Maryland, USA, and Yerevan, Armenia
MARY JANE ASHLEY
Toronto, Ontario, Canada
JOHN BAILAR III
Chicago, Illinois, USA
MICHAEL BAKER
Wellington, New Zealand
OLGA BASSO
Aarhus, Denmark
RENALDO BATTISTA
Montreal, Quebec, Canada
ROBERT BEAGLEHOLE
Auckland, New Zealand, and Geneva, Switzerland
SOLOMON BENATAR
Cape Town, South Africa
YOAV BEN-SHLOMO
Bristol, England, UK
ROGER BERNIER
Atlanta, Georgia, USA
RAJ BHOPAL
Edinburgh, Scotland, UK
NICHOLAS BIRKETT
Ottawa, Ontario, Canada
DANKMAR BÖHNING
Berlin, Germany
JEAN-FRANÇOIS BOIVIN
Montreal, Quebec, Canada
DAVID BONIFACE
London, England, UK
KNUT BORCH-JOHNSEN
Horsholm, Denmark
RIC BOUVIER
Kew, Victoria, Australia
ANNETTE BRAUNACK-MAYER
Adelaide, South Australia, Australia
CLIVE BROWN
Port of Spain, Trinidad and Tobago
ROSS BROWNSON
St. Louis, Missouri, USA
JIM BUTLER
Canberra, ACT, Australia
LEE CAPLAN
Atlanta, Georgia, USA
IAIN CHALMERS
Oxford, England, UK
YUE CHEN
Ottawa, Ontario, Canada
BERNARD CHOI
Ottawa, Ontario, Canada
STELLA CHUNGONG
Geneva, Switzerland
MIKE CLARKE
Oxford, England, UK
TAMMY CLIFFORD
London, Ontario, Canada

Philip Cole
Birmingham, Alabama, USA
Deborah Cook
Hamilton, Ontario, Canada
Doug Coyle
Ottawa, Ontario, Canada
Andrew Creese
Geneva, Switzerland
George Davey Smith
Bristol, England, UK
Silvia Declich
Rome, Italy
Del De Hart
Saginaw, Michigan, USA
Julia del Amo
Madrid, Spain
N. S. Deodhar
Pune, India
Bob Douglas
Canberra, ACT, Australia
Gerard Dubois
Amiens, France
John Duffus
Edinburgh, Scotland, UK
Kate Dunn
Keele, Newcastle, UK
Mark Elwood
Melbourne, Victoria, Australia
Leon Epstein
Jerusalem, Israel
Alvan Feinstein
New Haven, Connecticut, USA
Charles Florey
Sidmouth, England, UK
Erica Frank
Atlanta, Georgia, USA
Rayner Fretzel-Behme
Bremen, Germany
Gary Friedman
Oakland, California, USA
B. Burt Gerstman
San Jose, California, USA
Alan Gibbs
Manchester, England, UK
Philippe Grandjean
Odense, Denmark
Nicola Grandy
Paris, France
Sander Greenland
Los Angeles, California, USA
Duane Gubler
Atlanta, Georgia, USA
Charles Guest
Canberra, ACT, Australia
Tee Guidotti
Washington, DC, USA
Gordon Guyatt
Hamilton, Ontario, Canada
Philip Hall
Winnipeg, Manitoba, Canada
Philip Hannaford
Aberdeen, Scotland, UK
Susan Harris
Boston, Massachusetts, USA
Maureen Hatch
New York, New York, USA
Brian Haynes
Hamilton, Ontario, Canada
Miguel Hernán
Boston, Massachusetts, USA
Ildefonso Hernández
Maó, Menorca, Spain
Andrew Herxheimer
Edinburgh, Scotland, UK
Basil Hetzel
Adelaide, South Australia, Australia
Alan Hinman
Decatur, Georgia, USA
Walter Holland
London, England, UK
María-Graciela Hollm-Delgado
Montreal, Quebec, Canada
D'Arcy Holman
Perth, Western Australia, Australia
Ernest Hook
Berkeley, California, USA
Jeffrey House
San Francisco, California, USA
Konrad Jamrozik
Perth, Western Australia, Australia
Mohsen Janghorbani
Isfahan, Iran

TOM JEFFERSON
Camberley, England, UK
MILOS JENICEK
Rockwood, Ontario, Canada
MUSTAFA KHOGALI
Beirut, Lebanon
DANIEL KIM
Boston, Massachusetts, USA
MAURICE KING
Leeds, England, UK
TORD KJELLSTRÖM
Auckland, New Zealand
DAN KREWSKI
Ottawa, Ontario, Canada
NINO KÜNZLI
Barcelona, Catalonia, Spain
DIANA KUH
London, England, UK
CHANDRAKANT LAHARIYA,
New Delhi, India
STEPHEN LAMBERT
Melbourne, Victoria, Australia
HENK LAMBERTS
Amsterdam, Netherlands
RON LAPORTE
Pittsburgh, Pennsylvania, USA
JOHN LAST
Ottawa, Ontario, Canada
DIANA LAUDERDALE
Chicago, Illinois, USA
ABBY LIPPMAN
Montreal, Quebec, Canada
IRVINE LOUDON
Oxford, England, UK
SHI LUYAN
Wuhan, China
JOHAN MACKENBACH
Rotterdam, Netherlands
AHMID MANDIL
Dammam, Saudi Arabia
ARTURO MARTÍ-CARVAJAL
Valencia, Venezuela
JOHN MCCALLUM
Canberra, ACT, Australia
IAN MCDOWELL
Ottawa, Ontario, Canada
ROBERT MCKEOWN
Columbia, South Carolina, USA
RICK MCLEAN
Melbourne, Victoria, Australia
TONY MCMICHAEL
Canberra, Australia
CURTIS MEINERT
Baltimore, Maryland, USA
JAIME MIRANDA
London, England, UK
DAVID MOHER
Ottawa, Ontario, Canada
ALFREDO MORABIA
New York, New York, USA
SALAH MOSTAFA
Cairo, Egypt
NORMAN NOAH
London, England, UK
PATRICIA O'CAMPO
Baltimore, Maryland, USA
JØRN OLSEN
Aarhus, Denmark
NIGEL PANETH
Ann Arbor, Michigan, USA
SKIP PAYNE
Tiffin, Ohio, USA
NEIL PEARCE
Wellington, New Zealand
DIANA PETITTI
Sierra Madre, California, USA
AILEEN PLANT
Perth, Western Australia, Australia
MIQUEL PORTA
Barcelona, Catalonia, Spain
ZORAN RADOVANOVIC
Safat, Kuwait and Belgrade, Yugoslavia
MATI RAHU
Tallinn, Estonia
GLORIA RAMIREZ
Santiago de Chile, Chile
JOSE RIGAU
Atlanta, Georgia, USA
CHRIS RISSELL
Sydney, New South Wales, Australia
KEN ROTHMAN
Boston, Massachusetts, USA

MICHAEL RYAN
Geneva, Switzerland
LUCIE RYCHETNIK
Sydney, New South Wales, Australia
RODOLFO SARACCI
Lyon, France
DAVID SAVITZ
New York, New York, USA
PATHOM SAWANPANYALERT
Bangkok, Thailand
SABINE SCHIPF
Hamburg, Germany
FRAN SCOTT
Hamilton, Ontario, Canada
JACK SIEMIATYCKI
Laval, Quebec, Canada
CHITR SITTHI-AMORN
Bangkok, Thailand
BJÖRN SMEDBY
Uppsala, Sweden
CYNTHIA SONICH-MULLIN
Paris, France
COLIN SOSKOLNE
Edmonton, Alberta, Canada
BOB SPASOFF
Ottawa, Ontario, Canada
HANS STORM
Copenhagen, Denmark
DAVID STREINER
Hamilton, Ontario, Canada
EZRA SUSSER
New York, New York, USA
MERVYN SUSSER
New York, New York, USA
KAZUO TAJIMA
Nagoya, Japan
JOSÉ A. TAPIA
Ann Arbor, Michigan, USA
MICHEL THURIAUX
Geneva, Switzerland
KAREN TROLLOPE-KUMAR
Hamilton, Ontario, Canada
ELENA TSCHISHOWA
Berlin, Germany
JAN VANDENBROUCKE
Utrecht, Netherlands
HECTOR VELASCO
Baltimore, Maryland, USA, and Cuernavaca, Mexico
SALLY VERNON
Houston, Texas, USA
VASILY VLASSOV
Moscow, Russia
DOUGLAS L. WEED
Washington, DC, USA
DENISE WERKER
Ottawa, Ontario, Canada
CLAES-GÖRAN WESTRIN
Uppsala, Sweden
FRANK WHITE
Karachi, Pakistan
KERR WHITE
Charlottesville, Virginia, USA
P. AUKE WIEGERSMA
Groningen, The Netherlands
DON WIGLE
Ottawa, Ontario, Canada
ALLEN WILCOX
Research Triangle Park, North Carolina, USA
MICHAEL WOLFSON
Ottawa, Ontario, Canada
HIROSHI YANAGAWA
Jiichi, Japan
KUE YOUNG
Winnipeg, Manitoba, Canada

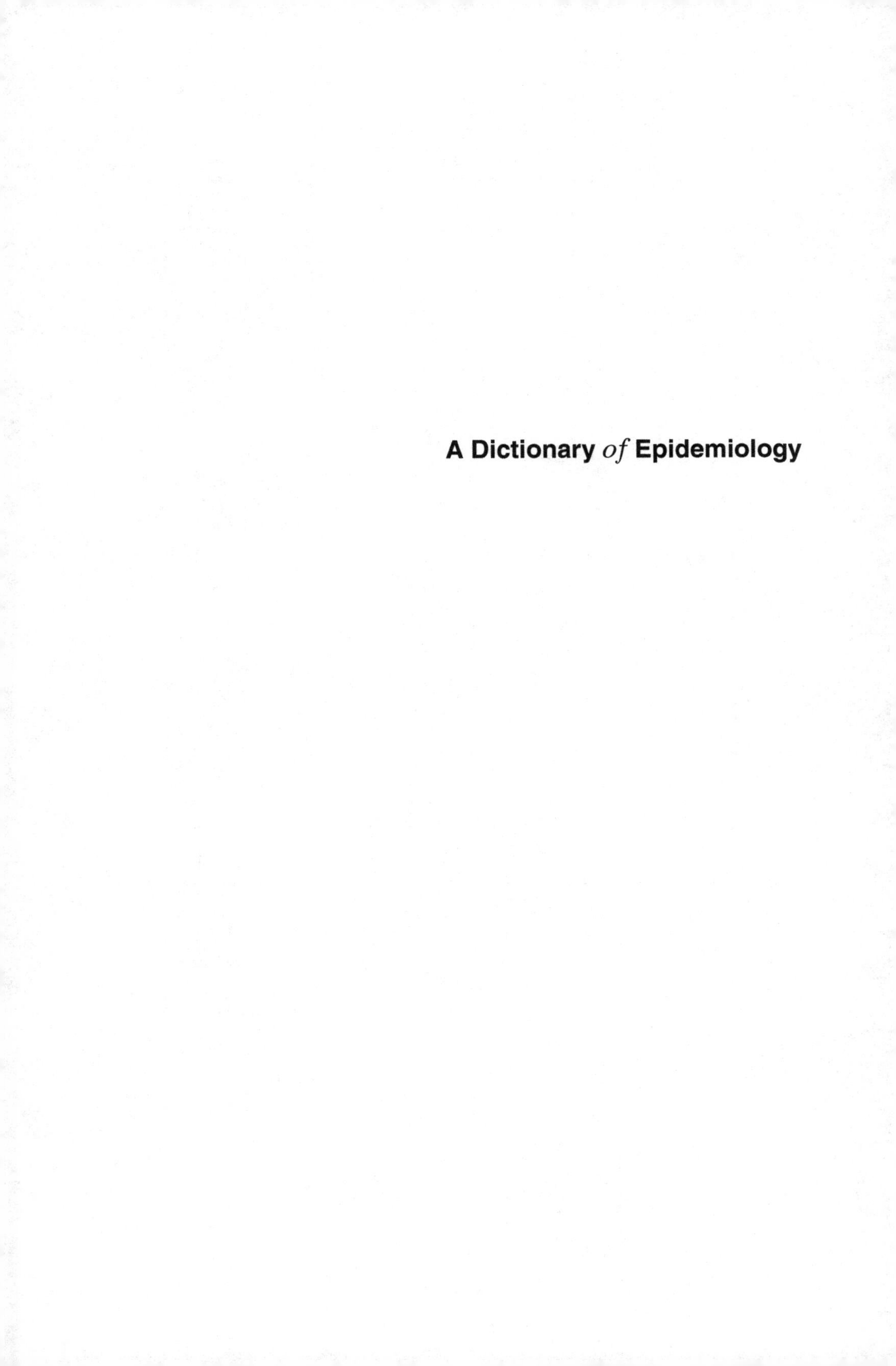

A Dictionary *of* Epidemiology

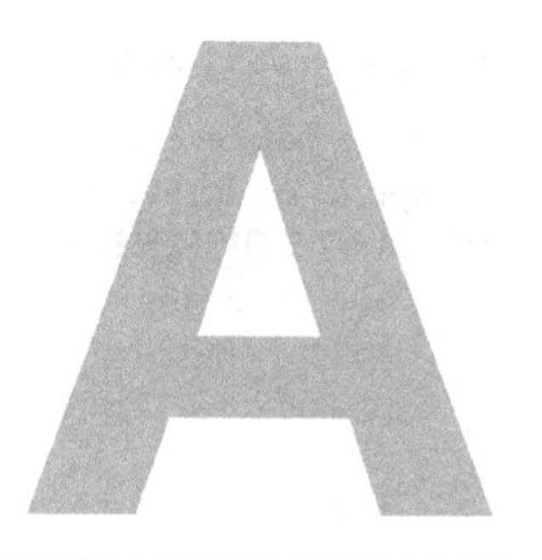

ABATEMENT The process of reducing or minimizing public health dangers and nuisances, usually supported by regulation or legislation; e.g., noise abatement, pollution abatement.

ABC APPROACH "Abstinence, Be faithful, use Condoms." ABC strategies are promoted to combat, foremost, infection with HIV and the HIV/AIDS pandemic as well as other sexually transmitted diseases. These are pragmatic sex education policies that aim at balancing abstinence-only sex education by including education about safe sex and birth control methods. Excessive emphasis on ABC strategies may marginalize broader, integrated programs in which all components are mutually reinforcing. See also CNN APPROACH.

ABORTION RATE The estimated annual number of abortions per 1000 women of reproductive age (usually defined as ages 15–44).

ABORTION RATIO The estimated number of abortions per 100 live births in a given year.

ABSCISSA The distance along the horizontal coordinate, or *x* axis, of a point *P* from the vertical or *y* axis of a graph. See also AXIS; GRAPH; ORDINATE.

ABSOLUTE EFFECT The effect of an exposure (expressed as the difference between rates, proportions, means), of the outcome, etc., as opposed to the ratio of these measures.[12] See also RISK DIFFERENCE.

ABSOLUTE POVERTY LEVEL Income level below which a minimum nutritionally adequate diet plus essential nonfood requirements is not affordable.[13] The amount of income a person, family, or group needs to purchase an absolute amount of the basic necessities of life. See also RELATIVE POVERTY LEVEL.

ABSOLUTE RATE The number of specified health events (disease onset, death, etc.) divided by the time at risk in a defined population over a specified time interval.[12] See also EVENT RATE; RATE RATIO.

ABSOLUTE RISK (AR) The probability of an event (usually adverse, but it may also be beneficial) in the population under study. Contrast with RELATIVE RISK. The number of events in a group divided by the total number of subjects in that group. Sometimes AR is wrongly used as a synonym for ATTRIBUTABLE FRACTION; EXCESS RISK; OR RISK DIFFERENCE.

ABSOLUTE RISK INCREASE (ARI) The absolute risk of adverse events in the treatment group (ART) minus the absolute risk of events in the control group (ARC): ARI = ART—ARC. Same as the RISK DIFFERENCE. Also, the proportion of treated persons who experience an adverse event minus the proportion of untreated persons who experience the event. See also NUMBER NEEDED TO HARM (NNH).

ABSOLUTE RISK REDUCTION (ARR)

1. The arithmetic difference between two event rates. The amount by which the risk of an undesirable event is reduced by elimination or control of a particular exposure. It enables an estimate of the number of people spared the consequences of an exposure.
2. The absolute risk of events in the control group (ARC) minus the absolute risk of events in the treatment group (ART): ARR = ARC—ART. The negative of the RISK DIFFERENCE. Also, the proportion of untreated persons who experience an adverse event minus the proportion of treated persons who experience this event.

The reciprocal of the ARR is the NUMBER NEEDED TO TREAT (NNT). The ARR is one measure of the strength of an association. It varies with the underlying risk of an event; e.g., it becomes smaller when EVENT RATES are low. The ARR is higher and the NNT lower in groups with higher absolute risks.[14, 15] See also EVENT RATE; HILL'S CRITERIA OF CAUSATION; MEASURE OF ASSOCIATION; PROBABILITY OF CAUSATION; RELATIVE RISK REDUCTION.

ACCEPTABLE RISK Risk that appears tolerable to some group. Risk that has minimal or long-term detrimental effects or for which the benefits outweigh the potential hazards. EPIDEMIOLOGICAL RESEARCH has provided data for calculation of risks increased by many medical procedures as well as by occupational and environmental exposures; these data are used, for instance, in CLINICAL DECISION ANALYSIS and HEALTH TECHNOLOGY ASSESSMENT.

ACCEPTANCE SAMPLING (Syn: stop-or-go sampling) Sampling method that requires division of the "universe" population into groups or batches as they pass a specified time point (e.g., age), followed by sampling of individuals within the sampled groups.

ACCIDENT An unanticipated event—commonly leading to INJURY or other harm—in traffic, the workplace, or a domestic or recreational setting. The primary event in a sequence that leads ultimately to injury if that event is genuinely not predictable. Epidemiological studies have demonstrated that the risk of accidents is often predictable and that accidents are preventable. This word is preferably avoided in many types of scientific works.

ACCUMULATION OF RISK The extent of cumulative damage to biological systems as the number, duration, or severity of exposures increases and as body systems age and become less able to repair damage. The notion that LIFE COURSE exposures or insults gradually accumulate through episodes of illness and injury, adverse environmental conditions, and health damaging behaviors. Exposures increasing risk of disease may be independent or clustered; in the latter case an accumulation model with risk clustering is used.[16] See also DEVELOPMENTAL AND LIFE COURSE EPIDEMIOLOGY; THRIFTY PHENOTYPE HYPOTHESIS.

ACCURACY

1. The degree to which a measurement or an estimate based on measurements represents the true value of the attribute that is being measured. Relative lack of ERROR. See also MEASUREMENT, TERMINOLOGY OF; VALIDITY, STUDY.
2. The ability of a diagnostic test to correctly classify the presence or absence of the target disorder. The diagnostic accuracy of a test is usually expressed by its SENSITIVITY and SPECIFICITY.

ACE American College of Epidemiology.

ACQUAINTANCE NETWORK A group of persons in contact or communication among whom transmission of an infectious agent and of knowledge, behavior, and values is possible and whose social interaction may have health implications. See also CONTEXT; TRANSMISSION OF INFECTION.

ACQUIRED IMMUNODEFICIENCY SYNDROME (AIDS) (Syn: acquired immune deficiency syndrome) The late clinical stage of infection with HUMAN IMMUNODEFICIENCY VIRUS (HIV), recognized as a distinct syndrome in 1981. The opportunistic or indicator diseases associated with AIDS include certain protozoan and helminth infections, fungal infections, bacterial infections, viral infections, and some types of cancer. The role of AIDS as an indicator in SURVEILLANCE has diminished since the advent of HIGHLY ACTIVE ANTIRETROVIRAL THERAPY (HAART). See also HUMAN IMMUNODEFICIENCY VIRUS (HIV).

ACTIVE LIFE EXPECTANCY See DISABILITY-FREE LIFE EXPECTANCY.

ACTIVITIES OF DAILY LIVING (ADL) SCALE A scale devised by Katz and others[17] to score physical ability/disability; used to measure outcomes of interventions for various chronic, disabling conditions, such as arthritis. The scale is based on scores for responses to questions about mobility, self-care, grooming, etc. This was the first widely used scale of this type; others, mostly refinements or variations of the ADL scale, have since been developed.

ACTIVITY SETTING The places, events, routines, and patterns that structure the experience of everyday life; e.g., a classroom, a neighborhood resident meeting, a commuter train, family meals, a waiting room in a hospital. The unit by which culture and community are propagated across time.[18] See also BEHAVIOR SETTING; CONTEXT.

ACTUARIAL RATE See FORCE OF MORTALITY.

ACTUARIAL TABLE See LIFE TABLE.

ACUTE

1. Referring to a health effect: sudden onset, often brief; sometimes loosely used to mean severe.
2. Referring to an exposure: brief, intense, or short-term; sometimes specifically referring to a brief exposure of high intensity. See also CHRONIC.

ADAPTATION

1. The process by which organisms surmount environmental challenges. See also RESILIENCE.
2. A heritable component of the phenotype that confers an advantage in survival and reproductive success.

ADDITIVE MODEL A model in which the combined effect on the risks or rates of several factors is the sum of the effects that would be produced by each of the factors in the absence of the others. For example, if factor X adds x to risk in the absence of Y and factor Y adds y to risk in the absence of X, an additive model states that the two factors together will add $(x + y)$ to risk. See also INTERACTION; LINEAR MODEL; MATHEMATICAL MODEL; MULTIPLICATIVE MODEL.

ADELF Association des Épidémiologistes de Langue Française (Association of Epidemiologists of French Language).

ADHERENCE Health-related behavior that adheres to the recommendations of a doctor, other health care provider, or investigator in a research project. The word *adherence* aims to avoid the authoritarian associations of COMPLIANCE, formerly used to describe this behavior. *Concordance* is another alternative to *compliance*.[19]

ADJUSTMENT A summarizing procedure for a statistical measure in which the effects of differences in composition of the populations being compared have been minimized by statistical methods.[20] Examples are adjustment by regression analysis, by inverse-probability weighting, and by standardization. Adjustment is often performed on a rate or on an EFFECT MEASURE, commonly because of differing age and sex distributions in the populations being compared. The mathematical procedure commonly used to adjust rates for age differences is (direct or indirect) STANDARDIZATION.

ADULT LITERACY RATE The percentage of persons 15 years of age and over who can read and write.[21]

ADVERSE REACTION An undesirable or unwanted consequence of a preventive, diagnostic, or therapeutic procedure. See also SIDE EFFECT.

AES American Epidemiological Society.

AETIOLOGY, AETIOLOGICAL See ETIOLOGY.

AGE The WHO recommends that age should be defined by completed units of time, counting the day of birth as zero.

AGE DEPENDENCY RATIO See DEPENDENCY RATIO.

AGENT (OF DISEASE) A factor—such as a microorganism, chemical substance, or form of radiation—whose presence, excessive presence, or (in deficiency diseases) relative absence is essential for the occurrence of a disease. A disease may have a single agent, a number of independent alternative agents (at least one of which must be present), or a complex of two or more factors whose combined presence is essential for the development of the disease. See also CAUSALITY; NECESSARY CAUSE.

AGE-PERIOD COHORT ANALYSIS See COHORT ANALYSIS.

AGE-SEX PYRAMID See POPULATION PYRAMID.

AGE-SEX REGISTER A list of all clients or patients of a medical practice or service, classified by age (birthdate) and sex; it provides denominators for calculating age- and sex-specific rates.

AGE-SPECIFIC FERTILITY RATE The number of live births occurring during a specified period to women of a specified age group divided by the number of person-years lived during that period by women of that age group. When an age-specific fertility rate is calculated for a calendar year, the number of live births to women of the specified age is usually divided by the midyear population of women of that age.

AGE-SPECIFIC RATE A rate for a specified age group. The numerator and denominator refer to the same age group.

Example:

$$\text{Age-specific death rate [age (25–34)]} = \frac{\begin{array}{c}\text{number of deaths among residents}\\ \text{age 25–34 in an area in a year}\end{array}}{\begin{array}{c}\text{average (for midyear) population}\\ \text{age 25–34 in the area in that year}\end{array}} \times 100{,}000$$

The multiplier (usually 100,000 or 1 million) is chosen to produce a rate that can be expressed as a convenient number.

AGE STANDARDIZATION A procedure for adjusting rates (e.g., death rates) designed to minimize the effects of differences in age composition in comparing rates for different populations. See also ADJUSTMENT; STANDARDIZATION.

AGGREGATION BIAS (Syn: ecological bias) See AGGREGATIVE FALLACY; ECOLOGICAL FALLACY; ATOMISTIC FALLACY.

AGGREGATE SURVEILLANCE The surveillance of a disease or health event by collecting summary data on groups of cases (e.g., general practitioners taking part in surveillance schemes are asked to report the number of cases of specified diseases seen over a specified period of time).

AGGREGATIVE FALLACY An erroneous application to individuals of a causal relationship observed at the group level. A type of ECOLOGICAL FALLACY (sometimes just a synonym) and an antonym of the ATOMISTIC FALLACY.[22]

AGING OF THE POPULATION An increase over time in the proportion of older persons in a defined population. It does not necessarily imply an increase in life expectancy or that people are living longer than they used to. In the past, the principal cause of aging of populations has been a decline in the birth rate: in the absence of a rise in the death rate at higher ages, when fewer children are born than in prior years, the proportion of older persons in the population increases. Nowadays, in developed societies, little further mortality reduction can occur in the first parts of life; thus, reductions in mortality that occur in the third and fourth quarters of life are leading to a rise in the proportion of older persons. See also DEMOGRAPHIC TRANSITION.

AIRBORNE INFECTION An infection whose agent is transmitted by particles, dust, or DROPLET NUCLEI suspended in the air. The infective agent may be transmitted by a patient or carrier in airborne droplets expelled during coughing and sneezing. See also TRANSMISSION OF INFECTION.

ALGORITHM Any systematic process that consists of an ordered sequence of steps with each step depending on the outcome of the previous one. The term is commonly used to describe a structured process—for instance, relating to computer programming or health planning. See also DECISION TREE.

ALGORITHM, CLINICAL (Syn: clinical protocol) An explicit description of steps to be taken in patient care in specified circumstances. This approach makes use of branching logic and of all pertinent data, both about the patient and from epidemiological and other sources, to arrive at decisions that yield maximum benefit and minimum risk.

ALLELE Alternative forms of a gene occupying the same locus on a chromosome. Each of the different states found at a polymorphic site.[23]

ALLOCATION BIAS An error in the estimate of an effect caused by failure to implement valid procedures for random allocation of subjects to intervention and control groups in a CLINICAL TRIAL.

ALLOCATION CONCEALMENT A method of generating a sequence that ensures random allocation between two or more arms of a study without revealing this to study subjects or researchers. The quality of allocation concealment is enhanced by computer-based random allocation and other procedures to make the process impervious to ALLOCATION BIAS. See also BLIND(ED) STUDY; RANDOM ALLOCATION.

ALMA-ATA DECLARATION See HEALTH CARE; HEALTH FOR ALL; PRIMARY HEALTH CARE.

ALPHA ERROR See ERROR, TYPE I.

AMBIENT Surrounding; pertaining to the environment in which events are observed.

AMES TEST A BIOASSAY for mutagenesis, using bacteria as target, to detect and screen for potentially CARCINOGENIC compounds. Developed from the early 1970s by Bruce Ames and colleagues at the University of California, Berkeley. See CARCINOGEN.

ANALYSIS OF VARIANCE (ANOVA) A statistical technique that isolates and assesses the contribution of categorical independent variables to the variance of the mean of a continuous dependent variable. The observations are classified according to their categories for each of the independent variables, and the differences between the categories in their mean values on the dependent variable are estimated and tested for STATISTICAL SIGNIFICANCE.

ANALYTICAL STUDY A study designed to examine putative or hypothesized causal relationships; hence, most such studies can be conceptualized as ETIOLOGICAL STUDIES. An analytical study is usually concerned with identifying or measuring the effects of RISK FACTORS or with the health effects of specific exposure(s) or interventions. Contrast DESCRIPTIVE STUDY, which usually does not test hypotheses. The common types of analytical study are CROSS-SECTIONAL, COHORT, and CASE-CONTROL. In an analytical study, individuals in the study population may be classified according to the absence or presence (or future development) of specific disease and according to "attributes" that may influence disease occurrence. Attributes may include age; race; sex; other disease(s); genetic, biochemical, and physiological characteristics; social position, economic status; occupation; residence; and various aspects of the environment or personal behavior. See also RESEARCH DESIGN.

ANECDOTAL EVIDENCE Evidence derived from descriptions of cases or events rather than systematically collected data that can be submitted to formal epidemiological and statistical analysis. Such evidence must be viewed with caution but sometimes is useful to raise a warning of danger or to generate hypotheses (e.g., as shown by voluntary reporting of adverse drug events). See also CASE REPORTS.

ANEUGENIC An agent that affects cell processes and structures resulting in the loss or gain of whole chromosomes. See also MUTAGENIC; CLASTOGENIC.

ANIMAL MODEL A study in a population of laboratory animals that uses conditions of animals analogous to conditions of humans to model processes comparable to those that occur in human populations. See also EXPERIMENTAL EPIDEMIOLOGY.

ANTAGONISM (Opposite: SYNERGISM)

1. One of two types of *effect modification* or INTERACTION: the EFFECT MODIFIER diminishes the effect of the putatively causal variable. The situation in which the combined effect of two or more factors is smaller than that expected from the effect of one factor in the absence of the other factors.[24]
2. In BIOASSAY, the situation when a specified response is produced by exposure to either of two factors but not to both together. Antagonism exists if there are persons who will get the disease when exposed to one of the factors alone but not when exposed to both.

ANTHROPOMETRY The technique dealing with the measurement of the size, weight, and proportions of the human body.

ANTHROPOPHILIC (adj.) Pertaining to an insect's preference for feeding on humans even when nonhuman hosts are available.

ANTIBODY Protein molecule produced in response to exposure to a "foreign" or extraneous substance (e.g., invading microorganisms responsible for infection) or active IMMUNIZATION. May also be present as a result of passive transfer from mother to infant, via immune globulin, etc. Antibody has the capacity to bind specifically to the foreign substance (antigen) that elicited its production, thus supplying a MECHANISM for protection against infectious diseases. Antibody is epidemiologically important because its concentration (titer) can be measured in individuals and therefore, in populations. See also SEROEPIDEMIOLOGY.

ANTIGEN A substance (protein, polysaccharide, glycolipid, tissue transplant, etc.) that is capable of inducing specific immune response. Introduction of antigen may be by the invasion of infectious organisms, immunization, inhalation, ingestion, etc.

ANTIGENIC DRIFT The "evolutionary" changes that take place in the molecular structure of DNA/RNA in microorganisms during their passage from one host to another. It may be due to recombination, deletion, or insertion of genes, to point mutations, or to several of these events. This process has been studied in common viruses, notably the influenza virus.[25] It leads to alteration (usually slow and progressive) in the antigenic composition and thus in the immunological responses of individuals and populations to exposure to the microorganisms concerned. See also ANTIGENIC SHIFT.

ANTIGENICITY (Syn: immunogenicity) The ability of agent(s) to produce a systemic or a local immunological reaction in the host.

ANTIGENIC SHIFT A mutation, or sudden change in molecular structure of DNA/RNA, in microorganisms, especially viruses, that produces new strains of the microorganism. Hosts previously exposed to other strains have little or no acquired immunity. Antigenic shift is believed to be the explanation for the occurrence of strains of the influenza A virus associated with large-scale epidemic and pandemic spread. See also ANTIGENIC DRIFT.

APACHE Acronym for Acute Physiology and Chronic Health Evaluation, a scoring system used to predict the outcome of critical illness or injury. This system and its variations (APACHE II, etc.) assign scores for state of consciousness, eye movements, reflexes, and physiological data such as blood pressure.[26]

APGAR SCORE A composite index used to evaluate neonatal status by assigning numerical scores (0–2) to heart rate, respiration, muscle tone, skin color, and response to stimulation. Developed by Virginia Apgar (1909–1974) a U.S. pediatrician/anesthetist. Low scores are associated with a poor prognosis.

APHA American Public Health Association.

APPLIED EPIDEMIOLOGY The application and evaluation of epidemiological knowledge and methods (e.g., in public health or in health care). It includes applications of etiological research, priority setting and evaluation of health programs, policies, technologies, and services. It is epidemiological practice aimed at protecting and/or improving the health of a defined population. It usually involves identifying and investigating health problems, MONITORING changes in health status, and/or evaluating the outcomes of interventions. It is generally conducted in a time frame determined by the need to protect the health of an exposed population and an administrative context that results in public health action.[27] See also FIELD EPIDEMIOLOGY; HOSPITAL EPIDEMIOLOGY.

ARBOVIRUS An arthropod-borne virus. Various RNA viruses transmitted principally by arthropods, including the causative agents of encephalitis, yellow fever and dengue. A group of taxonomically diverse animal viruses that are unified by an epidemiological concept, i.e., transmission between vertebrate host organisms by bloodfeeding (hematophagous) arthropod vectors such as mosquitoes, ticks, sand flies, and midges. The interaction of arbovirus, vertebrate host, and arthropod vector gives this class of infections unique epidemiological features. See VECTOR-BORNE INFECTION for terms that describe these features.

AREA SAMPLING A method of sampling that can be used when the numbers in the population are unknown. The total area to be sampled is divided into subareas (e.g., by means of a grid that produces squares on a map); these subareas are then numbered and sampled using a table of random numbers. Depending upon circumstances, the population in the sampled areas may first be enumerated, and then a second stage of sampling may be conducted.

ARITHMETIC MEAN See MEAN, ARITHMETIC; AVERAGE.

ARM (of a trial) A group of persons whose outcome in a study is compared with that of another group or groups; commonly the arms of a trial are categorized as *experimental* and *control* groups.

ARMITAGE-DOLL MODEL A model of carcinogenesis in which time elapsed since exposure, not age, is a prime determinant of cancer.[28] The model postulates three phases:

1. A normal cell develops into a cancer cell after a small number of transition stages.
2. Initially the number of normal cells at risk is very large, and for each cell transition is a rare event.
3. The transitions are independent of each other. There are no presumptions about precipitating causes of the transition from normal to cancerous cell. Named for the statistician Peter Armitage (1924–) and the epidemiologist Richard Doll (1912–2005).

ARTIFICIAL INTELLIGENCE A branch of computer science in which attempts are made to duplicate human intellectual functions. One application is in diagnosis, in which computer programs are based upon epidemiological analyses of data abstracted from clinical records.

ASCERTAINMENT The process of determining what is happening in a population or study group—e.g., family and household composition, occurrence of cases of specific diseases; the latter is also known as case finding.

ASCERTAINMENT BIAS Systematic failure to represent equally all classes of cases or persons supposed to be represented in a sample. This bias may arise because of the nature of the sources from which persons come (e.g., a specialized clinic); from a diagnostic process influenced by culture, custom, or idiosyncracy; or, in genetic studies, from the statistical CHANCE of selecting from large or small families.

ASSAY The quantitative or qualitative evaluation of a (hazardous) substance in water food, soil, air, etc; the results of such an evaluation. See also BIOASSAY.

ASSOCIATION [Syn: (statistical) dependence, relationship; sometimes *correlation* is used synonymously.]

1. Statistical dependence between two or more events, characteristics, or other variables. An association is present if the probability of occurrence of an event or characteristic, or the quantity of a variable, varies with the occurrence of one or more other events, the presence of one or more other characteristics, or the quantity of one or more other variables. The association between two variables is described as positive when higher values of a variable are associated with higher values of another variable. In a negative or inverse association, the occurrence of higher values of one variable is associated with lower values of the other variable. An association may be fortuitous or may be produced by various other circumstances; the presence of an association does not necessarily imply a causal relationship. In epidemiological and clinical research, the terms *association* and *relationship* may often be used interchangeably.

2. One of three properties David Hume, in his *Treatise of Human Nature* of 1739, deemed necessary (but insufficient standing alone) for assigning cause; the other two properties of a cause are CONNECTION and TIME ORDER.[9,10,71]

ASSOCIATION, FORTUITOUS A relationship between two variables that occurs by CHANCE and is thought to need no further explanation. See also RANDOM; CORRELATION, NONSENSE.

ASSOCIATION, SPURIOUS An ambiguous term used with different meanings by different authors. It may refer to artifactual, fortuitous, false, secondary, or many kinds of noncausal associations owing to CHANCE, BIAS, or CONFOUNDING.

ASSORTATIVE MATING Selection of a mate with preference (or aversion) for a particular genotype (i.e., nonrandom mating).

ASYMPTOTIC Pertaining to a limiting value, for example, of a dependent variable, when the independent variable approaches zero or infinity. See LARGE SAMPLE METHOD.

ASYMPTOTIC CURVE A curve that approaches but never reaches zero or infinity (e.g., an exponential or reciprocal exponential curve).

ASYMPTOTIC METHOD See LARGE SAMPLE METHOD.

ATOMISTIC FALLACY An erroneous inference about causal relationships in groups made on the basis of relationships observed in individuals.[22] The counterpart of the ECOLOGICAL FALLACY. An automatic, literal, or mechanical translation of CAUSAL INFERENCES made in individuals to population groups may be wrong because different causal processes may operate when the individual is the unit of interest than when the unit is a population or group. The atomistic fallacy may occur when studies based on individuals (individual-level studies) are assumed to be valid and sufficient to make causal inferences at an upper level of aggregation (e.g., on the relationship between exposures and diseases at the group level). Relevant in particular when individual-level factors (e.g., income or gun ownership) and group-level factors (e.g., average income in the neighborhood or prevalence of gun holders in a city) capture or mediate different aspects of health risks. See also AGGREGATIVE FALLACY; ECOLOGICAL FALLACY; INDIVIDUAL THINKING; MULTIPLE CAUSATION; POPULATION THINKING.

ATTACK RATE The proportion of a group that experiences the outcome under study over a given period (e.g., the period of an epidemic). This "rate" can be determined empirically by identifying clinical cases and/or by means of seroepidemiology. It also applies in noninfectious settings (e.g., mass poisonings). Because its time dimension is uncertain or arbitrarily decided, it should probably not be described as a rate. See also INFECTION RATE; MASS ACTION PRINCIPLE; REED-FROST MODEL; SECONDARY ATTACK RATE.

ATTENUATION Weakening (dilution) of the concentration, as of an antigen in a vaccine; also of an effect, e.g., relative risk.

ATTRIBUTABLE BENEFIT Antonym of ATTRIBUTABLE RISK; a term that can be used when exposure is beneficial rather than harmful.

ATTRIBUTABLE FRACTION (Syn: attributable proportion) For a causal association, the proportion of the caseload that can be attributed to a particular exposure. It is the causal attributable difference (attributable risk) divided by the incidence rate in the group. It is the proportion by which the incidence rate would be reduced if the exposure were eliminated.[29,30] The attributable fraction may apply to exposed individuals [ATTRIBUTABLE FRACTION (EXPOSED)] or to the whole population [ATTRIBUTABLE FRACTION (POPULATION)].

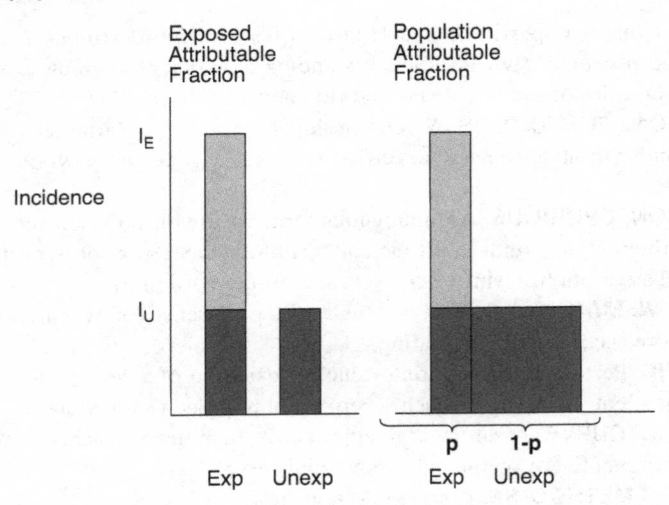

Attributable fractions. I_E and I_U are the incidence in the exposed and unexposed groups, p is the proportion of the population that is exposed, and 1-p the proportion not exposed. The lighter area represents cases that are attributable to the exposure (attributable risk, AR) and that would not have occurred in the absence of the exposure. It is assumed that in the absence of this hazardous exposure, the incidence would be I_U in the whole population. From Spasoff R, 1999. With permission.

ATTRIBUTABLE FRACTION (EXPOSED) [Syn: attributable proportion (exposed), attributable risk, etiological fraction (exposed), relative attributable risk]. With a given outcome, exposure factor, and population, the attributable fraction among the exposed is the proportion by which the incidence rate of the outcome among those exposed would be reduced if the exposure were eliminated. If there is no bias or confounding, it may be estimated by the formula

$$AF_e = \frac{I_e - I_u}{I_e}$$

where I_e is the incidence rate (proportion) among the exposed, I_u is the incidence rate (proportion) among the unexposed; or by the formula

$$AF_e = \frac{RR-1}{RR}$$

where RR is the rate ratio, I_e / I_u. It should not be confused with the ETIOLOGICAL FRACTION and the PROBABILITY OF CAUSATION.

ATTRIBUTABLE FRACTION (POPULATION) [Syn: attributable proportion (population), etiological fraction (population), population attributable risk proportion, Levin's attributable risk]. With a given outcome, exposure factor, and population, the attributable fraction for the population incidence rate is the proportion by which the incidence rate of the outcome in the entire population would be reduced if the exposure was eliminated. If there is no bias or confounding, it may be estimated by the formula

$$AF_p = \frac{I_p - I_u}{I_p}$$

where I_p is the incidence rate (proportion) in the total population and I_u is the incidence rate (proportion) among the unexposed.

The formula

$$AF_p = \frac{P_e(RR-1)}{1+P_e(RR-1)}$$

(where *RR* is the rate ratio, I_e/I_u and P_e is the proportion exposed in the entire population) is often cited, but it is biased if the RR is adjusted for confounders, as is normally the case. A formula that does not suffer from this problem is

$$AF_p = \frac{P_c(RR-1)}{RR}$$

(where P_c is the exposure prevalence among cases).

Attributable fractions may also be calculated for other measures of disease frequency; e.g., the attributable fraction for the caseload over a defined time period is

$$(A_p - A_u)/A_p$$

where A_p is the caseload in the population and A_u is what the caseload would be if everyone were not exposed. This is not the same as the quantity computed by rates because the rate fraction does not account for the effect of exposure on person time.

ATTRIBUTABLE NUMBER The excess caseload of a specific outcome attributable to an exposure over a defined time period. If there is no bias or confounding and the exposure has negligible effect on the person-time at risk, it may be estimated using the formula

$$AN = T_e(I_e - I_u)$$

where I_e is the incidence rate among the exposed, I_u is the incidence rate among the unexposed, and T_e is the person-time in the exposed population during the period in question.

ATTRIBUTABLE PROPORTION See ATTRIBUTABLE FRACTION

ATTRIBUTABLE RATE, ATTRIBUTABLE RISK (Syn: causal rate difference, causal risk difference) The proportion of the rate (risk) of a disease or other outcome in exposed individuals that can be attributed to the exposure. This measure is estimated by subtracting the rate (risk) of the outcome (usually, incidence or mortality) among the unexposed from the rate (risk) among the exposed individuals; this estimate assumes that causes other than the one under investigation have had equal effects on the exposed and unexposed groups. Unfortunately, this term has been used to denote a number of different concepts, including the ATTRIBUTABLE FRACTION in the population, the attributable fraction among the exposed, the POPULATION EXCESS RATE, and the RATE DIFFERENCE. See also ABSOLUTE RISK REDUCTION; IMPACT NUMBERS.

ATTRIBUTABLE RISK (EXPOSED) This term has been used with different connotations to denote the attributable fraction among the exposed and the excess risk among the exposed. See also ATTRIBUTABLE FRACTION (EXPOSED); RATE DIFFERENCE.

ATTRIBUTABLE RISK PERCENT Attributable fraction expressed as a percentage of the total rate or risk rather than as a proportion.

ATTRIBUTABLE RISK PERCENT (EXPOSED) The attributable fraction among the exposed, expressed as a percentage of the total rate or risk among the exposed. See also ATTRIBUTABLE FRACTION (EXPOSED).

ATTRIBUTABLE RISK PERCENT (POPULATION) The attributable fraction in the population, expressed as a percentage of the total rate or risk in the population. See also ATTRIBUTABLE FRACTION (POPULATION).

ATTRIBUTABLE RISK (POPULATION) This term has been used with different connotations to denote the attributable fraction in the population and the population excess risk. See also ABSOLUTE RISK REDUCTION; ATTRIBUTABLE FRACTION (POPULATION); POPULATION EXCESS RATE.

ATTRIBUTE A qualitative characteristic of an individual or an item.

ATTRITION Reduction in the number of participants in a study as it progresses (i.e., during FOLLOW-UP of a COHORT). Losses may be due to withdrawals, DROPOUTS, or protocol deviations.[31] See also CENSORING.

ATTRITION BIAS A type of SELECTION BIAS due to systematic differences between the study groups in the quantitative and qualitative characteristics of the processes of loss of their members during study conduct, i.e., due to ATTRITION among subjects in the study. Different rates of losses to follow-up in the exposure groups may change the characteristics of these groups irrespective of the studied intervention.[32,33]

AUDIT

1. An examination or review that establishes the extent to which a condition, process, or performance conforms to predetermined standards or criteria. Assessment or review of any aspect of HEALTH CARE to determine its quality; audits may be carried out on the provision of care, compliance with regulations, community response, completeness of records, etc.
2. An evaluation of the quality of health care, the use of resources, and outcomes. See also HEALTH SERVICES RESEARCH.
3. The process of checking whether the accounts of an institution, company, or association are complete, accurate, and consistent; whether they agree with other records of activity; and whether they comply with legal requirements and professional standards.

AUSTRALIA ANTIGEN Hepatitis B surface antigen (HBsAg). So called because it was first identified in an Australian aborigine. HBsAg is a BIOMARKER for the prevalence of infection with the virus of hepatitis B.

AUTONOMY, RESPECT FOR

1. In ETHICS, the principle of respect for human dignity and the right of individuals to decide things for themselves.
2. In epidemiological practice and research, this principle is central to the concept of INFORMED CONSENT. It can conflict with the need to protect the population from identified risks (e.g., risks related to contagious disease) and with the need for access to personally identifiable health-related data and information. See also CONFIDENTIALITY; CONSENT BIAS; PRIVACY.

AUTOPSY DATA Data derived from autopsied deaths; used, for instance, to study aspects of the natural history of disease or trends in frequency of disease. Autopsies are done on nonrandomly selected persons; findings should therefore be generalized only with great caution. See also BIAS IN AUTOPSY SERIES.

AUXILIARY HYPOTHESIS BIAS A form of RESCUE BIAS and thus of INTERPRETIVE BIAS, which occurs in introducing ad hoc modifications to imply that an unanticipated finding would have occurred otherwise had the experimental conditions been different. Because experimental conditions can easily be altered in many ways, adjusting a hypothesis is a versatile tool for saving a cherished theory.[34]

AVERAGE

1. In science, loosely, the ARITHMETIC MEAN. The arithmetic average of a set of n numbers is the sum of the numbers divided by n.
2. A measure of location, either the MODE or, in the case of numerical data, the MEDIAN or the MEAN.
3. Distribution of aggregate inequalities in a series among all the members of the series, so as to equalize them. See also MEASURE OF CENTRAL TENDENCY.
4. In everyday speech, ordinary, usual, or NORMAL; the normal or typical amount.

AVERAGE LIFE EXPECTANCY See EXPECTATION OF LIFE.

AXIS

1. One of the dimensions of a graph. A two-dimensional graph has two axes, the horizontal or x axis and the vertical or y axis. Mathematically, there may be more than two axes, and graphs are sometimes drawn with a third dimension. See also ABSCISSA; ORDINATE.
2. In NOSOLOGY, an axis of classification is the conceptual framework (e.g., etiological, topographical, psychological, sociological). The INTERNATIONAL CLASSIFICATION OF DISEASES, for example, is multiaxial: the primary axis is topographical (i.e., body systems), while secondary axes relate to etiology, manifestations of disease, detail of sites affected, severity, etc.

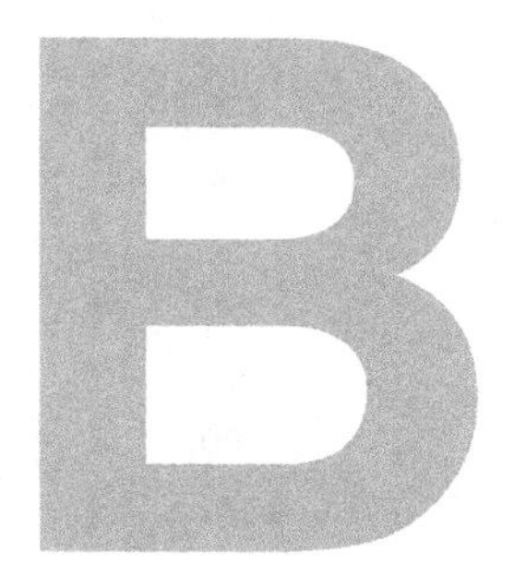

BACKGROUND LEVEL, RATE The concentration, often low, at which some substance, agent, or event is present or occurs at a particular time and place in the absence of a specific hazard or set of hazards under investigation. An example is the background level of the naturally occurring forms of ionizing radiation to which we are all exposed.

BACTERIA (singular: bacterium) Single-celled organisms found throughout nature, which can be beneficial or cause disease.

BAR CHART (Syn: bar diagram) A graphic technique for presenting DISCRETE DATA organized in such a way that each observation can fall into one and only one category of the variable. Frequencies are listed along one axis and categories of the variable along the other axis. The frequencies of each group of observations are represented by the lengths of the corresponding bars. See also HISTOGRAM.

BAR DIAGRAM See BAR CHART.

BARKER HYPOTHESIS See DEVELOPMENTAL ORIGINS HYPOTHESIS.

BARRIER METHOD Contraceptive method that interposes a physical barrier between sperm and ovum (e.g., condom, cervical cap, diaphragm).

BARRIER NURSING (Syn: bedside isolation) Nursing care of hospital patients that minimizes the risks of cross-infection by use of antisepsis, gowns, gloves, masks for nursing staff, and isolation of the patient, preferably alone in a single room. See also UNIVERSAL PRECAUTIONS.

BASELINE DATA A set of data collected at the beginning of a study.

BASE POPULATION See POPULATION, SOURCE.

BASE, STUDY See STUDY BASE.

BASIC REPRODUCTIVE RATE (R_0) A measure of the number of infections produced, on average, by an infected individual in the early stages of an epidemic, when virtually all contacts are susceptible. (Some authors use the symbol Z_0 for basic reproductive rate.)

BAYESIAN STATISTICS A method of statistical inference that begins with formulation of probabilities of hypotheses (called *prior probabilities*) before the data under analysis are taken into account. It then uses the data and a model for the data probability (usually the same model used by other methods, such as a LOGISTIC MODEL) to update the probabilities of the hypotheses. The resulting updated probabilities are called *posterior probabilities*. Central to this updating is BAYES' THEOREM,[35] although not all Bayesian methods require explicit use of the theorem and not all uses of the theorem are Bayesian methods. Bayesian statistics can be used alongside or in place of other methods for

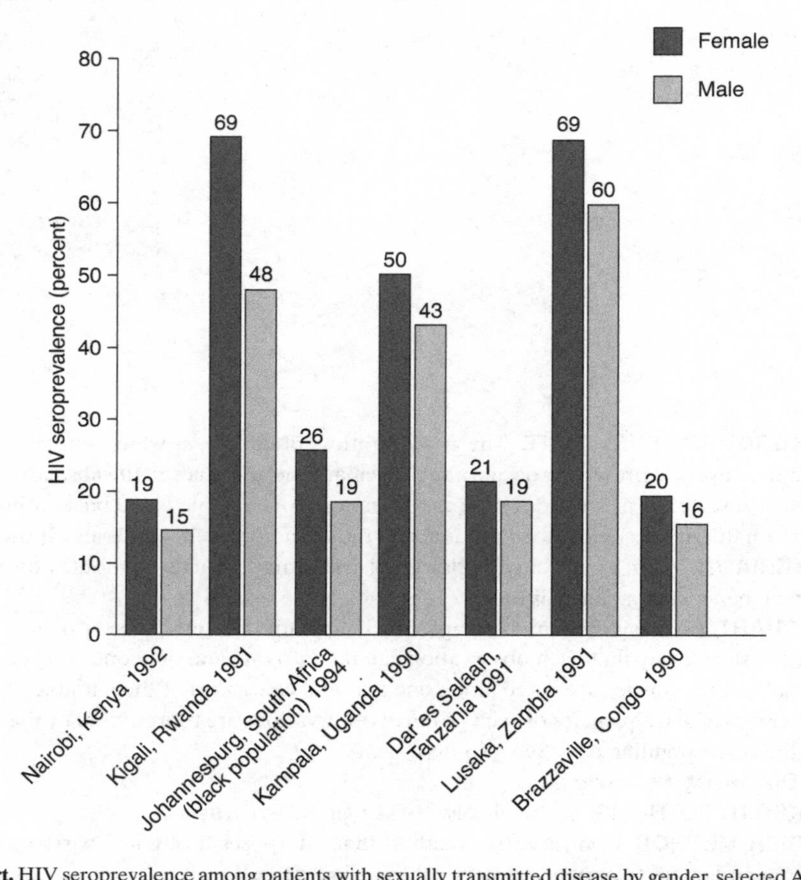

Bar chart. HIV seroprevalence among patients with sexually transmitted disease by gender, selected African countries, 1990–1993. From Mann J M, Tarantola D J M, eds. *AIDS in the World II.* New York: Oxford University Press, 1996, p. 47.

many purposes (e.g., evaluation of diagnostic tests, studies of disease progression, and analyses of geographic studies, clinical trials, cohort studies, and case-control studies).

BAYES' THEOREM A theorem of probability named for Thomas Bayes (1702–1761), an English clergyman and mathematician; his *Essay Towards Solving a Problem in the Doctrine of Chances* (1763, published posthumously) contained this theorem. In epidemiology, it is often used to obtain the probability of disease in a group of people with some characteristic on the basis of the overall rate of that disease (the prior probability of disease) and of the likelihoods of that characteristic in healthy and diseased individuals. The most familiar application is in CLINICAL DECISION ANALYSIS, where it is used for estimating the probability of a particular diagnosis given the appearance of some symptoms or test result. A simplified version of the theorem is

$$P(D|S) = \frac{P(S|D)P(D)}{P(S|D)P(D) + P(S|\bar{D})P(\bar{D})}$$

where D = disease, S = symptom, and $\bar{D}$ = no disease. The formula emphasizes what clinical intuition often overlooks—namely, that the probability of disease given this symptom depends not only on how characteristic of the disease that symptom is but also on how frequent the disease is among the population being served.

The theorem can also be used for estimating exposure-specific rates from case-control studies if there is added information about the overall rate of disease in that population.

Some of the terms in the theorem are named. The probability of disease given the symptom is the POSTERIOR PROBABILITY. It is an estimate of the probability of disease posterior to knowing whether or not the symptom was present. The overall probability of disease among the population or our guess of the probability of disease before knowing of the presence or absence of the symptom is the PRIOR PROBABILITY. The theorem is sometimes presented in terms of the odds of disease before knowing the symptom (PRIOR ODDS) and after knowing the symptom (POSTERIOR ODDS).

BEDSIDE ISOLATION See BARRIER NURSING.

BEHAVIORAL EPIDEMIC An epidemic attributable to the power of suggestion or to culturally determined behavioral patterns (as opposed to invading microorganisms or physical agents). Examples include the dancing manias of the Middle Ages, episodes of mass fainting or convulsions ("hysterical epidemics"), crowd panic, and waves of fashion or enthusiasm. The communicable nature of the behavior is dependent not only on person-to-person transmission of the behavioral pattern but also on group reinforcement (as with smoking, alcohol, and drug use). Behavioral epidemics may be difficult to differentiate from outbreaks of organic disease (e.g., due to CONTAMINATION of the environment by a toxic substance) or may complicate them.

BEHAVIORAL RISK FACTOR A characteristic or behavior that is associated with increased probability of a specified outcome; the term does not imply a causal relationship.

BEHAVIOR SETTING The place where a pattern or sequence of behavior regularly occurs; it includes the ordinary events of daily life.[18] A forerunner of the concept of ACTIVITY SETTING.

BENCHMARK A slang or jargon term, usually meaning a measurement taken at the outset of a series of measurements of the same variable, sometimes meaning the best or most desirable value of the variable.

BENEFICENCE Literally, doing good. In bioethics, a principle underlying utilitarian approaches. It implies a certain obligation to promote benefits of things judged to be good, typically balancing potential or produced goods against risks. In public health, it implies acting in the best interest of the population at stake.[36,37]

BENEFIT Advantage or improvement resulting from an intervention.

BENEFIT-COST RATIO See COST-BENEFIT ANALYSIS.

BERKSONIAN BIAS (Syn: Berkson's bias, Berkson fallacy) A form of SELECTION BIAS arising when both the exposure and the disease under study affect selection. In its classical form, it causes hospital cases and controls in a case-control study to be systematically different from one another.[38] This occurs when the combination of exposure and disease under study increases the probability of admission to hospital, leading to a systematically higher exposure rate among hospital cases than among hospital controls; the process hence biases the odds ratio.

BERNOULLI DISTRIBUTION The probability distribution associated with two mutually exclusive and exhaustive outcomes—e.g., death or survival; a Bernoulli variable is one that has only two possible values—e.g., death or survival. See also BINOMIAL DISTRIBUTION.

BERTILLON CLASSIFICATION The first numerically based NOSOLOGY in which disease entities were arranged in chapters, developed by Jacques Bertillon (1851–1922).[39] It descended from a nosology proposed in 1853 by Marc d'Espigne and William Farr. Bertillon's classification was adopted at the International Statistical Institute (conference) in Chicago in 1893 and was the progenitor of the INTERNATIONAL CLASSIFICATION OF DISEASES (ICD).

BETA ERROR See ERROR, TYPE II.

BIAS Systematic deviation of results or inferences from truth. Processes leading to such deviation. An error in the conception and design of a study—or in the collection, analysis, interpretation, reporting, publication, or review of data—leading to results or conclusions that are systematically (as opposed to randomly) different from truth.[5–12,14,31–34]

Ways in which deviation from the truth can occur include:

1. Systematic variation of measurements from the true values (syn: systematic measurement error).
2. Variation of statistical summary measures (means, rates, measures of association, etc.) from their true values as a result of systematic variation of measurements, other flaws in study conduct and data collection, flaws in study design, or analysis.
3. Deviation of inferences from truth as a result of conceptual or methodological flaws in study conception or design, data collection, or the analysis or interpretation of results.
4. A tendency of procedures (in study design, data collection, analysis, interpretation, review, or publication) to yield results or conclusions that depart from the truth.
5. Prejudice leading to the conscious or unconscious selection of research hypotheses or procedures that depart from the truth in a particular direction or to one-sidedness in the interpretation of results.

The term *bias* does not necessarily carry an imputation of prejudice or any other subjective factor, such as the experimenter's desire for a particular outcome. This differs from conventional usage, in which *bias* refers to a partisan point of view—to prejudice or unfairness.

BIAS, ASCERTAINMENT See ASCERTAINMENT BIAS.

BIAS, BERKSON'S See BERKSON'S BIAS.

BIAS, CONFOUNDING See CONFOUNDING BIAS.

BIAS, WORKUP See WORKUP BIAS.

BIAS DUE TO DIGIT PREFERENCE See DIGIT PREFERENCE.

BIAS DUE TO INSTRUMENT ERROR Systematic error due to faulty CALIBRATION, inaccurate measuring instruments, contaminated reagents, incorrect dilution or mixing of reagents, etc. See also CONTAMINATION, DATA.

BIAS DUE TO WITHDRAWALS A difference between the true effect and the association observed in a study due to characteristics of subjects who choose to withdraw. See also ATTRITION; CENSORING; DROPOUT.

BIAS IN ASSUMPTIONS (Syn: conceptual bias) Error arising from faulty logic or premises or mistaken beliefs on the part of the investigator. False conclusions about the explanation for associations between variables. Example: Having correctly deduced the mode of transmission of cholera, John Snow concluded that yellow fever was transmitted by similar means. In fact, the "miasma" theory would have been a better fit for the facts of yellow fever transmission. See also BIOLOGICAL PLAUSIBILITY; COHERENCE.

BIAS IN AUTOPSY SERIES Systematic errors resulting from the fact that autopsies represent a nonrandom sample of all deaths.

BIAS IN HANDLING OUTLIERS Error arising from biased discarding of unusual values or due to exclusion of unusual values that should be included.

BIAS IN THE PRESENTATION OF DATA Error due to irregularities produced by DIGIT PREFERENCE, incomplete data, poor techniques of measurement, technically poor laboratory procedures, or intentional attempts to mislead.

BIAS IN PUBLICATION See PUBLICATION BIAS.

BIAS OF AN ESTIMATOR The difference between the expected value of an estimator of a parameter and the true value of this parameter. See also UNBIASED ESTIMATOR.

BIAS OF INTERPRETATION See INTERPRETIVE BIAS.

BIBLIOGRAPHIC IMPACT FACTOR (BIF) In SCIENTOMETRICS, a useful measure of the "average" frequency with which articles in a scientific periodical are cited by articles in journals that are chosen by the Thomson Corporation to be indexed in the Science Citation Index (SCI) and related databases.[40,41]

Given the limited properties of the BIF, even when properly applied to journals, and the well-known fact that scientific articles may have a wide spectrum of impacts (or none),[41] it is clear that the cultural impact of the "impact factor" in the academic community has less to do with scientific rationality than with the SOCIOLOGY OF SCIENTIFIC KNOWLEDGE (and human nature). Attributing bibliometric indicators for *journals* to *articles* or to individual *authors* is a form of the ECOLOGICAL FALLACY.

The BIF has virtues and limitations. Main reasons why, even for a given journal, BIF is often not the scientometric indicator of choice include the following: BIF is extremely influenced by the number of "source items" or "citeable articles" chosen as the denominator of the BIF (i.e., by the number of articles chosen by Thomson among articles published in the journal in the previous 2 years); such articles are not disclosed; criteria used by Thomson to decide which articles are included and excluded in the denominator of the BIF are unknown, and so is the consistency of their application across journals; citations to articles excluded from the denominator of the BIF are nevertheless counted in the numerator.

If the *journal* is the unit of analysis, the total number of citations received by all articles published by such journal may be a better indicator. If the bibliographic "impact" of an *article* is of interest, the total number of citations received by the article may the best place to start.[41]

BILLS OF MORTALITY Weekly and annual abstracts of christenings and burials compiled from parish registers in England, especially London, that date from 1538. Beginning in 1629, the annual bills were published and included a tabulation of deaths from plague and other causes. These were the basis for the earliest English vital statistics, compiled, analyzed, and discussed by John Graunt (1620–1674) in *Natural and Political Observations ... on the Bills of Mortality* (London, 1662).

BIMODAL DISTRIBUTION A distribution with two regions of high frequency separated by a region of low frequency of observations. A two-peak distribution.

BINARY VARIABLE A variable having only two possible values (e.g., *on* or *off*, 0 or 1). See also MEASUREMENT SCALE.

BINOMIAL DISTRIBUTION A probability distribution associated with two mutually exclusive outcomes (e.g., presence or absence of a clinical or laboratory sign, death or survival). The probability distribution of the number of occurrences of a binary event in a sample of n independent observations. The binomial distribution may be used to model CUMULATIVE INCIDENCE rates and PREVALENCE. The BERNOULLI DISTRIBUTION is a special case of the binomial distribution with $n = 1$.

BIOACCUMULATION Progressive increase in the concentration of a chemical compound in an organism, organ, or tissue when the rate of uptake exceeds the rate of excretion or metabolism. In humans, exposure to and bioaccumulation of persistent chemical agents occurs largely through the fatty components of animal foods, including recycled animal fats from slaughterhouses, which are used as components of food products and animal feed ingredients. Bioaccumulation occurs within a trophic (food chain) level. See also BIOMAGNIFICATION.

BIOASSAY The quantitative evaluation of the potency of a substance by assessing its effects on tissues, cells, live experimental animals, or humans. Bioassay may be a direct method of estimating relative potency: groups of subjects are assigned to each of two (or more) preparations, the dose that is just sufficient to produce a specified response is measured, and the estimate is the ratio of the mean doses for the two (or more) groups. In this method, the death of the subject may be used as the "response." The indirect method (more commonly used) requires study of the relationship between the magnitude of a dose and the magnitude of a quantitative response produced by it. See also INTERACTION.

BIODIVERSITY (Syn: biological diversity) The variety of species of plants, animals, and microorganisms in a natural community, of communities within a particular environment, and of genetic variation within a species (GENETIC DIVERSITY). Biodiversity is important for the stability of ecosystems. To many individuals worldwide it is also a cultural value.

"BIOLOGICAL AGE"

1. An attribute of body tissue that is relevant in PATHOGENESIS; e.g., "age" of breast tissue, which develops after puberty, in relation to breast cancer risk.[42] See also ARMITAGE-DOLL MODEL.
2. People age with different "speed" at equal "calendar age." Some people are physically older than others, and this is expressed in external appearance, body characteristics, or physical and social functioning. The concept is applied in the form of the calculation of the biological age of the subject by multiple regression.

BIOLOGICAL MONITORING (Syn: biomonitoring) Performance, analysis, and interpretation of biological measurements aimed at detecting changes (often adverse) in the health status of populations, in an environmental compartment (including water, air or soils), or in other health DETERMINANTS (e.g., food samples, animal feed). Monitoring of concentrations of suspected or known toxic or hazardous substances using biological means in well-defined populations (e.g., analyses of concentrations of environmental chemical agents in samples of urine, blood, or adipose tissue). Examples include the U.S. National Reports on Human Exposure to Environmental Chemicals (www.cdc.gov/exposurereport) and the German Environmental Surveys (www.umweltbundesamt.de/survey-e). See also MONITORING; SURVEILLANCE.

BIOLOGICAL PLAUSIBILITY The CAUSAL CRITERION or consideration that an observed, presumably causal ASSOCIATION is plausible on the basis of existing biomedical knowledge.

On a schematic continuum including *possible, plausible, compatible*, and *coherent*, the term *plausible* is not a demanding or stringent requirement, given the many biological mechanisms that often may underlie clinical and epidemiological observations; hence, in assessing CAUSALITY, it may be logically more appropriate to require COHERENCE (biological as well as clinical and epidemiological). The criterion of *biological plausibility* should hence be used cautiously, since it could impede development of new knowledge that does not fit existing biological evidence or pathophysiological reasoning. Innovative, valid, and relevant clinical and epidemiological discoveries may precede the acquisition of knowledge on their biological mechanisms; i.e., biologically relevant epidemiological evidence may precede biological evidence. In evaluating associations between genetic variants and common complex diseases, we should fully expect biologically meaningful associations with small clinical or epidemiological effects.[43] See also COHERENCE; HILL'S CRITERIA OF CAUSATION.

BIOLOGICAL TRANSMISSION See VECTOR-BORNE INFECTION.

BIOMAGNIFICATION (Syn: biological magnification, bioamplification) Sequence of processes in an ecosystem by which higher concentrations (e.g., of a persistent toxic substance) are attained in organisms at higher levels in the food chain. The increase in concentration of an element or compound, such as a pesticide, that occurs in a food chain. Biomagnification occurs across trophic (food chain) levels. See also BIOACCUMULATION.

BIOMARKER, BIOLOGICAL MARKER A cellular, biochemical, or molecular indicator of exposure; of biological, subclinical, or clinical effects; or of possible susceptibility (e.g., biomarkers of internal dose, biologically effective dose, early biological response, altered structure, altered function). It is occasionally an ambiguous term that suggests insufficient understanding of the pathophysiological or mechanistic role of the "marker." See also MOLECULAR EPIDEMIOLOGY.

BIOMETRY Literally, measurement of life. The application of statistical methods to the study of numerical data based on observation of biological phenomena. The term was made popular by Karl Pearson (1857–1936), who founded the journal *Biometrika*. The British biologist Francis Galton (1822–1911) has been described as the founder of biometry, but others—e.g., the Frenchman Pierre-Charles-Alexandre Louis (1787–1872)—preceded him.

BIOMONITORING See BIOLOGICAL MONITORING.

BIOSTATISTICS Application of STATISTICS to biological problems. The term should not be restricted to mean the application of statistics to medical problems (MEDICAL STATISTICS), since its real meaning is broader, subsuming agricultural statistics, forestry, and ecology, among other applications.

BIRTH CERTIFICATE Official, legal document recording details of a live birth, usually comprising name, date, place, identity of parents, and sometimes additional information such as birth weight. It provides the basis for vital statistics of birth and birthrates in a political or administrative jurisdiction and for the DENOMINATOR for infant mortality and certain other vital rates.

BIRTH COHORT The location of a person in historical time as indexed by his or her year of birth. Birth cohorts are often differentially affected by social events. Numerous COHORT variations in factors that have long-term effects on health (e.g., childbearing, smoking, physical activity) have been documented. Cohort effects are easiest to distinguish when disease trends have accelerated, decelerated, or changed direction; where they are steady and linear, they can hardly be distinguished reliably from period effects.[16,31] See also DEVELOPMENTAL AND LIFE COURSE EPIDEMIOLOGY; LIFE COURSE.

BIRTH COHORT ANALYSIS See COHORT ANALYSIS.

BIRTH INTERVAL Time interval between termination of one completed pregnancy and the termination of the next. Time interval between the birth of one offspring and the birth of the next offspring of the same mother.

BIRTH INTERVAL, CLOSED This applies to the population of women who gave birth to two or more living children: it counts only birth intervals between two completed pregnancies (i.e., the interval is closed by next pregnancy).

BIRTH INTERVAL, OPEN This applies also to the population of women who gave birth to two or more living children, but it counts only birth intervals after completed pregnancies.

BIRTH ORDER The ordinal number of a given live birth in relation to all previous live births of the same woman. Thus, 4 is the birth order of the fourth live birth occurring to the same woman. This strict demographic definition may be loosened to include all births, i.e., stillbirths as well as live births. More loosely, the ranking of siblings according to age, starting with the eldest in a family.

BIRTHRATE A summary rate based on the number of live births in a population over a given period, usually 1 year.

$$\text{Birthrate} = \frac{\begin{array}{c}\text{number of live births to residents}\\ \text{in an area in a calendar year}\end{array}}{\begin{array}{c}\text{average or midyear population}\\ \text{in the area in that year}\end{array}} \times 1000$$

Demographers refer to this as the *crude birthrate*.

BIRTH WEIGHT Infant's weight recorded at the time of birth and, in some countries, entered on the birth certificate. Certain variants of birth weight are precisely defined. Low birth weight (LBW) is below 2500 g. Very low birth weight (VLBW) is below 1500 g. Ultra-low birth weight (ULBW) is below 1000 g. Large for gestational age (LGA) is birth weight above the 90th percentile. Average weight for gestational age (AGA) (syn: appropriate or adequate) is birth weight between the 10th and 90th percentiles. Small for gestational age (SGA) (syn: small for dates) is birth weight below the 10th percentile.

"BLACK BOX"

1. A method of reasoning or studying a problem in which the methods and procedures are not described, explained, or perhaps even understood. Nothing is stated or inferred about the method; discussion and conclusions relate solely to the empirical relationships observed.
2. A method of formally relating an input (e.g., quantity of a drug administered, exposure to a putative causal factor) to an output or an observed effect (e.g., amount of the drug eliminated, disease), without making detailed assumptions about the MECHANISMS that have contributed to the transformation of input to output within the organism (the "black box").

"BLACK-BOX EPIDEMIOLOGY" A common epidemiological approach, used both in research and in public health practice, in which the focus is on assessing putative causes and clinical effects (beneficial or adverse) rather than the underlying biological MECHANISMS. It is not a formal branch or specialty of epidemiology, nor is it an epidemiological method or philosophy. Loosely speaking, it is an opposite of MECHANISTIC EPIDEMIOLOGY.

BLIND(ED) STUDY (Syn: masked study) A study in which observer(s) and/or subjects are kept ignorant of the group to which the subjects are assigned, as in an EXPERIMENT, or of the population from which the subjects come, as in a nonexperimental study. When both observer and subjects are kept ignorant, we refer to a DOUBLE-BLIND trial or study. If the statistical analysis is also done in ignorance of the group to which subjects belong, the study is sometimes described as TRIPLE-BLIND. The intent of keeping subjects and/or investigators blinded (i.e., unaware of knowledge that might introduce a bias) is to eliminate the effects of such biases. To avoid confusion about the meaning of the word *blind*, some authors prefer to describe such studies as *masked*. See also ALLOCATION CONCEALMENT; PERFORMANCE BIAS.

BLOCKED RANDOMIZATION (Syn: restricted randomisation) A procedure used in a RANDOMIZED CONTROLLED TRIAL that helps achieve a similar number of subjects allocated to each group, often within defined baseline categories. For example, for allocation in two groups (A and B) in blocks of four, there are six variants: (1) A A B B; (2) A B A B; (3) A B B A; (4) B B A A; (5) B A B A; (6) B A A B. To create the allocation sequence, such blocks are used at random. As a result of this procedure, the number of subjects in two groups at any time differs by no more than half the block length. Block size is usually a multiple of the number of groups in the trial. Small blocks are used at the beginning of the trial to balance subjects in small participating clinics or centers. Large blocks control balance less well but mask the allocation sequence better. It may be seen as an analogue in a RANDOMIZED CONTROLLED TRIAL of individual matching in an observational study. See also RANDOM ALLOCATION; STRATIFIED RANDOMIZATION.

BLOT, WESTERN, NORTHERN, SOUTHERN Varieties of tests using electrophoresis, nucleic acid base pairing, and/or protein antibody interaction to detect and identify DNA or RNA samples. The *Southern blot*, named for its discoverer, E. Southern, is used to identify a specific segment of DNA in a sample. Molecular biologists named variations of the test for the points of the compass. The *Northern blot* detects and identifies samples of RNA. The *Western blot* is widely used in a test for HIV infection.

BODY BURDEN Total amount of a substance present in the body.

BODY MASS INDEX (BMI) (Syn: Quetelet's index) Anthropometric measure, defined as weight in kilograms divided by the square of height in meters. This measure, suggested by the Belgian scientist Lambert Adolphe Jacques Quetelet (1796–1857) and then known as Quetelet's index II, correlates closely with body density and skinfold thickness; in this respect it is superior to the PONDERAL INDEX. It is a standard measure for the purpose of detecting overweight and obesity.

BONFERRONI CORRECTION See MULTIPLE COMPARISON TECHNIQUES.

BOOKMARKING In GENETICS and EPIGENETICS, a biological phenomenon believed to function as an epigenetic mechanism for transmitting cellular memory of the pattern of GENE EXPRESSION in a cell, throughout mitosis, to its daughter cells. It is vital for maintaining the phenotype in a lineage of cells. See also EPIGENETIC INHERITANCE.

BOOTSTRAP (Syn: resampling) A technique for estimating the variance and the bias of an estimator by repeatedly drawing random samples with replacement from the observations at hand. One applies the estimator to each sample drawn, thus obtaining a set of estimates. The observed variance of this set is the bootstrap estimate of variance.

the bootstrap estimate of bias. Many more sophisticated uses of the repeated samples have been developed.[12]

The difference between the average of the set of estimates and the original estimate is the bootstrap estimate of bias. Many more sophisticated uses of the repeated samples have been developed.[12]

BOX-AND-WHISKERS PLOT (Syn: box plot, cat-and-whiskers plot) A graphical method of presenting the distribution of a variable measured on a numerical scale. The midpoint (or sometimes, the median) of the distribution is often represented by a horizontal line; the values above and below this line divided into quartiles by horizontal lines (the "hinges" of the box) are the two quartiles nearer the midpoint; values beyond the hinges are represented by lines (the "whiskers") extending to the extreme value in each direction. Both the box-and-whiskers plot and the STEM-AND-LEAF DISPLAY were developed by the statistician John Tukey.[44]

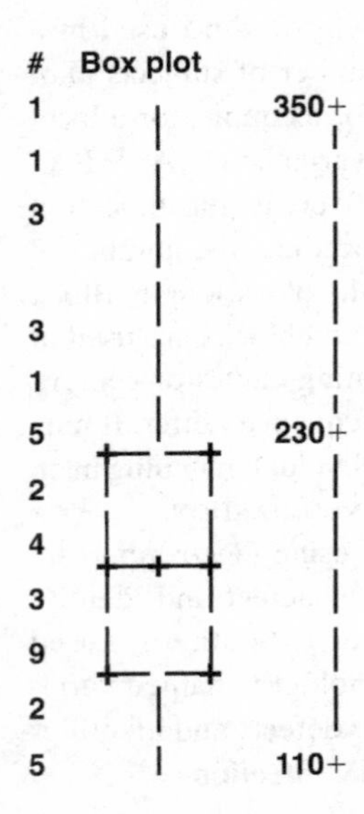

Box-and-whiskers plot. Four-week totals of reported cases of meningococcal infections, United States, 1987–1989. From Teutsch and Churchill, 1994.

"BRAIN SPARING" A human baby receiving an inadequate supply of nutrients or oxygen may protect its brain. One way in which it does this is by diverting more blood to the brain at the expense of the blood supply to the trunk. The growth of organs such as the liver is therefore "traded off" to protect growth of the brain. Brain sparing may also be effected through metabolic processes such as insulin resistance.[45] See also DEVELOPMENTAL ORIGINS HYPOTHESIS; PLASTICITY; THRIFTY PHENOTYPE.

BREAKPOINT In helminth epidemiology, the critical mean wormload in a community below which the helminth mating frequency is too low to maintain reproduction. A value exceeding the breakpoint of a wormload means that the wormload will increase until equilibrium is reached; a value less than or equal to the breakpoint means that the wormload will decrease progressively.

BUBBLE PLOT Display of three sets of variables, two of which form a scatter diagram while the third is represented by circles of varying diameter.

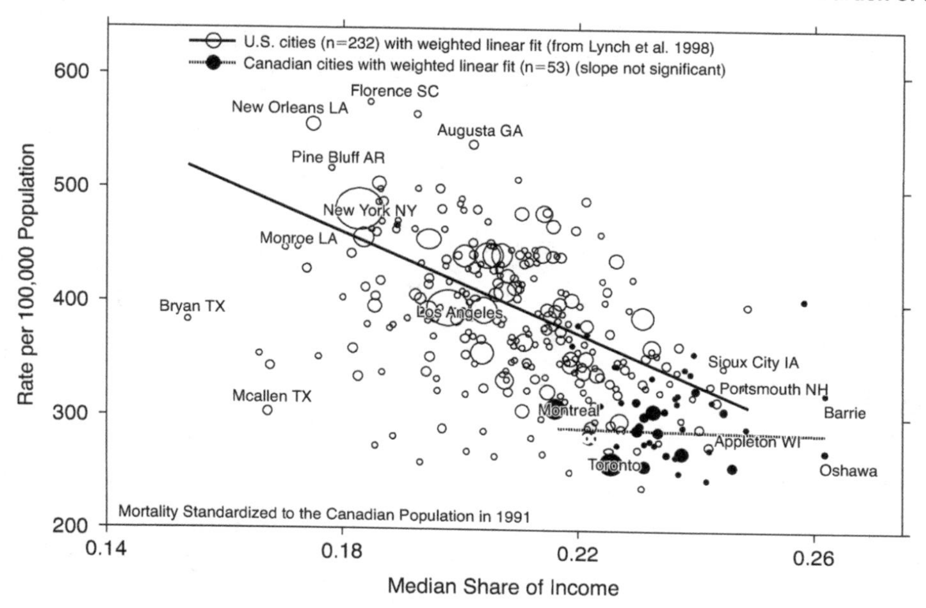

Bubble plot. Standardized mortality rates of working-age people by proportion of income of the less-well-off half of households, U.S. and Canadian cities, 1990–1991. U.S. cities open circles, Canadian cities solid circles. From Ross NA et al. *Br Med* J 2000; 320:898–902. With permission.

BURDEN OF DISEASE The impact of disease in a population. An approach to the analysis of health problems, including loss of healthy years of life. It is an important concept for public health and for other professions interested in the societal impact of ill-health, including injuries and disabilities. It may be expressed as lost HEALTHY LIFE YEARS (HEALYS), DISABILITY-ADJUSTED LIFE YEARS (DALYS), or QUALITY-ADJUSTED LIFE YEARS (QALYS). Use of indicators that integrate the societal burden caused by both death and morbidity allows for the comparison of the burden due to various risk factors or diseases. Sophisticated methodologies used in GLOBAL BURDEN OF DISEASE studies enable the combined measurement of mortality and non-fatal health outcomes, and provide comparable and comprehensive measures of population health across countries. They are also relevant to investigate the costs, efficacy, effectiveness, and other impacts of major health interventions applied in diverse settings.[30,46,47] The World Health Organization offers practical guidance for the estimation of disease burden at national or local levels for selected environmental and occupational risk factors.[48] These methodologies are somewhat controversial, however, because few diseases can be completely eradicated with most known interventions; it is therefore argued that disease burden provides a limited basis for policy, and that planning should be based on other considerations (e.g., the likely impact of interventions instead) and values. See also ATTRIBUTABLE FRACTION.

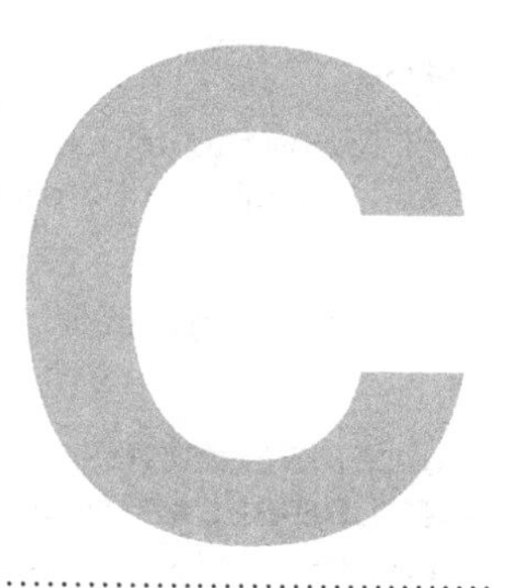

CALIBRATION Adjustment of an instrument or its measurements so the distribution of measurements matches a standard. In multicenter studies, calibration ensures a common standard and therefore comparability of measurements.

CALIPER MATCHING See MATCHING.

CAMPBELL COLLABORATION An independent international nonprofit organization that aims to help people make well-informed decisions about the effects of interventions in the social, behavioral, and educational arenas. An international network of social scientists that produces and disseminates systematic reviews of research evidence on the effectiveness of social interventions. Also known as "C2" because of its relationship with the COCHRANE COLLABORATION. www.campbellcollaboration.org.

CANADIAN MORTALITY DATABASE A large set of computer-stored death statistics; personal identifiers and causes of all deaths in Canada since 1950 have been computer-stored, with the death certificates preserved on microfiche. This database and record linkage have been used in some important historical cohort studies. See also NATIONAL DEATH INDEX.

CANCER EPIDEMIOLOGY A branch or subspecialty of epidemiology that studies factors influencing the occurrence (e.g., incidence, population distribution) of neoplastic and preneoplastic diseases and related disorders. Primary outcomes include incidence, prevalence, survival, and mortality from all types of cancers.

As mentioned below, EPIDEMIOLOGY studies *all types* of diseases and health-related events in populations; hence, this dictionary includes only a few examples of definitions of some disease-based subspecialties of epidemiology. See also CARCINOGENESIS; CARDIOVASCULAR EPIDEMIOLOGY; ENVIRONMENTAL EPIDEMIOLOGY; MOLECULAR EPIDEMIOLOGY; NEUROEPIDEMIOLOGY.

CANCER MORTALITY:INCIDENCE RATIO (Syn: cancer MIR, cancer mortality-to-incidence ratio) The ratio of mortality to incidence for each of several cancer sites being considered in a study. It is one diagnostic technique among several that can be used to gain some sense of cancer data quality; its main use is in studies of the natural history and survival rates of malignancies. Because not all patients with cancer die of cancer, the number of new cases in any one year should exceed cancer deaths in that same year, and—if cancer mortality and incidence are reported accurately—the ratio between the two should be proportional to the known survival for each specific site. For example, cancers with poor survival, such as pancreatic cancer, would be expected to have an

MIR closer to unity than cancers with better survival, such as testicular cancer. If MIR exceeds unity, concern should arise about the quality of the data.[49]

$$\text{Cancer MIR} = \frac{\text{no. of cancer-specific deaths over a specified length of time}}{\text{no. of cancer-specific new cases in the same time period}}$$

CANCER REGISTRY See REGISTER.

CAPTURE-RECAPTURE METHOD A method of estimating the size of a target population or a subset of this population that uses overlapping and presumably incomplete but intersecting sets of data about that population.[50,51] The method originated in wildlife biology, where it relied on tagging and releasing captured animals and then recapturing them. The method was adopted in veterinary epidemiology and later in vital statistics (census taking) and epidemiology. If two independent sources or population estimates are available, with (a) cases found by both, (b) cases found only by the first source, or (c) cases found only by the second source, the maximum likelihood population estimate is the product of the total in each source divided by the total found in both sources, i.e., $(a + b) \times (a + c) / a$. If the two sources are positively (negatively) dependent, the result will be biased toward an underestimate (overestimate). If three or more sources are available, log-linear methods can sometimes be used to model the degrees of dependency among the sources. Although the capture-recapture methods have some limitations, they are useful to estimate numbers of cases and numbers at risk in elusive populations, such as homeless people and sex workers. See also SNOWBALL SAMPLING.

CARCINOGEN A substance or agent that can cause cancer. Also, a physical, chemical, or biological agent that may induce or otherwise participate in the causation of cancer. A carcinogen may or may not be MUTAGENIC. Some compounds do not bind to DNA and are not mutagenic, yet they are carcinogenic in animal models and in humans. Carcinogens act through GENOTOXIC and NONGENOTOXIC mechanisms. "Complete carcinogens" [e.g., some polycyclic aromatic hydrocarbons (PAHs)] can induce both somatic (acquired) mutations in genes through DNA binding (tumor "initiation" phase) and subsequent outgrowth of irreversibly transformed cells (tumor "promotion" phase). In the early 1980s, carcinogenic PAHs were shown to induce activating mutations in *ras* genes. Today, about 200 different chemical compounds and mixtures are officially recognized as "known" or "anticipated to be" human carcinogens. See also PROCARCINOGEN; TCDD.

The International Agency for Research on Cancer (IARC) classifies carcinogens as follows:

Sufficient evidence. A positive causal relationship has been established between exposure and occurrence of cancer.

Limited evidence. A positive association has been observed between exposure to the agent and cancer for which a causal interpretation is credible, but chance, bias, or confounding cannot be ruled out.

Inadequate evidence. Available studies are of insufficient quality, consistency, or statistical power to permit a conclusion regarding the presence or absence of a causal relationship.

Evidence suggesting lack of carcinogenicity. Several adequate studies covering the full range of doses to which humans are known to be exposed are mutually consistent in not showing a positive association between exposure to the agent and any studied cancer at any level of exposure.

Overall evaluation: Taking all the evidence into account, the agent is assigned to one of the following categories:

Group 1: The agent is carcinogenic to humans.

Group 2: At one extreme, the evidence for human carcinogenicity is almost sufficient (group 2A, probably carcinogenic); at the other, there are no human data but there is experimental evidence of carcinogenicity (group 2B, possibly carcinogenic).

Group 3: The agent is not classifiable as to its human carcinogenicity.

Group 4: The agent is probably not carcinogenic to humans.

CARCINOGENESIS The process by which cancer is produced. Carcinogenesis is a multistage process driven by carcinogen-induced accumulation of genetic and EPIGENETIC damage in susceptible cells, which gain a selective growth advantage and undergo clonal expansion as the result of activation of (proto)oncogenes and inactivation of tumor suppressor genes. Accumulation of genetic and epigenetic alterations is hence a key causal process linking environment exposure and the occurrence of DISEASES OF COMPLEX ETIOLOGY.

The traditional stages of carcinogenesis are as follows:

Initiation. The primary step of tumor INDUCTION; the irreversible transformation of a cell's growth-regulatory processes whereby the potential for unregulated growth is established, usually through genetic damage by a chemical or physical CARCINOGEN.

Promotion. The second stage, in which a promoting agent induces an initiated cell to divide abnormally.

Progression. Transition of initiated promoted cells to a phase of unregulated growth and invasiveness, frequently with metastases and morphological changes in the cancer cells.

Research in MOLECULAR EPIDEMIOLOGY often generates evidence that clarifies aspects of the carcinogenic process (e.g., the mutational spectra of chemical and physical carcinogens in critical genes are of interest to define endogenous and exogenous carcinogenic mechanisms).

CARDIOVASCULAR EPIDEMIOLOGY A branch or subspecialty of epidemiology that studies factors influencing the occurrence of diseases that affect the cardiovascular system, like coronary heart disease and stroke. Primary outcomes include incidence, prevalence, survival, and mortality from cardiovascular diseases. Established and putative RISK FACTORS include individual-level behavioral factors (e.g., diet, smoking, physical activity) and psychosocial risk factors (e.g., social support, depression) as well as macro-, aggregate-, or higher-level socioeconomic factors and processes (e.g., geographic and economic characteristics of neighborhoods or cities).

As mentioned below, EPIDEMIOLOGY studies *all types* of diseases and health-related events in populations; hence, this dictionary includes just some examples of definitions for a few disease-based and exposure-based branches or subspecialties of epidemiology. See also CLINICAL EPIDEMIOLOGY; ENVIRONMENTAL EPIDEMIOLOGY; MOLECULAR EPIDEMIOLOGY; PHARMACOEPIDEMIOLOGY.

CARRIER A person or animal harboring a specific infectious agent in the absence of discernible clinical disease and serves as a potential source of infection. The carrier state may occur in an individual with an infection that is inapparent throughout its course (known as a healthy or asymptomatic carrier) or the carrier state may exist only during the incubation period, convalescence, and postconvalescence of an individual with a clinically recognizable disease (known as an incubatory carrier or convalescent carrier).

The carrier state may be of short or long duration (temporary or transient carrier or chronic carrier).[52]

CARRYING CAPACITY FOR HUMANS In a community of subsistence farmers, the carrying capacity denotes the maximum number of people that a hectare of land can support sustainably in an average year at a practicable level of technology and at a specified standard of living—commonly mere survival. For example, if a hectare of land grows 1 ton of maize and 250 kg will feed one person for a year, the carrying capacity of that land is four people to the hectare. There is uncertainty about the earth's carrying capacity: some experts argue that there is abundant unused capacity, while others believe that the earth is already exceeding its carrying capacity.

CARRYING CAPACITY FOR OTHER SPECIES The maximum sustainable size of a resident population in a given ecosystem.

CARRYOVER EFFECT

1. A BIAS that may occur when the effects of an exposure persist into a subsequent period when a second exposure of interest is acting.
2. In a CROSSOVER CLINICAL TRIAL the effect of the treatment given in the first period may continue ("carryover") into the second treatment period.
3. Treatments may be randomly allocated to paired organs (eyes, arms, hips, kidneys) if treatments act only locally. However, CONTAMINATION may occur if there is a carryover effect of the experimental treatment to the control organ of the pair.[14]

CARTOGRAM A diagrammatic map on which epidemiological or statistical information is presented visually; examples include ISODEMOGRAPHIC and CHOROPLETHIC maps.

CASE A particular disease, health disorder, or condition under investigation found in an individual or within a population or study group. As often non-strictly used in the health sciences, a person having a particular disease, disorder, or condition (e.g., a case of cancer, a case in a case-control study). A variety of criteria may be used to identify cases, e.g., individual physicians' diagnoses, registries and notifications, abstracts of clinical records, surveys of the GENERAL POPULATION, population screening, and reporting of defects, as in a dental record. The epidemiological definition of a case is not necessarily the same as the ordinary clinical definition.

CASE, AUTOCHTHONOUS In infectious disease epidemiology, a case of local origin. Literally, "native where it arises." See also CASE, IMPORTED; CASE, INDIGENOUS.

CASE-BASE STUDY A variant of the case-control design in which the controls are drawn from the same STUDY BASE as the cases, regardless of their disease status.[12,53] Cases of the disease of interest are identified, and a sample of the entire base population (cases and noncases) forms the controls. This design provides for estimation of the risk ratio or rate ratio without any RARE DISEASE ASSUMPTION. Specific examples include the CASE-COHORT STUDY and the DENSITY CASE-CONTROL STUDY.

CASE-CASE STUDY A type of study in which cases of a given disease with a specific characteristic are compared with other cases with the same disease but without the characteristic; the latter may be, for instance, an acquired (somatic) genetic alteration or an inherited genetic variant. The aim is to identify etiological or susceptibility factors specific to the subset of cases with the characteristic.[54] The design is also used in infectious disease epidemiology to detect different transmission ways between subtypes of one disease.[55–57] It is also useful to analyze infectious disease outbreaks: exposures of an outbreak cluster are compared with exposures among individuals infected by another subtype of the same disease. See also CASE-ONLY STUDY.

CASE-COHORT STUDY A variant of the case-control design in which the controls are drawn from the same COHORT as the cases regardless of their disease status. Cases of the disease of interest are identified, and a sample of the entire starting cohort (regardless of their outcomes) forms the controls. This design provides an estimate of the risk ratio without any RARE DISEASE ASSUMPTION.[12,31] A type of CASE-BASE STUDY. See also DENSITY CASE-CONTROL STUDY; NESTED CASE-CONTROL STUDY.

CASE, COLLATERAL A case occurring in the immediate vicinity of a case that has been the subject of an epidemiological investigation; a term used mainly in malaria control programs, equivalent to the term *contact* as used in infectious disease epidemiology.

CASE, IMPORTED In infectious disease epidemiology, a case that has entered a region by land, sea, or air transport, in contrast to one acquired locally. See also CASE, AUTOCHTONOUS.

CASE, INDIGENOUS In infectious disease epidemiology, a case in a person residing in the area.

CASE, INDUCED In malaria epidemiology, a case occurring in a person who has received a transfusion of blood containing malaria parasites; the term is generalizable to other conditions that can be transmitted by infected blood (e.g., HIV, hepatitis C).

CASE CLASSIFICATION In surveillance epidemiology, gradations in the likelihood of being a case (e.g., suspected/probable/confirmed); a useful method when early reporting of cases is important (e.g., Ebola hemorrhagic fever) and where there are difficulties in making a definitive diagnosis, (e.g., because specialized laboratory tests are required) or when the diagnosis is based on a scoring system, as with multiple sclerosis.

CASE-COMPARISON STUDY A term considered a synonym for CASE-CONTROL STUDY in the past.

CASE-COMPEER STUDY Another term that in the past was considered a synonym for CASE-CONTROL STUDY.

CASE-CONTROL STUDY (Syn: case-referent study) The observational epidemiological study of persons with the disease (or another outcome variable) of interest and a suitable control group of persons without the disease (comparison group, reference group). The potential relationship of a suspected RISK FACTOR or an attribute to the disease is examined by comparing the diseased and nondiseased subjects with regard to how frequently the factor or attribute is present (or, if quantitative, the levels of the attribute) in each of the groups (diseased and nondiseased).[12,31]

It is not correct to call "case-control study" any comparison of a group of people having a specific outcome with another group free of that outcome.[10] The case-control study used to be called "retrospective" because, conceptually, it goes from disease onset backwards to the postulated causal factors. Yet cases and controls in a case-control study are often accumulated prospectively: the conduct of the study starts before cases have been diagnosed and, as each new case is diagnosed and identified, it is entered in the study. Subjects in a RANDOMIZED CONTROLLED TRIAL should not be described as *cases* and *controls*.

CASE-CROSSOVER DESIGN A variant of the CASE-ONLY STUDY. An observational analogue of a CROSSOVER STUDY. It can be used when a brief exposure triggers an outcome or causes a transient rise in the risk of a disease with an acute onset (e.g., to assess the effect of medication use on the short-term risk of myocardial infarction). [12,58] One key difference between a traditional case-control study and the case-crossover design is that in the latter latter each case serves as its own matched control. The exposure status of each case is assessed during different time windows, and the exposure status at the time of case occurrence is compared to the status at other times. Conditions to be met include the following:

1. Acute cases are needed, an abrupt outcome applies best.
2. Crossover in exposure status. There must be a sufficient number of individuals who crossed from higher to lower exposure level and vice-versa.
3. Brief and transient exposures. The exposure or its effects must be short-lived.
4. Selection of control time periods must be unrelated to any general trends in exposure.

Properly applied, the design allows estimation of the rate ratio without need for a RARE DISEASE ASSUMPTION. See also CASE-TIME CONTROL STUDY.

CASE DEFINITION A set of criteria (not necessarily diagnostic criteria) that must be fulfilled in order to identify a person as representing a case of a particular disease. It is different from case diagnosis. Case definition can be based on geographic, clinical, laboratory, or combined clinical and laboratory criteria or on a scoring system with points for each criterion that matches the features of the disease. Where the diagnosis is based on a scoring system (e.g., multiple sclerosis), it is important to abide by the system for surveillance purposes and in deciding whether to include or exclude cases in an epidemiological study.[59]

CASE FATALITY RATE The proportion of cases of a specified condition that are fatal within a specified time.

$$\text{Case fatality rate (usually expressed as a percentage)} = \frac{\text{number of deaths from a disease (in a given period)}}{\text{number of diagnosed cases of that disease (in the same period)}} \times 100$$

This definition can lead to paradox when more persons die of the disease than develop it during a given period. For instance, chemical poisoning that is slowly but inexorably fatal may cause many persons to develop the disease over a relatively short period of time, but the deaths may not occur until some years later and may be spread over a period of years during which there are no new cases. Thus, in calculating the case fatality rate, it is necessary to acknowledge that the time dimension varies: it may be brief (e.g., covering only the period of stay in a hospital); of finite duration (e.g., 1 year); or of longer duration still. The term *case fatality rate* is then better replaced by a term such as *survival rate* or by the use of a survivorship table. See also ATTACK RATE; SURVIVORSHIP STUDY.

CASE FINDING

1. (Syn: Contact tracing). A standard procedure in the control of certain contagious diseases (e.g., tuberculosis and sexually transmitted diseases) whereby diligent efforts are made to locate and treat persons who have had close or intimate contact with a known case. Also, seeking persons who have been exposed to risk of other potentially harmful factors, like toxic substances, epidemic conditions, or outbreaks such as food poisoning.
2. SECONDARY PREVENTION through EARLY CLINICAL DETECTION of cases among persons using health services for other reasons (e.g., checking blood pressures of all patients who attend a physician's office).

CASE HISTORY STUDY

1. In clinical medicine, a CASE REPORT or a report on a CASE SERIES.
2. A term considered a synonym for CASE-CONTROL STUDY in the past.

CASE IMPACT NUMBER See IMPACT NUMBERS

CASE INVESTIGATION In surveillance epidemiology, examination to determine whether an individual is or is not involved in an epidemic, especially an INDEX CASE.

CASE-MIX INDEX (CMI) A measure of the complexity of illness. Among hospital patients, it is based on the relative severity indexes assigned to a DIAGNOSIS-RELATED GROUP. A high CMI indicates a high proportion of complex cases and justifies higher rates of reimbursement in medical care insurance systems such as Medicare.

CASE-ONLY STUDY A method that analyzes data from a case series. It may be seen as an epidemiological equivalent of the "thought experiment" used by theoretical physicists. It is used in the CASE-CROSSOVER STUDY, in CASE-SPECULAR designs, and in molecular and genetic epidemiology to assess relationships between environmental exposures and genotypes.[60] See also CASE-CASE STUDY.

CASE REFERENT STUDY See CASE-CONTROL STUDY.

CASE REPORTS Detailed descriptions of a few patients or clinical cases (frequently, just one sick person) with an unusual disease or complication, uncommon combinations of diseases, an unusual or misleading SEMIOLOGY, CAUSE or OUTCOME (maybe a surprising recovery ...). They often are preliminary observations that are later refuted. They cannot estimate disease frequency or risk (e.g., for lack of a valid DENOMINATOR). However, as Pierre Charles Alexandre Louis, Claude Bernard, Thomas Lewis, Austin Bradford Hill, and many others have shown (e.g., more recently, Jan P. Vandenbroucke or Gordon Guyatt, or organizations like the COCHRANE COLLABORATION), many problems worthy of investigation in medicine are first identified by observations at the bedside.[61] Indeed, case reports may thoughtfully integrate clinical, anatomopathological, genetic, pathophysiological, biochemical, or molecular information and reasoning; they may thus build a sound mechanistic or pragmatic hypothesis and help set the foundation for microbiological studies and for larger clinical and epidemiological studies. They may also properly raise a suspicion of a new adverse drug event, and they are an important means of surveillance for rare clinical events. They help us to reflect on and learn from medical error.[62,63]

CASE SERIES A collection of patients with common characteristics used to describe some clinical, pathophysiological, or operational aspect of a disease, treatment, or diagnostic procedure. Some are similar to the larger CASE REPORTS and share the virtues of this design. The number of subjects does not attenuate the limitations of the design. A case series does not include a comparison group and is often based on prevalent cases and on a SAMPLE of convenience.[62] Common selection biases and confounding severely limit their power to make CAUSAL INFERENCES. See also INCEPTION COHORT.

CASE-SPECULAR STUDY A type of CASE-ONLY STUDY that obtains the actual distribution of exposure among the dwellings of the cases and a reflected or "specular" exposure distribution, which is what the exposure distribution would have been if the dwellings had been placed on the opposite side of the street. From these two distributions (i.e., the actual and the specular distribution) and some assumptions, including a RARE DISEASE ASSUMPTION, a relative risk estimate for the effect of exposure can be calculated, much as it can for a case-control study, albeit with different assumptions. For example, the distance of each case's front door from an electrical wire is matched with the distance from the same wire of a hypothetical front door located exactly across the street.[64]

CASE STUDY A detailed analysis of the occurrence, development, and outcome of a particular problem or innovation, often over a period of time. A detailed description of a concrete situation requiring ethical analysis, judgment, and—sometimes—action.

CASE-TIME-CONTROL DESIGN A design in which exposure of cases and controls during one period is compared in matched-pair analyses to their own exposure during another period of similar length.[65] See also CASE-CROSSOVER STUDY.

CASUISTRY A method of reasoning and decision making, especially in ETHICS, based on experience with and decisions about similar cases in the past. This contrasts with ethical decision making that is more strongly based on ethical principles. Medical *casuistics* is the study of cases of disease.

CAT-AND-WHISKERS PLOT See BOX-AND-WHISKERS PLOT.

CATASTROPHE THEORY A branch of mathematics dealing with large changes in the total system that may result from small changes in a critical variable in the system. An example is the sudden change in the physical state of water into steam or ice with rise or fall of temperature beyond a critical level. Certain epidemics, gene frequencies, and behavioral phenomena in populations may abide by the same mathematical rule. Herd immunity is an example. See also CHAOS THEORY.

CATCHMENT AREA Region from which the clients of a particular health facility are drawn. Such a region may be well or ill defined.

CATEGORIZATION One way of organizing information on objects or ideas. The process of recognition, differentiation, and understanding of objects by grouping into categories, usually for statistical analysis or graphic representation. *Category* is from late Latin *categoria*—a division within a system of CLASSIFICATION. See also TAXONOMY; ONTOLOGY; DIRECTORY; CATALOGUING; CLUSTERING.

CAUSAL CRITERIA or **CAUSAL CONSIDERATIONS** Considerations (often called "criteria") that help to guide judgments about causality and to make causal inferences.[6,9,10,14,66,67] Examples close to epidemiology include John Stuart MILL'S CANONS, the "rules" of David Hume, EVANS'S POSTULATES, HENLE-KOCH POSTULATES, or HILL'S CRITERIA OF CAUSATION.

CAUSAL DIAGRAM (Syn: causal graph, path diagram) A graphical display of causal relations among variables, in which each variable is assigned a fixed location on the graph (called a *node*) and in which each direct causal effect of one variable on another is represented by an arrow with its tail at the cause and its head at the effect.[68] Direct noncausal associations are usually represented by lines without arrowheads. Graphs with only directed arrows (in which all direct associations are causal) are called *directed graphs*. Graphs in which no variable can affect itself (no feedback loop) are called *acyclic*. Algorithms have been developed to determine from causal diagrams which sets of variables are sufficient to control CONFOUNDING and for when control of variables leads to BIAS.[69,70]

CAUSAL INFERENCE The thought processes and methods that assess or test whether a relation of cause to effect does or does not exist. See also ASSOCIATION; HILL'S CRITERIA OF CAUSATION; PROBABILITY OF CAUSATION; PROPERTIES OF A CAUSE; VERIFICATION.

CAUSALITY The relating of causes to the effects they produce. The property of being causal. The presence of cause. Ideas about the nature of the relations of cause and effect. The potential for changing an outcome (the effect) by changing an antecedent

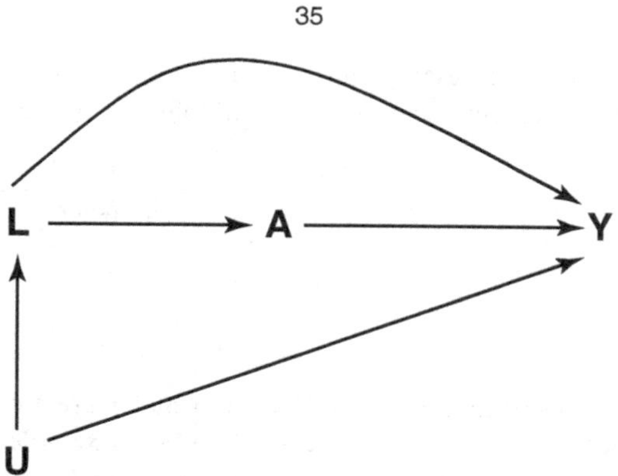

Causal diagram representing outcome Y, exposure A, their unmeasured common cause U, and risk factor L. Graph theory can be used to show that data on L are sufficient to eliminate the confounding, caused by the presence of U, for the effect of A on Y.

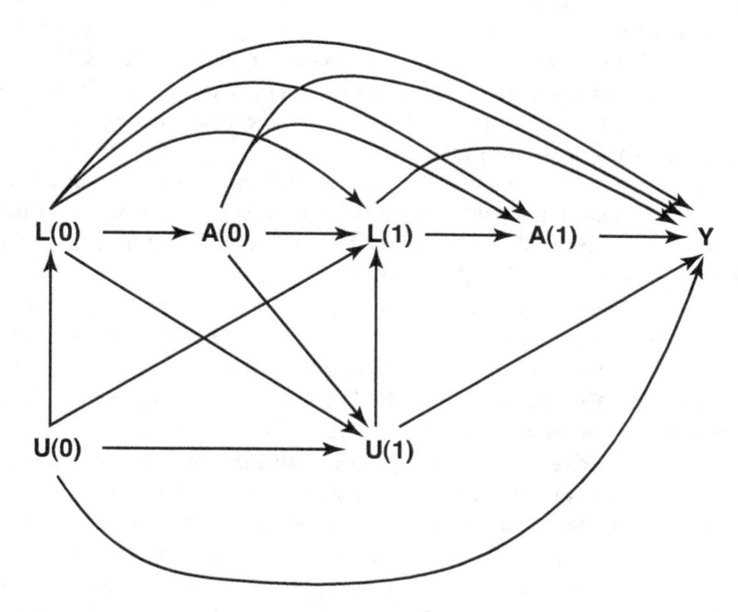

Causal diagram representing outcome Y and time-varying exposure A(t), their unmeasured common cause U(t), and risk factor L(t) at times t = 0 and t = 1. Graph theory can be used to show that data on L(0) and L(1) are sufficient to eliminate the confounding, caused by the presence of U(0) and U(1), for the joint effect of A(0) and A(1) on Y.

(the cause). Most of clinical, epidemiological, and public health research concerns causality. In the health and life sciences, causality is often established by integration of biological, clinical, epidemiological, and social evidence, as appropriate to the hypothesis at stake. Several types of causes can be distinguished.[66,67] A cause is termed "necessary" when it must always precede an effect. This effect need not be the sole result of the one cause. A cause is termed "sufficient" when it inevitably initiates or produces an effect.

Any given cause may be necessary, sufficient, neither, or both. Hence, there are four general conditions under which independent variable *X* may cause *Y*:

	X is necessary	*X* is sufficient
1.	+	+
2.	+	–
3.	–	+
4.	–	–

1. *X* is necessary and sufficient to cause *Y*. Both *X* and *Y* are always present together, and nothing but *X* is needed to cause *Y*; $X \rightarrow Y$. For example, the measles virus is necessary to cause measles in an unimmunized individual or population.
2. *X* is necessary but not sufficient to cause *Y*. *X* must be present when *Y* is present, but *Y* is not always present when *X* is. Some additional factor(s) must also be present; *X* and $Z \rightarrow Y$. *Mycobacterium tuberculosis* is the necessary cause of tuberculosis but often is not a sufficient cause without poverty, poor nutrition, overcrowding, etc.
3. *X* is not necessary but is sufficient to cause *Y*. *Y* is present when *X* is, but *X* may or may not be present when *Y* is present, because *Y* has other causes and can occur without *X*. For example, an enlarged spleen can have many separate causes that are unconnected with each other; $X \rightarrow Y$; $Z \rightarrow Y$. Lung cancer can be caused by cigarette smoking, asbestos fibers, or radon gas.
4. *X* is neither necessary nor sufficient to cause *Y*. Again, *X* may or may not be present when *Y* is present. Under these conditions, however, if *X* is present with *Y*, some additional factor must also be present. Here *X* is a contributory cause of *Y* in some causal sequences; *X* and $Z \rightarrow Y$; *W* and $Z \rightarrow Y$.

Necessary and *sufficient* were Galileo's descriptors of a true cause for the experimental science he advocated. See also ASSOCIATION; CAUSAL CRITERIA; DISEASES OF COMPLEX ETIOLOGY; HILL'S CRITERIA OF CAUSATION; NECESSARY CAUSE.

CAUSATION OF DISEASE, FACTORS IN The following factors have been differentiated, although they are not mutually exclusive:

1. PREDISPOSING FACTORS are those that prepare, sensitize, condition, or otherwise create a situation such as a level of immunity or state of susceptibility so that the host tends to react in a specific fashion to a disease agent, personal interaction, environmental stimulus, or specific incentive. Examples include age, sex, marital status, family size, educational level, previous illness experience, presence of concurrent illness, dependency, working environment, and attitudes toward the use of health services. These factors may be "necessary" but are rarely "sufficient" to cause the phenomenon under study.
2. ENABLING FACTORS are those that facilitate the manifestation of disease, disability, ill-health, or the use of services or conversely those that facilitate recovery from illness, maintenance or enhancement of health status, or more appropriate use of health services. Examples include income, health insurance coverage, nutrition, climate, housing, personal support systems, and availability of medical care. These factors may be "necessary" but are rarely "sufficient" to cause the phenomenon under study.
3. PRECIPITATING FACTORS are those associated with the definitive onset of a disease, illness, accident, behavioral response, or course of action. Usually one factor is more important or more obviously recognizable than others if several are involved and one may often be regarded as "necessary." Examples include exposure to specific disease,

amount or level of an infectious organism, drug, noxious agent, physical trauma, personal interaction, occupational stimulus, or new awareness or knowledge.

4. REINFORCING FACTORS are those tending to perpetuate or aggravate the presence of a DISEASE, DISABILITY, IMPAIRMENT, attitude, pattern of behavior, or course of action. They may tend to be repetitive, recurrent, or persistent and may or may not necessarily be the same or similar to those categorized as predisposing, enabling, or precipitating. Examples include repeated exposure to the same noxious stimulus (in the absence of an appropriate immune response) such as an infectious agent, work, household, or interpersonal environment, presence of financial incentive or disincentive, personal satisfaction or deprivation. See also PROBABILITY OF CAUSATION.

CAUSE-DELETED LIFE TABLE A life table constructed using death rates lowered by eliminating the risk of dying from a specified cause; its most common use is to calculate the gain in life expectancy that would result from the elimination of one cause. See also COMPETING RISK.

CAUSE, PROPERTIES See PROPERTIES OF A CAUSE.

CAUSES, COMPONENTS See COMPONENT CAUSES.

CAUSES IN PUBLIC HEALTH SCIENCES In epidemiology and other population sciences, causes include contextual factors, even if such factors can seldom be manipulated experimentally to produce change,[71,72] given the following facts: causes operate at upper, aggregate, and distal levels as well as across macro- and micro-levels (climate, geographic location, diet); some causes are fairly constant or inmutable conditions (as gender); others show large variations across time and space in the extent to which they change in an individual's lifecourse (educational and occupational achievement, social mobility and status, income, living arrangements).[16] Hence, causes of individual and population health often change with global and local societal processes, and many act in specific periods of susceptibility (as in utero), often with long latencies, or throughout life. None of these characteristics per se excludes or refutes CAUSALITY. Research on the causes of diseases is a "natural meeting place" for basic science (whose focus is knowledge on biological mechanisms), clinical sciences, and epidemiology (which aims at generating knowledge useful for primary prevention). See also STRATEGY, "POPULATION."

CAUSES OF DEATH See DEATH CERTIFICATE.

CAUSE-SPECIFIC RATE A rate that specifies events, such as deaths, according to their cause.

CCS See CASE-CONTROL STUDY.

CDC Centers for Disease Control and Prevention. An agency of the U.S. Public Health Service (www.cdc.gov).

CENSORING

1. Loss or ATTRITION of subjects from a follow-up study; the occurrence of the event of interest among such subjects is uncertain after a specified time when it was known that the event of interest had *not* occurred; it is not known, however, if or when the event of interest occurred subsequently. Such subjects are described as *censored*. For example, in a follow-up study with myocardial infarction as the outcome of interest, a subject who has not had an infarct but is killed in a traffic crash in year 6 is described as censored as of year 6, since it cannot be known when, if ever, he might have had an infarct at a later year of follow-up. This is censoring by competing risk; other varieties include loss to follow-up and termination of the study. Examination of data for censoring requires the use of special analytical methods, such as life table analysis.[12,31]

2. Observations with unknown values from one end or a particular interval of a frequency distribution. Left-censored data come from the left-hand portion, or low end, and right-censored data come from the right-hand portion, or high end, of the distribution.

CENSUS An enumeration of a population, originally intended for purposes of taxation and military service. Ancient civilizations such as the Romans conducted censuses; Jesus of Nazareth was born in Bethlehem because Mary and Joseph had gone there to be counted in a Roman census. Census enumeration of a population usually records identities of all persons in every place of residence, with age or birth date, sex, occupation, national origin, language, marital status, income, and relationship to head of household in addition to information on the dwelling place. Many other items of information may be included, e.g., educational level (or literacy) and health-related data such as permanent disability. A de facto census allocates persons according to their location at the time of enumeration. A de jure census assigns persons according to their usual place of residence at the time of enumeration.

CENSUS TRACT An area for which details of population structure are separately tabulated at a periodic census; normally it is the smallest unit of analysis of census tabulations. Census tracts are chosen because they have well-defined boundaries, sometimes the same as local political jurisdictions, sometimes defined by conspicuous geographical features such as main roads or rivers. In urban areas census tracts may be further subdivided (e.g., into city blocks), but published tables do not contain details to this level. Census tracts are usually relatively homogenous in demographic, socioeconomic, and ethnic composition.

CENTILE See QUANTILES.

CESSATION EXPERIMENT Controlled study in which an attempt is made to evaluate the termination of an exposure to risk such as a living habit that is considered to be of etiological importance.

CHAINS OF RISK A sequence of linked exposures that increase (or decrease) disease risk because one negative (or positive) experience or exposure tends to lead to another and then another. See also LIFE COURSE.

CHANCE

1. Frequency PROBABILITY.
2. Accidental, unanticipated, unplanned, fortuitous, serendipitous (e.g., a chance finding during DATA DREDGING). See also FORTUITOUS.
3. In ordinary use, the possibility that an event will happen (e.g., "There is a chance that she will survive"). Prospect, probability, likelihood. An opportunity.

CHAOS THEORY Branch of mathematics dealing with events and processes that cannot be predicted by conventional mathematical theorems or laws because small, localized perturbations have widespread general consequences. Examples include long-range weather changes and turbulence in fast-flowing water. The unpredictable course of some epidemics and metastases in many kinds of cancer accord with chaos theory.

CHART The medical dossier of a patient. See also INFORMATION SYSTEM; MEDICAL RECORD.

CHECK DIGIT A single digit, derived from a multidigit number such as a case identification number, that is used as a screening test for transcription errors.

CHEMOPROPHYLAXIS The administration of a chemical, including antibiotics, to prevent the development of an infection or to slow progression of the disease to a clinically manifest form. Applicable to infectious and noninfectious diseases.

CHEMOTHERAPY The use of a chemical to treat a clinically recognizable disease or to limit its further progress.

CHILD DEATH RATE The number of deaths of children age 1–4 years in a given year per 1000 children in this age group. This is a useful measure of the burden of preventable communicable diseases in the child population.

CHILD MORTALITY RATE (Syn: under-5 mortality rate) Health indicator used by the United Nations Children's Fund (formerly the United Nations International Children's Emergency Fund, or UNICEF), the United Nationd Development Programme (UNDP), and other international agencies. It is computed as an annual rate, dividing the death count of children under age 5 by the count of live births in the same year and expressing the result per thousand. Therefore it is not an age-specific mortality rate, since the denominator is not the size of the child population under age 5. This rate is preferable to the child death rate, which is more difficult to determine in communities where the age of young children may not be known precisely.

CHILD NUTRITION, MEASURES OF UNCF defines several aspects of infant and child nutrition:

Stunting A measure of protein-energy malnutrition, indicated by low height for age or failure to achieve expected stature.

Underweight A composite measure of protein-energy malnutrition, indicated by low weight for age.

Wasting A measure of protein-energy malnutrition that occurs when a child's weight for height falls significantly below what is expected in the reference population; an indicator of current malnutrition.

CHI-SQUARE (χ^2) DISTRIBUTION A variable is said to have a chi-square distribution with K degrees of freedom if it is distributed like the sum of the squares of K independent random variables, each of which has a normal distribution with mean zero and variance one.

CHI-SQUARE (χ^2) TEST Any statistical test based on comparison of a test statistic to a chi-square distribution. The oldest and most common chi-square tests are for detecting whether two or more population distributions differ from one another; these tests usually involve counts of data and may involve comparison of samples from the distributions under study or the comparison of a sample to a theoretically expected distribution. The Pearson chi-square test is probably the best known; another is the MANTEL-HAENSZEL TEST. (Statisticians disagree about the terminal letter; most of those who contributed to the discussion of this entry prefer *chi-square* rather than *chi-squared*. Either usage is acceptable.)

CHOROPLETHIC MAP A method of mapping to display quantitative information (e.g., rates) in defined jurisdictions such as counties or states; an example is a color-coded atlas of cancer mortality.

CHRISOMS This word, which appears in BILLS OF MORTALITY, means infants who die before formal baptism: therefore the number recorded in Bills of Mortality can be used to estimate (albeit inaccurately) neonatal death rates in studies of historical demography and epidemiology.

CHRONIC

1. Referring to a health-related state, lasting a long time.
2. Referring to exposure, prolonged or long-term, often with specific reference to low intensity.

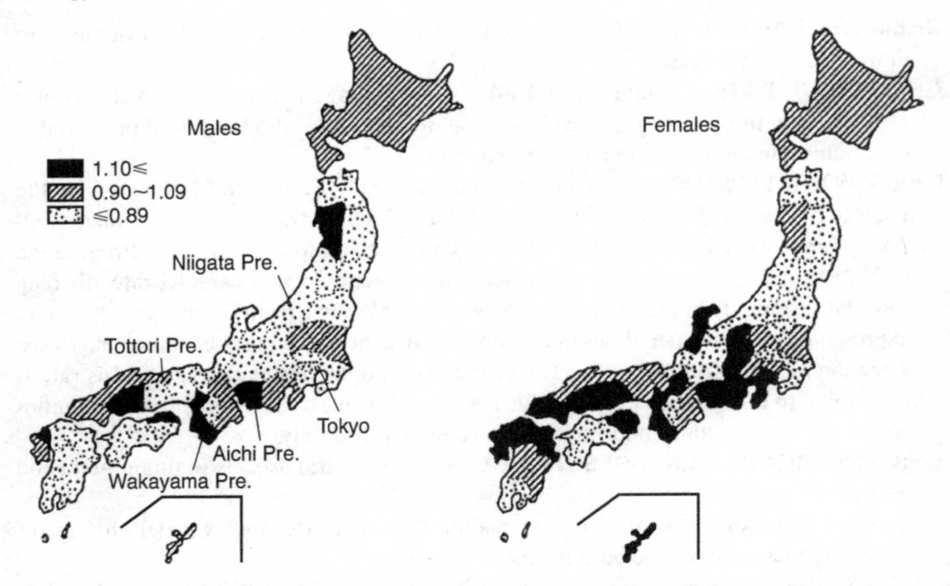

Choroplethic map. Regional differences of hip fracture incidence in Japan. From Hosoda et al. *Jpn J Epidemiol*, 1992; 2(Suppl 2): S205–S213. With permission.

3. The U.S. National Center for Health Statistics defines a "chronic" condition as one of 3 months' duration or longer.

CHRONOBIOLOGY The study of biological processes that possess periodicity (e.g., circadian rhythms, the menstrual cycle).

CIOMS Council for International Organizations of the Medical Sciences. See also COHORT STUDY, HISTORICAL.

CIRCULAR EPIDEMIOLOGY Needlessly repetitive epidemiological studies that merely reiterate what has already been done and demonstrated unequivocally.[73]

CIRCULAR REASONING

1. Reasoning that requires that the conclusion be used to support one of the premises. Circularity may be a problem in definitions.[74]
2. An argument whose conclusion is implicitly assumed in one of the premises.

As with the assessment of a TEMPORAL RELATIONSHIP, detection of circular reasoning in a research study may need to be based on a complex and subtle assessment of the study design, conduct, and analysis.

CLASS A term used in the theory of frequency distributions. The total number of observations made upon a particular variate may be grouped into classes according to convenient divisions of the variate range in order to make subsequent analyses less laborious or for other reasons. A group so determined is called a *class*. The variate values that determine the upper and lower limits of a class are called *class boundaries*, the interval between them is the *class interval*, and the frequency falling into the class is the *class frequency*. See also SET; SOCIAL CLASS.

CLASSIFICATION

1. Assignment to predesignated classes on the basis of perceived common characteristics.
2. A means of giving order to a group of disconnected facts.

Ideally, a classification should be characterized by (1) naturalness—the classes correspond to the nature of the thing being classified, (2) exhaustiveness—every member of the group will fit into one (and only one) class in the system, (3) usefulness—the classification is practical, (4) simplicity—the subclasses are not excessive, and (5) constructability—the set of classes can be constructed by a demonstrably systematic procedure. See also CATEGORIZATION; TAXONOMY.

CLASSIFICATION OF DISEASES Arrangement of diseases into groups having common characteristics. Useful in efforts to achieve standardization, and therefore comparability, in the methods of presentation of mortality and morbidity data from different sources. May include a systematic numerical notation for each disease entry. Examples include the INTERNATIONAL CLASSIFICATION OF DISEASES (ICD) and the See INTERNATIONAL CLASSIFICATION OF PRIMARY CARE, SECOND EDITION REVISED (ICPC-2-R). See also FAMILY OF CLASSIFICATIONS.

CLASS INTERVAL The difference between the lower and upper limits of a class.

CLASTOGENIC That causes damage to chromosomes. See also MUTAGENIC; ANEUGENIC.

CLINICAL DECISION ANALYSIS Application of DECISION ANALYSIS in a clinical setting, often to assess probabilities of outcomes of alternative decisions (e.g., surgical procedures or drug treatment for myocardial ischemia). It considers three aspects of the decision: choices (options available to the patient), chances (probabilities of outcome for each choice), and values (quantitative expression of the desirability of different outcomes). It can be applied to small numbers of cases and even to a single patient. A method to systematically assess available treatment options, possible outcomes, and the desirability of each possible outcome. See also DECISION ANALYSIS; N-OF-ONE STUDY.

CLINICAL ECOLOGY An outdated term for the study of ENVIRONMENTAL HYPERSENSITIVITY. Also an earlier name for environmental medicine.

CLINICAL ECONOMICS The application of cost-benefit and cost-effectiveness analytic techniques in a clinical setting or to clinical problems.

CLINICAL EPIDEMIOLOGY The application of epidemiological knowledge, reasoning, and methods to study clinical issues and improve clinical care. In practice, unfortunately, "clinical" is often restricted to "medical" ("medical epidemiology" is also a completely acceptable and commonly used term). Research often addresses etiological, mechanistic, diagnostic, therapeutic, and prognostic medical issues, is conducted in clinical settings, is led by clinicians, and has patients as the subjects of study. Clinical epidemiology uses epidemiological principles mostly to aid decision making involving sick individuals, although the wider CONTEXT is also considered.[9,10,14,61–63,75] See also CLINICAL DECISION ANALYSIS; N-OF-ONE STUDY.

CLINICAL IMPORTANCE See SIGNIFICANCE, CLINICAL.

CLINICAL PREDICTION RULE A set of criteria used to estimate the probability of a specific outcome or outcomes, particularly in a group of patients.[62] See also CLINICAL DECISION ANALYSIS.

CLINICAL SIGNIFICANCE See SIGNIFICANCE, CLINICAL.

CLINICAL STUDY (Syn: clinical investigation) An investigation involving persons and aiming to understand or control disease and other HEALTH states in persons. Often—but not exclusively—carried out on patients, by physicians, and in a health care setting. Problems found worthy of investigation in caring for patients are frequently taken to the laboratories; yet the nature and purpose of the investigation often remains clinical, and the laboratory results must be tested again on actual persons—eventually by integrating epidemiological and statistical reasoning with clinical, pathophysiological, and microbiological (e.g., genetic) reasoning.[61] See also CASE REPORTS; CLINICAL EPIDEMIOLOGY; INDIVIDUAL THINKING; INTEGRATIVE RESEARCH.

CLINICAL TRIAL (Syn: therapeutic trial) A research activity that involves the administration of a test regimen to humans to evaluate its efficacy and safety. The term is subject to wide variation in usage, from the first use in humans without any control treatment to a rigorously designed and executed experiment involving RANDOM ALLOCATION of test and control treatments. Four phases of clinical trials are distinguished:

Phase I trial It is the first test of a drug (or a candidate vaccine) in a small group of humans to determine its safety and mode of action. It usually involves fewer than 100 healthy volunteers. The focus is on safety and pharmacological profiles; it may also assess dose and route of administration.

Phase II trial Pilot efficacy studies. Initial trial to examine efficacy, usually in 200 to 500 volunteers; with vaccines, the focus is on immunogenicity, and with drugs, on demonstration of safety and efficacy in comparison to existing regimens. Usually but not always, subjects are randomly allocated to the study and control groups.

Phase III trial Extensive clinical trial. This phase is intended for complete assessment of safety and efficacy. It involves larger numbers of patients with the disease or condition of interest, sometimes thousands: it uses random allocation to study and control groups.

Phase IV trial Conducted after the regulatory authority has approved registration and marketing begins. The common aim is to estimate the incidence of rare adverse reactions and other potential effects of long-term use in real life; it may also study new uses and indications. It is part of POSTMARKETING SURVEILLANCE, which also includes OBSERVATIONAL STUDIES. See also COMMUNITY TRIAL.

CLINICAL TRIAL, NEGATIVE See NEGATIVE STUDY; NULL STUDY.

CLINICAL TRIAL, SPLIT-MOUTH A design used frequently in oral research: the mouth is divided into two or more subunits. Active and control (comparison) treatments are applied to the subunits (e.g., to the left and right sides). Treatments are compared within each patient. The design may reduce interpatient variability, much as in a CROSSOVER CLINICAL TRIAL. See also CARRYOVER EFFECT.

CLINIMETRICS The domain concerned with indexes, rating scales, and other expressions used to describe or measure symptoms, physical signs, and other distinctly clinical phenomena in clinical medicine.[75] Such measurements are an essential part of many microbiological, clinical, and epidemiological studies. See also CLINICAL EPIDEMIOLOGY.

CLOSED COHORT A population in which membership begins at a defined time or with a defined event and ends only through occurrence of the study outcome or the end of eligibility for membership. An example is a population of women in labor being studied to determine the vital status of their offspring (i.e., whether live or stillborn).

CLOSED POPULATION A population that gains no new members and loses members only to death. Compare CLOSED COHORT.

CLUSTER Aggregations of relatively uncommon events or diseases in space and/or time in amounts that are believed or perceived to be greater than could be expected by chance. Putative disease clusters are often perceived to exist on the basis of ANECDOTAL EVIDENCE, and much effort may be expanded by epidemiologists and biostatisticians in assessing whether a treu cluster of disease exists

CLUSTER ANALYSIS A set of statistical methods used to group variables or obser-vations into interrelated subgroups (e.g., to detect clusters in routine surveillance of disease).

CLUSTERING (Syn: disease cluster, time cluster, time-place cluster) A closely grouped series of events or cases of a disease or other health-related phenomena with well-defined distribution patterns in relation to time or place or both. The term is normally used to describe aggregation of relatively uncommon events or diseases (e.g., leukemia, multiple sclerosis).

CLUSTER SAMPLING A sampling method in which each unit selected is a group of persons (all persons in a city block, a family, etc.) rather than an individual.

CNN APPROACH "Condoms, Needle exchange, Negotiation." A set of strategies aiming to combat the HIV/AIDS pandemic, other sexually transmitted diseases, and other blood-borne infections. Harm reduction approaches to reducing the rate of HIV transmission through the adoption of safer sex and through risk reduction in intravenous drug users by provision of clean needles. See also ABC APPROACH.

COCARCINOGEN A substance that enhances the effect of a CARCINOGEN.

COCHRANE COLLABORATION An international organization of clinicians, epidemiologists, patients, and others that aims to help health professionals make well-informed decisions about HEALTH CARE by preparing, maintaining, disseminating, and promoting the accessibility of systematic reviews of the effects of health care interventions. *Cochrane Reviews* are prepared and updated by collaborating authors working in a *Cochrane Collaborative Review Group* and using explicitly defined methods to minimize the effects of bias; where appropriate and feasible, META-ANALYSIS is used to reduce imprecision. The collaboration honors Archibald L. Cochrane, who advocated preference (including financial advantage) for interventions that have been assessed and found to be effective and efficient (www.cochrane.org). See also EFFECTIVENESS.

COCHRAN-MANTEL-HAENSZEL TEST See MANTEL-HAENSZEL TEST.

CODE A numerical and/or alphabetical system for classifying information (e.g., about diagnostic categories).

CODING Translation of information (e.g., questionnaire responses) into numbered categories for entry in a data processing system.

CODE OF CONDUCT A formal statement of desirable conduct that research workers and/or practitioners are expected to honor; there may be penalties for violation. Examples include the Hippocratic Oath, the Nürnberg (Nuremberg) Code, and the Helsinki Declaration, which govern requirements for research on human subjects. See also GUIDELINES.

COEFFICIENT OF CONCORDANCE A measure of the agreement among several rankings or categories.

COEFFICIENT OF VARIATION The ratio of the standard deviation to the mean. This is meaningful only if the variable is measured on a ratio scale. See MEASUREMENT SCALE.

COERCION Excessive pressure or influence to force or entice a person to act in a given way (e.g., to enroll in a research study or a public health program). May be exercised by offering excessive incentives, applying social pressure, using authority figures, or otherwise manipulating the vulnerable person or group.[37] See also INFORMED CONSENT.

COGNITIVE DISSONANCE The state of having inconsistent thoughts, beliefs, perceptions (i.e., cognitions), or attitudes, especially as relating to behavioral decisions and attitude change.[76] The drive to reduce *dissonance* in one's system of beliefs may lead to surprising strategies of belief formation and retention.[77] A theory that addresses competing or contradictory elements of cognition and behavior (e.g., why do people continue smoking when they know that smoking damages health?). Dissonance reduction may be attained through a change in behavior (e.g., quit smoking), in attitude or in beliefs.[78]

COGNITIVE DISSONANCE BIAS A form of INTERPRETIVE BIAS that occurs when the belief in a given mechanism increases rather than decreases in the face of contradictory evidence.[79] See also CONFIRMATION BIAS.

COHERENCE The extent to which a hypothesized causal ASSOCIATION fits with preexisting theory and knowledge.[67] Biological coherence requires more than just biological plausibility or compatibility with biological knowledge derived from studies of nonhuman species or experimental systems.

COHERENCE, EPIDEMIOLOGICAL The extent to which a biological, clinical, or social observation is coherent with epidemiological evidence. A criterion for causal inference in the biological and clinical sciences, approximately but not fully reciprocal to the criterion of BIOLOGICAL PLAUSIBILITY in epidemiological causal inference.[80]

COHORT (From Latin *cohors*, warriors, the tenth part of a legion)

1. The component of the population born during a particular period and identified by period of birth so that its characteristics (e.g., causes of death and numbers still living) can be ascertained as it enters successive time and age periods.
2. The term "cohort" has broadened to describe any designated group of persons who are followed or traced over a period of time, as in COHORT STUDY (prospective study). See also BIRTH COHORT; HISTORICAL COHORT STUDY.

COHORT ANALYSIS The tabulation and analysis of morbidity or mortality rates in relation to the ages of a specific group of people (COHORT) identified at a particular period of time and followed as they pass through different ages during part or all of their life span. In certain circumstances (e.g., studies of migrant populations), cohort analysis may be performed according to duration of residence of migrants in a country, rather than year of birth, in order to relate health or mortality experience to duration of exposure. The aim is to detect age, period, and generation effects. Age-period-cohort models can be fitted to distinguish these effects; because of the dependency among the three factors, they require assumptions in order to estimate the parameters of the model. See also ACCUMULATION OF RISK; BIRTH COHORT; DEVELOPMENTAL AND LIFE COURSE EPIDEMIOLOGY.

COHORT COMPONENT METHOD A method of population projection that takes the population distributed by age and sex at a base date and carries it forward in time on the basis of separate allowances for fertility, mortality, and migration.

COHORT EFFECT See GENERATION EFFECT.

COHORT INCIDENCE See INCIDENCE.

COHORT SLOPES (Syn: graphical cohort analysis) Arrangement of data so that when plotted graphically, lines connect points representing the age-specific rates for population segments from the same generation of birth (see diagram). These slopes represent changes in rates with age during the life experience of each cohort.

COHORT STUDY (Syn: concurrent, follow-up, incidence, longitudinal, panel, prospective study) The analytic epidemiological study in which subsets of a defined population can be identified who are, have been, or in the future may be exposed or not exposed, or exposed in different degrees, to a factor or factors hypothesized to influence the occurrence of a given disease or other outcome.[9–12] The main feature of cohort study is observation of large numbers over a long period (commonly years), with comparison of incidence rates in groups that differ in exposure levels. The alternative terms for a cohort study (i.e., follow-up, longitudinal, and prospective study) describe an essential feature of the method, which is observation of the population for a sufficient number of person-years to generate reliable incidence or mortality rates in the population subsets.

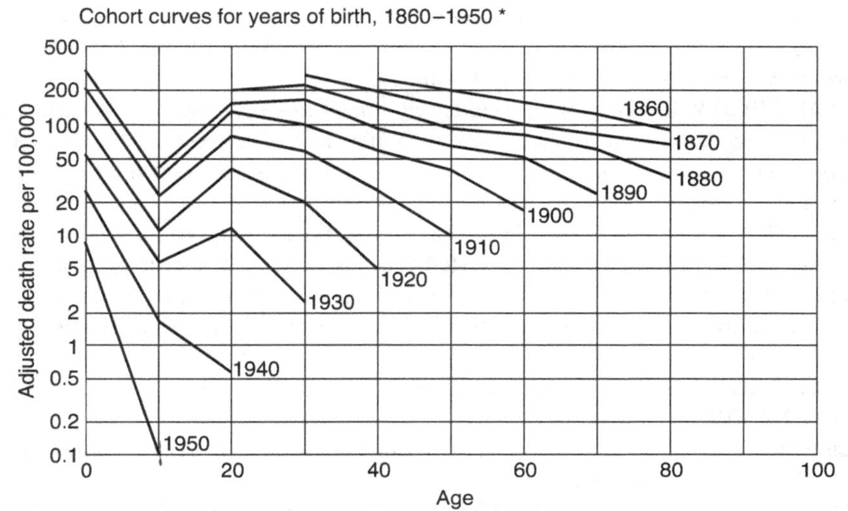

Cohort slopes. Tuberculosis mortality rates of successive birth generations; death rates for tuberculosis by age, United States, 1900–1960, per 100,000 population, logarithmic scale. From Susser, Watson, Hopper, 1985.

This generally implies study of a large population, study for a prolonged period (years), or both. The denominators used for analysis may be persons or person-time.[81] See also COHORT ANALYSIS.

COHORT STUDY, HISTORICAL (Syn: historical prospective study, nonconcurrent prospective study, prospective study in retrospect) A COHORT STUDY conducted by reconstructing data about persons at a time or times in the past. This method uses existing records about the health or other relevant aspects of a population as it was at some time in the past and determines the current (or subsequent) status of members of this population with respect to the condition of interest. Different levels of past exposure to risk factor(s) of interest must be identifiable for subsets of the population. RECORD LINKAGE systems are often used in historical cohort studies. Growing public concern about protection of PRIVACY threatens such studies, which in the past have often made very valuable contributions to scientific understanding of disease causation. Ethical reviewers of research proposals for historical cohort studies increasingly require the investigators to obtain the informed consent of persons whose archived records are to be used in the study. If the study involves very large numbers and/or some or all of the persons are dead or cannot be traced, it is obviously not feasible to obtain their informed consent. Guidelines such as those composed by the Council for International Organizations of Medical Sciences (CIOMS) recommend that the informed consent requirement be waived in such circumstances.

COINTERVENTION In a RANDOMIZED CONTROLLED TRIAL, the application of additional diagnostic or therapeutic procedures to members of either or both the experimental and the control groups.

COLD CHAIN A system of protection against high environmental temperatures for heat-labile vaccines, sera, and other active biological preparations. Unless the cold chain is preserved, such preparations are inactivated and IMMUNIZATION procedures, etc., will be ineffective. Preservation of the cold chain is an integral part of the WHO expanded program on immunization in tropical countries.

COLLAPSIBILITY Equality of stratum-specific measures of association or effect with the crude (collapsed), unstratified measure. Often, lack of collapsibility is equated with CONFOUNDING but may instead signal inappropriate stratification (as in BERKSON'S BIAS and some forms of SELECTION BIAS). See CONFOUNDING BIAS.

COLLIDER A variable directly affected by two or more other variables in the CAUSAL DIAGRAM.[68,69,82] In the following "inverted fork" $X \rightarrow C \leftarrow Y$ the arrow represents a direct effect of the tail variable on the head variable; C is then called a collider on the X-C-Y pathway in the graph, and stratifying on C will tend to change the association of X and Y.

COLLINEARITY Very high correlation among variables.

COLONIZATION See INFECTION.

COMMENSAL Literally, eating together (sharing the same table). An organism that lives harmlessly in the gut. See also XENOBIOTIC.

COMMON DISEASE GENETIC AND EPIGENETIC HYPOTHESIS The CDGE hypothesis argues that in addition to genetic variation, EPIGENETICS provides an added layer of variation that might mediate the relationship between GENOTYPE and internal and external environmental factors. This epigenetic component may help to explain the marked increase in common diseases with age as well as the frequent discordance of diseases between monozygotic twins.[83]

COMMON GOOD Shared values or benefits deemed to be good, either explicitly or tacitly, for individuals and for society. Although the definition is critical for public health, in complex democratic societies it may be difficult to achieve consensus on certain "goods." For epidemiological and public health practice, elements of the larger public good include health itself as social value, and the broader value of "assuring conditions under which people can be healthy."[37] See also PUBLIC HEALTH.

COMMON SOURCE EPIDEMIC (Syn: common vehicle epidemic) See EPIDEMIC, COMMON SOURCE.

COMMON VEHICLE SPREAD Transmission of a disease agent (infectious pathogen, toxic chemical, etc.) from a source that is common to those who acquire the disease. Common vehicles include air, water, food, injected substances. Legionellosis is an example of common vehicle spread in air that has passed through air conditioning equipment contaminated by the causal organism. HIV disease and hepatitis B and C can be spread among illicit drug users by the common vehicle of contaminated needles and syringes. Cholera and many other waterborne diseases are spread by the common vehicle of contaminated water. The principal modes of foodborne common vehicle spread were sonorously summarized by an anonymous author (probably Sir Andrew Balfour) in *Memoranda on Medical Diseases in Tropical and Subtropical Areas*,[84] published by the British War Office in 1914–1918: ". . . careless carriers, contact cases, chiefly cooks, dirty drinking water, the dust of dried dejecta and the repulsive regurgitation, dangerous droppings, and filthy feet of faecal-feeding flies fouling food." The work has not lacked chances to be revised often in later wars.

COMMUNICABLE DISEASE (Syn: infectious disease) An illness due to a specific infectious agent or its toxic products that arises through transmission of that agent or its products from an infected person, animal, or reservoir to a susceptible host, either directly or indirectly through an intermediate plant or animal host, vector, or the inanimate environment. See also TRANSMISSION OF INFECTION.

COMMUNICABLE PERIOD The time during which an infectious agent may be transferred directly or indirectly from an infected person to another person, from an infected animal to humans, or from an infected person to an animal, including arthropods. See also TRANSMISSION OF INFECTION.

COMMUNITARIAN ETHICS An approach to ethics emphasizing communal values, the COMMON GOOD, or social goals. Closely aligned with the cooperative virtues and a community's shared understanding of life. Need not be pitted against individual rights.[36,85,86]

COMMUNITY A group of individuals organized into a unit or manifesting some unifying trait or common interest; loosely, the locality or catchment area population for which a service is provided or, more broadly, the state, nation, or body politic.

COMMUNITY DIAGNOSIS The process of appraising the health status of a community, including assembly of vital statistics and other health-related statistics and of information pertaining to DETERMINANTS of health, such as prevalence of tobacco smoking, and examination of the relationships of these determinants to health in the specified community. The term may also denote the findings of this diagnostic process. Community diagnosis may attempt to be comprehensive or may be restricted to specific health conditions, determinants, or subgroups. J. N. Morris identified community diagnosis as one of the uses of epidemiology.[87]

COMMUNITY HEALTH See PUBLIC HEALTH.

COMMUNITY MEDICINE

1. The study of health and disease in the population of a specified community. The goal is to identify health problems and needs, to identify means by which these needs may be met, and to evaluate the extent to which health services meet these needs.
2. The practice of medicine concerned with communities (or specified populations) rather than individuals; this includes the above elements and the organization and provision of HEALTH CARE at a community (or specified population) level.

COMMUNITY NEED ASSESSMENT A method of identifying the needs of the community so that corrective measures can be taken.

COMMUNITY-ORIENTED PRIMARY HEALTH CARE Integration of community medicine with the primary health care of individuals. The PRIMARY HEALTH CARE practitioner or team is responsible for health care both at the individual and the community or population levels. See also PUBLIC HEALTH; SOCIAL MEDICINE.

COMMUNITY TRIAL Experiment in which the unit of allocation to receive a preventive, therapeutic, or social intervention is an entire community or political subdivision. Examples include the trials of fluoridation of drinking water and of heart disease prevention in North Karelia (Finland) and California. See also CLINICAL TRIAL; EXPERIMENT; EXPERIMENTAL EPIDEMIOLOGY.

COMORBIDITY Disease(s) that coexist(s) in a study participant in addition to the index condition that is the subject of study.

COMPARISON GROUP Any group to which the index group is compared. Usually synonymous with *control group*. Use of this term is preferably restricted to randomly allocated groups.

COMPETING CAUSE In considering a particular cause of death (or other inevitable outcome), one must take account of other causes, which are commonly called competing causes. When a previously common cause of death becomes rare, competing causes must become more prominent. For instance, among young adults, pneumonia and other infections were a common cause of death until about midway through the twentieth century; their control has brought to prominence some competing causes of death, such as cancers and suicide.

COMPETING RISK An event that removes a subject from being at risk for the outcome under investigation. For example, in a study of smoking and cancer of the lung, a subject who dies of coronary heart disease is no longer at risk of lung cancer; in this situation, coronary heart disease is a competing risk.

COMPLETED FERTILITY RATE The number of children born alive per woman in a cohort of women by the end of their childbearing years. See also TOTAL FERTILITY RATE.

COMPLETING THE CLINICAL PICTURE The use of epidemiology to define all modes of presentation of a disease and all possible outcomes. One of the "uses of epidemiology" identified by J. N. Morris.[87]

COMPLETION RATE The proportion or percentage of persons in a SURVEY for whom complete data are available for analysis. See also RESPONSE RATE.

COMPLEX TRAIT (Syn: polygenic trait, multifactorial trait) Any PHENOTYPE that results from the effect of multiple genes at two or more loci, often from environmental influences as well.[23]

COMPLIANCE See ADHERENCE.

COMPONENT CAUSES Multiple causes (not necessarily RISK FACTORS) that act jointly to cause a given effect. They do so in different combinations, each combination of component causes capable of giving rise to particular effects. No component cause is sufficient to produce the effect. In some processes (e.g., diseases), one of the component causes is necessary, but in other instances this is not so (i.e., none of the component causes may be necessary). The frequency of the components of a SUFFICIENT CAUSE influences their relative strength. This heuristic model is useful when it also integrates the analysis of antecedent causes, the sequence and TIME ORDER of causal events, and causal processes that operate at different levels.[12,66–69,88]

COMPOSITE INDEX An index, such as the APGAR SCORE or the tumor/nodes/metastases (TNM) system to stage cancer, that contains contributions from categories of several different variables.

COMPOSITIONAL EFFECTS Effects of individual-level factors (i.e., characteristics of individuals within a group or area, such as individual income) on individual-level outcomes after accounting for the effects of relevant group- or area-level factors (referred to as CONTEXTUAL EFFECTS). They are estimated using MULTILEVEL ANALYSIS.[89] See also CAUSES IN PUBLIC HEALTH SCIENCES.

COMPRESSION OF MORBIDITY A term describing abbreviation of the average period of life when chronic illness or disability affects physical, mental, or social function. In theory, as health promotion and disease prevention become more efficacious, this period of long-term morbidity is compressed into a smaller proportion of the total life span. Empirical observations in several countries have failed to demonstrate the phenomenon. Others envisage an EXPANSION OF MORBIDITY or a state of balance. See also RECTANGULARIZATION OF MORTALITY.

CONCORDANCE Pairs or groups of individuals of identical phenotype. In twin studies, a condition in which both twins exhibit or fail to exhibit a trait under investigation.

CONCORDANT A term used in TWIN STUDY to describe a twin pair in which both twins exhibit a certain trait and in matched pair analysis when the pairs match.

CONCURRENT STUDY See COHORT STUDY.

CONDITIONAL PROBABILITY The probability of an event given that another event has occurred. If D and E are two events and P (...) is "the probability of (...)," the conditional probability of D given that E occurs is denoted $P(D|E)$, where the vertical slash is read "given" and is equal to $P(D \text{ and } E)/P(E)$. The event E is the "conditioning event." Conditional probabilities obey all the axioms of probability theory. See also BAYES' THEOREM; PROBABILITY THEORY.

CONFIDENCE INTERVAL (CI) The conventional form of an INTERVAL ESTIMATE, computed in statistical analyses, based on the theory of frequency PROBABILITY. If the underlying statistical model is correct and there is no bias, a confidence interval derived from a valid analysis will, over unlimited repetitions of the study, contain the true parameter with a frequency no less than its confidence level (often 95% is the stated level, but other levels are also used).[12]

CONFIDENCE LIMITS The upper and lower boundaries of the confidence interval.

CONFIDENTIALITY The obligation not to disclose information; the right of a person to withhold information from others. Information in medical records, case registries, and other data files and bases is generally confidential, and epidemiologists are required to obtain permission before being given access to it. This may be the INFORMED CONSENT of the person to whom the records relate or the permission of an INSTITUTIONAL REVIEW BOARD. Epidemiologists have an obligation to preserve confidentiality of information they obtain during their studies. See also INFORMED CONSENT; PRIVACY.

CONFIRMATION BIAS A form of BIAS that may occur when evidence that supports one's preconceptions is evaluated differently from evidence that challenges these convictions.[34] The tendency to test one's beliefs or conjectures by seeking evidence that might confirm or verify them and to ignore evidence that might disconfirm or refute them.[90] See also CONSISTENCY.

CONFLICT OF INTEREST Compromise of a person's objectivity when that person has a vested interest (e.g., in peer review, in the outcome of a study). It occurs when the person could benefit financially or in other ways (e.g., promotion, tenure, prestige) from some aspect of a study, report, or other professional activity. Conflicts of interest are not limited to research settings. See also DISCLOSURE OF INTERESTS.

CONFOUNDING (From the Latin *confundere*, to mix together) Loosely, the distortion of a measure of the effect of an exposure on an outcome due to the association of the exposure with other factors that influence the occurrence of the outcome. Confounding occurs when all or part of the apparent association between the exposure and outcome is in fact accounted for by other variables that affect the outcome and are not themselves affected by exposure.[5–12] See also CONFOUNDING BIAS.

CONFOUNDING BIAS (Syn: confounding)

1. Bias of the estimated effect of an exposure on an outcome due to the presence of a common cause of the exposure and the outcome. Example: The effect of aspirin use on the risk of stroke will be confounded if aspirin is more likely to be prescribed to individuals with heart disease, which is hence both an indication for treatment and a risk factor for the disease. Heart disease may be a risk factor for stroke if it has a direct causal effect on stroke (heart disease is then the common cause of aspirin use and stroke) or if atherosclerosis causes both heart disease and stroke (atherosclerosis is then the common cause).
2. Bias of the estimated effect of an exposure on an outcome due to baseline differences among exposure groups in the risk factors for the outcome, or differences in POTENTIAL

OUTCOMES.[91] Unlike the first definition, this definition includes biases produced by selection when the selection occurred prior to the exposure of interest (e.g., M-BIAS[82] and CONFOUNDING BY INDICATION). Confounding bias is often equated with lack of COLLAPSIBILITY, but the latter concept is purely numerical, not causal.

CONFOUNDING BY INDICATION A type of CONFOUNDING BIAS that occurs when a symptom or sign of disease is judged as an indication (or a contraindication) for a given therapy and is therefore associated both with the intake of a drug or medical procedure (or its avoidance) and with a higher probability of an outcome. The reason to initiate treatment, assessed by a health professional or by the patient, is thus associated both with the prescription of a drug (or with self-medication) and with a higher probability of a particular outcome—usually adverse. Confounding by indication generally arises in a common clinical situation and in full coherence with clinical logic: before beginning to take a given drug patients who are prescribed the drug have a poorer prognosis (or a higher risk of a disease-related adverse outcome) than patients who do not receive the drug. Confounding by indication stems from an initial lack of similarity in the prognostic expectations of treated and nontreated subjects.[92] It shares some features with "susceptibility bias," "procedure selection bias," PROTOPATHIC BIAS, and SELECTION BIAS.

CONFOUNDING, NEGATIVE Confounding that produces a downward bias in the effect estimate. Alternatively, confounding that dilutes, underestimates, obscures, or attenuates (rather than exaggerates or overestimates) the estimated effect of an exposure on an outcome. These alternative definitions often coincide for causal factors but are opposites for preventive factors; hence the term can be confusing.

CONFOUNDING, POSITIVE Confounding that produces an upward bias in the effect estimate. Alternatively, confounding that creates, overestimates, or exaggerates (rather than underestimates) the estimated effect of an exposure on an outcome. These alternative definitions often coincide for preventive factors but are opposites for causal factors; hence the term can be confusing.

CONFOUNDING VARIABLE, CONFOUNDER A variable that can be used to decrease CONFOUNDING BIAS when properly adjusted for. The identification of confounders requires expert or substantive knowledge about the causal network of whichexposure and outcome are part (e.g., pathophysiological and clinical knowledge). Attempts to select confounders solely based on observed statistical associations may lead to bias.[12,31,69,93]

CONNECTION Something that can be shown to make a difference: an observed change in state (the effect) is consequent on change in an independent antecedent state (the cause) and not vice versa. One of the three essential properties of a cause specified by David Hume, along with ASSOCIATION and TIME ORDER. It requires the elimination of alternative explanations (e.g., confounding).[9,71] See also DIRECTION.

CONSANGUINE Related by a common ancestor within the previous few generations.

CONSENT BIAS A type of SELECTION BIAS in epidemiological and clinical studies caused by the process of asking for INFORMED CONSENT (e.g., to be interviewed for the study, to access medical records, to store biological specimens). The sample of subjects, records, or specimens included in the study is systematically different from the original sample.

CONSISTENCY

1. Close conformity between the findings in different samples, strata, or populations, or at different times or in different circumstances, or in studies conducted by different methods or investigators. Consistency may be examined in order to study an EFFECT

MODIFIER. Consistency of results on replication of studies is an important criterion in judgments of causality. See also CONFIRMATION BIAS; HILL'S CRITERIA OF CAUSATION.

2. In statistics, an estimator is said to be consistent if the probability of its yielding estimates close to the true value approaches 1 as the sample size grows larger.
3. A potential or counterfactual outcome under exposure level *a* is said to be consistent when, for each individual actually exposed to level *a*, its value equals that of the observed outcome.

CONSORT Consolidated Standards of Reporting Trials. An evidence-based and structured approach to reporting CLINICAL TRIALS. Its central features include a checklist and a flow diagram spelling out the important features of the trial [i.e., protocol, methods, participant (subject) assignment, masking procedures, details of analysis, participant flow, results, and follow-up]. The aim is to improve the quality of reporting of randomized trials (www.consort-statement.org and www.cochrane.dk).[94,95] See also MOOSE; QUOROM; STARD; STROBE.

CONTACT, DIRECT A mode of transmission of infection between an infected host and a susceptible host. Direct contact occurs when skin or mucous surfaces touch, as in shaking hands, kissing, and sexual intercourse. See also CONTAGION; TRANSMISSION OF INFECTION.

CONTACT, INDIRECT A mode of transmission of infection involving FOMITES or VECTORS. Vectors may be mechanical (e.g., filth flies) or biological (when the disease agent undergoes part of its life cycle in the vector species). See also TRANSMISSION OF INFECTION.

CONTACT, PRIMARY Person(s) in direct contact or associated with a communicable disease case.

CONTACT, SECONDARY Person(s) in contact or associated with a primary contact.

CONTACT (OF AN INFECTION) A person or animal that has been in such association with an infected person or animal or a contaminated environment as to have had opportunity to acquire the infection.

CONTACT TRACING See CASE FINDING.

CONTAGION The transmission of infection by direct contact, droplet spread, or contaminated FOMITES. These are the modes of transmission specified by Fracastorius (1484–1553) in *De Contagione* (1546). Contemporary usage is sometimes looser, but use of this term is best restricted to description of infection transmitted by direct contact.

CONTAGIOUS Transmitted by contact; in common usage, "highly infectious."

CONTAINMENT The concept of regional eradication of communicable disease, first proposed by Soper in 1949 for the elimination of smallpox.[96] Containment of a worldwide communicable disease demands a globally coordinated effort, so that countries that have effected an interruption of transmission do not become reinfected following importation from neighboring endemic areas.

CONTAMINATION

1. The presence of an infectious, toxic, or otherwise harmful agent (radioactive material, biological or chemical compounds) on or in the body—also on or in clothes, bedding, toys, medical devices, surgical instruments or dressings, other objects; in air, water, and food; or on buildings or land. POLLUTION may be deemed distinct from contamination: the agent causing the pollution or present in the polluted environment is noxious but not necessarily infectious. Contamination of a body surface does not imply a carrier state. See also SOURCE OF INFECTION; TRANSMISSION OF INFECTION.

2. The situation that exists when a population being studied for one condition or factor also possesses other conditions or factors that modify results of the study. In a RANDOMIZED CONTROLLED TRIAL, the application of the experimental procedure to members of the control group or failure to apply the procedure to members of the experimental group.

CONTAMINATION, DATA In computing, the intentional or accidental alteration of data (e.g., in a computer system).

CONTEXTUAL ANALYSIS Analysis of CONTEXTUAL EFFECTS.

CONTEXT

1. The location of a person by time and place; the latter refers to both geographical location and to group membership (e.g., in terms of family, friends, age, class, ethnicity, residence, gender). Context may affect exposure to risk and the individual's response strategies.[16]
2. In linguistics, the text surrounding a word; knowledge of the context allows the reader to gain a better understanding of what the word means.

CONTEXTUAL EFFECTS Effects of group- or area-level factors (e.g., neighborhood poverty) on individual-level outcomes after accounting for the effects of relevant individual-level confounders (referred to as COMPOSITIONAL EFFECTS). They are estimated using MULTILEVEL ANALYSIS.[89] See also INTEGRATIVE RESEARCH.

CONTINGENCY TABLE A tabular cross-classification of data such that subcategories of one characteristic are indicated horizontally (in rows) and subcategories of another characteristic are indicated vertically (in columns). Tests of association between the characteristics in the columns and rows can be readily applied. The simplest contingency table is the fourfold or 2 × 2, table. Contingency tables may be extended to include several dimensions of classification.

CONTINGENT VARIABLE See INTERMEDIATE VARIABLE.

CONTINUING SOURCE EPIDEMIC (OUTBREAK) An epidemic in which new cases of disease occur over a long period, indicating persistence of the disease source.

CONTINUOUS DATA, CONTINUOUS VARIABLE Data (variable) with a potentially infinite number of possible values along a continuum (e.g., height, weight, enzyme output).

CONTOUR PLOT Diagrammatic presentation, usually computer-generated, of data involving three variables, one each on the horizontal and vertical axes and a third represented by lines of constant value. It can be used in epidemiology to show the distribution of concentration of environmental contaminants. See also PERSPECTIVE PLOT.

CONTROL

1. (v.) To regulate, restrain, correct, restore to normal.
2. (v.) To adjust for or take into account extraneous influences or observations.
3. (n. or adj.) Applied to many communicable and some noncommunicable conditions, *control* means ongoing operations or programs aimed at reducing incidence and/or prevalence, or eliminating such conditions.
4. (n.) As used in the expressions *case-control study* and *randomized control(led) trial*, *control* means person(s) in a group that is used for reference in comparison to a case group or a treated group, respectively. See CONTROL GROUP.
5. (adj.) The expression *control variable* refers to an independent variable other than the hypothetical causal variable that has a potential effect on the dependent variable and is subject to control by analysis.

CONTROL GROUP, CONTROLS Subjects with whom comparison is made in a case-control study, a randomized controlled trial, or other epidemiological study. The use of the noun *control* to describe the reference group in a case-control study and in a randomized controlled clinical trial may be confusing. One essential distinction is that there is no intervention in the lives of the controls in a case-control study, whereas controls in a RANDOMIZED CONTROLLED TRIAL may be asked to undergo a procedure or regimen that may affect their health; their informed consent is therefore essential. Consent may not be required (save to gain access to medical records) to study controls in a case-control study. Another essential difference is that controls in a case-control study are often defined as noncases or by other postexposure events, making them especially susceptible to SELECTION BIAS. Selection of appropriate controls is crucial to the VALIDITY of epidemiological and clinical studies.

CONTROLS, HISTORICAL Persons or patients used for comparison who had the condition or treatment under study at a different time, generally at an earlier period than the study group or cases. Historical controls are often unsatisfactory because other factors affecting the condition under study may have changed to an unknown extent in the time elapsed.

CONTROLS, HOSPITAL Persons used for comparison who are drawn from the population of patients in a hospital. If wrongly chosen, hospital controls may be a source of SELECTION BIAS.

CONTROLS, MATCHED Controls who are selected so that they are similar to the study group, or cases, in specific characteristics. Some commonly used matching variables are age, sex, race, and socioeconomic status.[5,12,97] See also MATCHING.

CONTROLS, NEIGHBORHOOD Persons used for comparison who live in the same locality as cases and therefore may resemble cases in environmental and socioeconomic criteria.

CONTROLS, SIBLING Persons used for comparison who are the siblings of cases and therefore share genetic makeup.

CONVENIENCE SAMPLE See SAMPLE.

COORDINATES In a two-dimensional graph, the values of ordinate and abscissa that define the locus or position of a point.

CORDON SANITAIRE The barrier erected around a focus of infection. Used mainly in the isolation procedures applied to exclude cases and contacts of life-threatening communicable diseases from society. Mainly of historical interest.

CORRELATION The degree to which variables change together. How closely two (or more) variables are related.

CORRELATION COEFFICIENT A measure of association that indicates the degree to which two variables have a linear relationship. This coefficient, represented by the letter r, can vary between +1 and –1; when $r = +1$, there is a perfect positive linear relationship in which one variable varies directly with the other; when $r = -1$, there is a perfect negative linear relationship between the variables. The measure can be generalized to quantify the degree of linear relationship between one variable and several others, in which case it is known as the multiple correlation coefficient. Kendall's tau, Spearman's rank correlation, and Pearson's product moment correlation tests are special varieties with applications in clinical and epidemiological research.[98,99] Lack of correlation does not imply lack of relation, only lack of linear relation on the scale used to assess the correlation; therefore the use of correlation as a synonym for relation or association can be misleading. There are also several problems associated with attempting to interpret correlation coefficients as MEASURES OF EFFECT, among them that the correlation coefficient depends on the standard deviations of the causal and outcome variable. It can therefore vary greatly across populations and subgroups, even if the increase in the mean outcome, risk, or rate produced by exposure is identical across populations and subgroups.

CORRELATION, INTRACLASS A measure of the degree of relationship between two variables that presents the proportion of intersubject variance with respect to total variance (e.g., it compares the variance between patients to the total variance, including both between- and within-patient variance). It is used, for example, to assess interrater reliability or the reproducibility of a diagnostic test.

CORRELATION, NONSENSE A meaningless correlation between two variables. Nonsense correlations sometimes occur when social, environmental, or technological changes have the same trend as incidence or mortality rates. An example is the correlation between the birthrate and the density of storks in parts of Holland. See also ASSOCIATION, FORTUITOUS; CONFOUNDING BIAS; ECOLOGICAL FALLACY.

COST The value of resources engaged in a service.[100]

COST, AVERAGE The average cost per unit; equals the total costs divided by the units of production.

COST, AVOIDED Costs caused by a health problem that are avoided by a health care intervention. Estimating avoided costs is one way to assess the value of benefits of health care interventions; sometimes known as benefits.

COST-BENEFIT ANALYSIS An analysis of the economic and social costs of medical care and the benefits of reduced loss of net earnings owing to the prevention of premature death or disability. The general rule for the allocation of funds in a cost-benefit analysis is that the ratio of marginal benefit (the benefit of preventing an additional case) to marginal cost (the cost of preventing an additional case) should be equal to or greater than 1. The benefit-cost ratio is the ratio of net present value of measurable benefits to costs. Calculation of a benefit-cost ratio is used to assess the economic feasibility or success of a public health program.

COST, DIRECT Those costs borne by the health care system, the community, and patients' families (e.g., costs of diagnosis and treatment).

COST-EFFECTIVENESS ANALYSIS This form of analysis seeks to determine the costs and effectiveness of an activity or to compare similar alternative activities to determine the relative degree to which they will obtain the desired objectives or outcomes. The preferred action or alternative is one that requires the least cost to produce a given level of effectiveness or that provides the greatest effectiveness for a given level of cost. In the health care field, outcomes are measured in terms of health status.

COST, FIXED Costs that, within a defined period, do not vary with the quantity produced (e.g., overhead costs of maintaining a building).

COST, INCREMENTAL The difference between marginal costs of alternative interventions.

COST, INDIRECT Lost productivity caused by disease and borne by the individual, the family, society, or the employer.

COST, INTANGIBLE Costs of pain, grief, suffering, loss of leisure time; the cost of a life is usually included in case of death.

COST, OPPORTUNITY See OPPORTUNITY COST.

COST, TOTAL All costs incurred in producing a set quantity of service.

COSTS, MARGINAL The additional costs from an increase in an activity. The additional cost incurred as a result of the production of one extra unit of output; the increase is equal to the cost of the next unit produced.

COST-UTILITY ANALYSIS A form of economic evaluation in which the outcomes of alternative procedures or programs are expressed in terms of a single "utility-based" unit of measurement. A widely used utility-based measure is the QUALITY-ADJUSTED LIFE YEAR (QALY). See also UTILITY.

COUNTERFACTUAL DEFINITION A measure of effect in which at least one of two circumstances in the definition of variables must be contrary to fact.[12] An example is a hypothetical control group that represents what the distribution of exposure would have been if past events had been different from what they actually were. In a CASE-SPECULAR study design, the counterfactual control group comprises (imaginary) dwellings on the opposite side of the street from the dwellings occupied by the cases. The purpose is to assess what the exposure would have been in these hypothetical dwellings. The counterfactual difference in past exposure must be defined precisely to facilitate unambiguous calculation of variables in the hypothetical control group.[101]

COUNTERFACTUAL LOGIC Deductive reasoning that involves counterfactual premises or conditions (premises or conditions that are known to be contrary to fact). For example, in a thought experiment, an entity imagining that it had been exposed to the change agent is compared with the same entity had there been no exposure; or an entity that had no exposure to the change agent is compared with the same entity imagining that it had been exposed.[102] See also POTENTIAL OUTCOME.

COUNTERMATCHING A matching procedure for case-control studies nested within a cohort when exposure status is known for all cohort members and information about confounders is acquired only on a sample of paired cases and controls; "countermatching" to each exposed case an unexposed control, and vice versa, may improve the efficiency of the study.[103]

COVARIATE A variable that is possibly predictive of the outcome under study. A covariate may be of direct interest to the study or may be a confounding variable or effect modifier.

COVERAGE A measure of the extent to which the services rendered cover the potential need for these services in a community. It is expressed as a proportion in which the numerator is the number of services rendered and the denominator is the number of instances in which the service should have been rendered. Example:

$$\text{Annual obstetric coverage in a community} = \frac{\text{number of deliveries attended by a qualified midwife or obstetrician}}{\text{expected number of deliveries during the year in a given community}}$$

COX MODEL See PROPORTIONAL HAZARDS MODEL.

CREATIVITY

1. The ability to produce ideas, policies and objects (including "knowledge objects") that are both novel or original and worthwhile or appropriate (i.e., useful, attractive, meaningful, and valid).[90]
2. In EPIDEMIOLOGICAL RESEARCH, the capacity of a set of studies to harmonize relevance, validity, meaning, innovation, feasibility, and precision—ideally, beauty

and simplicity as well. An epidemiological study reflects creativity to the extent that it generates knowledge that is relevant, new, valid, practical, and precise. Complexity may be a plus; it need not clash with simplicity and elegance. Relevance may be social, environmental, sanitary, clinical, biological, methodological, ethical, technological, intellectual.... Studies may blend, weave, knit, or weld such qualities in extraordinarily different ways.

3. A public health policy or program shows creativity when it is relevant, meaningful, useful, and attractive for populations, persons, and institutions... when it is innovative, imaginative, simple... if effective and efficient in abating harmful determinants of health and significantly improving important health indicators. It may be morally and socially relevant if it increases freedom, justice, education, equity, or social cohesion. It needs be culturally, environmentally, and economically sustainable... Creativity is an importat value for epidemiology and the other health, life, and social sciences.[104]

CRITERION A principle or standard by which something is judged. See also STANDARD.

CRITICAL APPRAISAL Application of rules of evidence to a study to assess the VALIDITY of the data, completeness of reporting, methods and procedures, conclusions, compliance with ethical standards, etc. The rules of evidence vary with circumstances. See also HIERARCHY OF EVIDENCE.

CRITICAL PERIOD See SENSITIVE PERIOD.

CRITICAL TIME WINDOW (Syn: etiologically relevant exposure period) The period during which exposure to a causal factor is relevant to causation of a disease.

CRITICAL POPULATION SIZE The theoretical minimum host population size required to maintain an infectious agent. This size varies depending on the agent and demographic, social, and environmental conditions (hygiene, ambient temperature, etc.) and, in the case of vector-borne diseases, the conditions required for survival and propagation of the vector species.

CRONBACH'S ALPHA (Syn: internal consistency reliability) An estimate of the correlation between the total score across a series of items from a rating scale and the total score that would have been obtained had a comparable series of items been employed.

CROSS-CULTURAL STUDY A study in which populations from different cultural backgrounds are compared.

CROSS-DESIGN SYNTHESIS A method for evaluating outcomes of medical interventions developed by the U.S. General Accounting Office (GAO).[105] It is conducted by pooling databases such as the results of a RANDOMIZED CONTROLLED TRIAL (RCT) and of routinely treated patients; the latter databases may come from hospital discharge statistics and other sources. Thus it is a variation of META-ANALYSIS.[106] This method is claimed to be more relevant to daily practice than some RCTs because it includes outcomes of patients in categories not included in RCTs; however, the validity of the databases should be carefully assessed.

CROSS–INFECTION Infection of one person with pathogenic organisms from another and vice versa. Not the same as NOSOCOMIAL INFECTION, which occurs in a health care setting; cross-infection can occur anywhere (e.g., in military barracks, schools, workplaces).

CROSS-LEVEL BIAS Biases occurring in ecological studies owing to aggregation at the population level of causes and/or effects that do not aggregate, operate, or interact at the individual level.[107] See also ECOLOGICAL FALLACY, AGGREGATIVE FALLACY, ATOMISTIC FALLACY.

CROSSOVER CLINICAL TRIAL, CROSSOVER EXPERIMENT A method of comparing two (or more) treatments or interventions in which subjects, upon completion of one treatment, are switched to the other. In the case of two treatments, A and B, half the patients are randomly allocated to receive these in the order "A first, then B," and half to receive them in the order "B first, then A." The outcomes cannot be permanent changes (e.g., they can be symptoms, functional capacity). A "washout" phase is often needed before beginning the second treatment. The analysis will have to check whether a CARRYOVER EFFECT was present. If the biological and clinical bases of the trial are coherent, the results will be unbiased and the design will help reduce "noise" and sample size requirements. See also CASE-CROSSOVER STUDY; N-OF-ONE STUDY.

CROSS-PRODUCT RATIO See ODDS RATIO.

CROSS-SECTIONAL STUDY (Syn: disease frequency survey, prevalence study) A study that examines the relationship between diseases (or other health-related characteristics) and other variables of interest as they exist in a defined population at one particular time. The presence or absence of disease and the presence or absence of the other variables (or, if they are quantitative, their level) are determined in each member of the study population or in a representative sample at one particular time. The relationship between a variable and the disease can be examined (1) in terms of the prevalence of disease in different population subgroups defined according to the presence or absence (or level) of the variables and (2) in terms of the presence or absence (or level) of the variables in the diseased versus the nondiseased. Note that disease PREVALENCE rather than incidence is normally recorded in a cross-sectional study.[31] The temporal sequence of cause and effect cannot necessarily be determined in a cross-sectional study. See also MORBIDITY SURVEY.

CROSS-VALIDATION A statistical method for model development and testing based on splitting the data set into a *training sample* to which a model is fit, and *test sample* on which the model is tested. In modern applications, this process is repeated many times using different (possibly random) splits of the data, and the final model is derived by synthesizing over the results from each split. Cross-validated models tend to exhibit far better generalizability (out-of-sample performance) than conventionally fitted models. See also JACKNIFE; MACHINE LEARNING; OVERFITTING.

CRUDE DEATH RATE See DEATH RATE.

CULTURE

1. In microbiology, the growth of an organism in or on a nutrient medium.
2. In social science, a set of beliefs; values; intellectual, artistic, and religious characteristics; customs, etc., common to and characteristic of a community or nation. Culturally determined characteristics include language, acceptable gender roles and occupations, and much health-related behavior.[108]

CUMULATIVE DEATH RATE The proportion of a group that dies over a specified time interval. It is the INCIDENCE PROPORTION of death. This may refer to all deaths or to deaths from a specific cause or causes. If follow-up is not complete on all persons, the proper estimation of this rate requires the use of methods that take account of CENSORING. Distinct from FORCE OF MORTALITY.

CUMULATIVE INCIDENCE, CUMULATIVE INCIDENCE RATE (Syn: incidence proportion, average risk) The number or proportion of a group (cohort) of people who experience the onset of a health-related event during a specified time interval; this interval is generally the same for all members of the group, but, as in lifetime incidence, it may vary from person to person without reference to age.

CUMULATIVE INCIDENCE RATIO The ratio of the cumulative incidence rate in the exposed to the cumulative incidence rate in the unexposed.

CUSUM Acronym for cumulative sum (of a series of measurements). A way to demonstrate a change in trend or direction of a series of measurements.[109] Calculation begins with a reference figure (e.g., the expected average measurement). As each new measurement is observed, the reference figure is subtracted, and a cumulative total is produced by adding each successive difference; this cumulative total is the CUSUM.

CUT POINT An arbitrarily chosen point or value in an ordered sequence of values used to separate the whole into parts. Commonly the cut point divides a distribution of values into parts that are arbitrarily designated as within or beyond the range considered normal. For example, a cut point of 85, 90, or 95 mm Hg differentiates normal from high blood pressure. Synonym: cutoff point.

CYCLICITY, SEASONAL The annual cycling of incidence on a seasonal basis. Certain acute infectious diseases, if of greater than rare occurrence, peak in one season of the year and reach the low point 6 months later (or in the opposite season). The onset of some symptoms of some chronic diseases also may show this amplitudinal cyclicity. Demographic phenomena, such as marriages, births, and mortality from all causes and certain specific causes may also exhibit seasonal cyclicity. See also CHRONOBIOLOGY.

CYCLICITY, SECULAR Fluctuation in disease incidence over a period longer than a year. For instance, in large, unimmunized populations, measles tends to have a 2-year cycle of high and low incidence. Empirical observations of secular and seasonal cycles of infectious diseases were the basis for epidemic theory (e.g., the MASS ACTION PRINCIPLE). Mass immunization programs, by raising herd immunity levels, have eliminated many such cycles.

CYST COUNT See WORM COUNT.

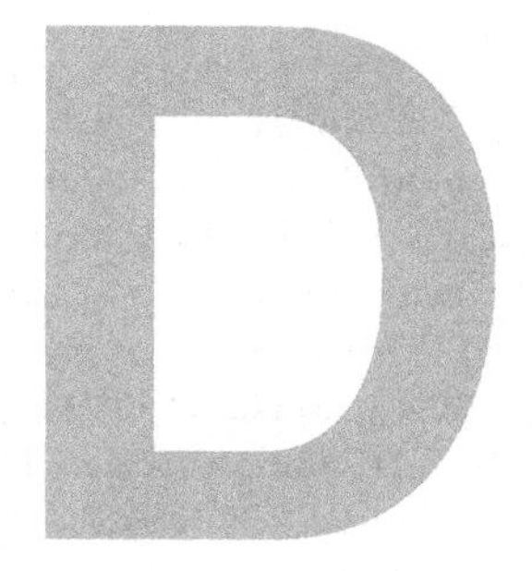

DAG See DIRECTED ACYCLIC GRAPH.

DALY See DISABILITY-ADJUSTED LIFE YEARS.

DATA A collection of items of information. Note: The singular of *data* is *datum;* the plural noun should not be accompanied by a singular verb.

DATA CONTAMINATION See CONTAMINATION, DATA.

DATABASE An organized set of data or collection of files that can be used for a specified purpose.

DATA CLEANING The process of excluding the information in incomplete, inconsistent records or irrelevant information collected in a survey or other form of epidemiological study before analysis begins. This may mean excluding information that would distort the results if an attempt were made to edit and include it in the analysis, but it can also introduce biases. The fact that this step has been taken should be reported, along with the results of the study of analyzed data. See also RAW DATA.

DATA DREDGING A jargon term meaning analyses done on a post hoc basis without benefit of prestated hypotheses as a means of identifying noteworthy differences. Such analyses are sometimes done when data have been collected on a large number of variables and unanticipated hypotheses are suggested by hypothesis-free analyses. The scientific validity of data dredging is dubious, usually unacceptable. See also CHANCE; CROSS VALIDATION; OVERFITTING; RANDOM.

DATA MINING The extraction of information from large databases or files, often with the use of artificial intelligence technology and sophisticated statistical and bioinformatics methods. An important exploratory approach in "–omics" research (e.g., genomics, peptidomics).

DATA PROCESSING Conversion of items of information into a form that permits storage, retrieval, and analysis.

DATA REDUCTION The process of summarizing a set or sets of data in the form of an index, such as life expectancy or gross domestic product.

DEATH CERTIFICATE A vital record signed by a licensed physician or another designated health worker that includes cause of death, decedent's name, sex, birth date, places of residence and of death, and whether the deceased had been medically attended before death. Occupation, birthplace, and other information may be included. Immediate cause of death is recorded on the first line, followed by conditions giving rise to the immediate cause; the underlying cause is entered last.

The underlying cause is coded and tabulated in official publications of cause-specific mortality. Other significant conditions may also be recorded separately, as is the mode of death, whether accidental or violent, etc. The most important entries on a death certificate are underlying causes of death and cause of death. These are defined in the tenth (1990) revision of the INTERNATIONAL STATISTICAL CLASSIFICATION OF DISEASES AND RELATED HEALTH PROBLEMS (ICD-10) as follows:

"*Causes of death:* The causes of death to be entered on the medical certificate of cause of death are all those diseases, morbid conditions, or injuries that either resulted in or contributed to death and the circumstances of the accident or violence which produced any such injuries.

Underlying cause of death: The underlying cause of death is (1) the disease or injury that initiated the train of events leading to death or (2) the circumstances of the accident or violence that produced the fatal injury."

Personal identifying information such as birthplace, parents' names (last name at birth), birth date, and personal identifying numbers are included on death certificates in some jurisdictions; this extra information makes possible a range of RECORD LINKAGE studies. See also INTERNATIONAL FORM OF MEDICAL CERTIFICATE OF CAUSES OF DEATH.

DEATH RATE An estimate of the portion of a population that dies during a specified period. The numerator is the number of persons dying during the period; the denominator is the

INTERNATIONAL FORM OF MEDICAL CERTIFICATE OF CAUSE OF DEATH

Cause of death		Approximate interval between onset and death
I Disease or condition directly leading to death*	(a)	....
	due to (or as a consequence of)	
Antecedent causes Morbid conditions, if any, giving rise to the above cause, stating the underlying condition last	(b)	....
	due to (or as a consequence of)	
	(c)	....
	due to (or as a consequence of)	
	(d)	....
II Other significant conditions contributing to the death, but not related to the disease or condition causing it	....	....
	....	....

* *This does not mean the mode of dying, e.g. heart failure, respiratory failure. It means the disease, injury, or complication that caused death.*

Death certificate. The International Standard Form. From *International Statistical Classification of Diseases and Related Health Problems*, 10th rev. (ICD-10), vol. 2. Geneva: World Health Organization, 1991. With permission.

number in the population, usually estimated as the midyear population. The death rate in a population is generally calculated by the following formula:

$$\frac{\text{Number of deaths during a specified period}}{\text{Number of persons at risk of dying during the period}} \times 10^n$$

This rate is an estimate of the person-time death rate, i.e., the death rate per 10^n person-years. If the rate is low, it is also a good estimate of the cumulative death rate. This rate is also called the crude death rate.

DEATH REGISTRATION AREA A geographic area for which mortality data are collected, and often published.

DECISION ANALYSIS A derivative of OPERATIONS RESEARCH and GAME THEORY to identify all available choices, and POTENTIAL OUTCOMES of each, in a series of decisions that have to be made (e.g., about aspects of patient care as diagnostic procedures, preventive and therapeutic regimens, prognosis). Epidemiological data play a large part in analyzing the probabilities of outcomes following each potential choice. The range of choices can be plotted on a DECISION TREE; at each branch of the tree, or decision node, the probabilities of each outcome that can be predicted are displayed. The decision tree thus portrays the choices available to those responsible for patient care and the probabilities of each outcome that will follow the choice of a particular action or strategy. The relative worth of each outcome is preferably described as a UTILITY or quality-of-life measure (e.g., a probability of life expectancy or of freedom from disability, often expressed as quality-adjusted life years, or QALYs). See also CLINICAL DECISION ANALYSIS.

DECISION TREE The alternative choices expressed, in quantitative terms, available at each stage in the process of thinking through a problem may be likened to branches and the hierarchical sequence of options to a tree. Hence, *decision tree*. It is a graphic device used in DECISION ANALYSIS in which a series of decision options are represented as branches and subsequent possible outcomes are represented as further branches. The decisions and the eventualities are presented in the order in which they are likely to occur. The junction where a decision must be taken is called a *decision node*.

DECOMPOSITION METHOD Comparison of groups by analyzing mathematical functions of rates, incidence densities, and exposure prevalence. This simplifies identification of relevant contributing factors in risk analysis.[110]

DEDUCTION Reasoned argument proceeding from the general to the particular.

DEDUCTIVE LOGIC Logic that predicts specific outcomes from prior general hypotheses—that is, it proceeds from the general to the particular. Logic based on derivation of necessary conclusions implied by explicit assumptions (premises), as in mathematics. See also HYPOTHETICO-DEDUCTIVE METHOD; INDUCTIVE LOGIC.

DEGREES OF FREEDOM *(df)* The number of independent comparisons that can be made between the members of a sample. Roughly, it refers to the number of independent dimensions of variation in a sample under an assumed sampling model. More specifically, it is the number of independent contributions to a sampling distribution (such as χ^2, t, and F distribution) from the data-generating mechanism. For example, in a CONTINGENCY TABLE with fixed margins, the total degrees of freedom is one less than the

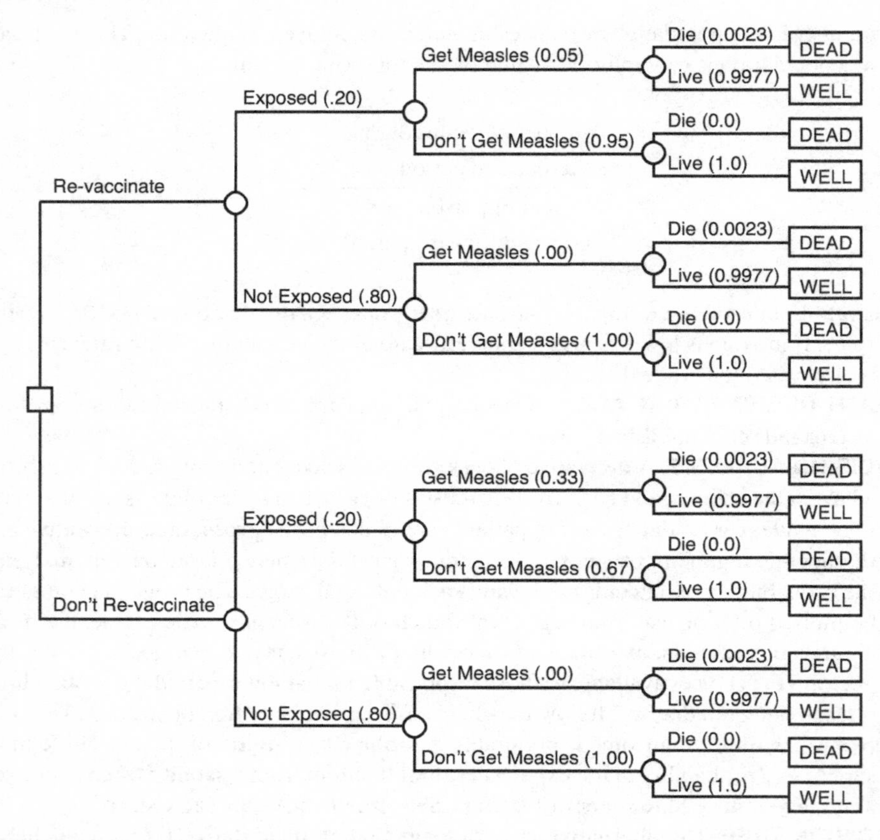

Decision tree. Probabilities of different outcomes with and without revaccination against measles. From Petitti DB. *Meta-Analysis, Decision Analysis and Cost-Effectiveness Analysis*. New York: Oxford University Press, 1994. With permission.

number of row categories multiplied by one less than the number of column categories. See also DIMENSIONALITY.

DELPHI METHOD Iterative circulation to a panel of experts of questions and responses that are progressively refined in light of responses to each round of questions; preferably participants' identities should not be revealed to each other. The aim is to reduce the number of viable options or solutions, perhaps to arrive at a consensus judgment on an issue or problem, or a set of issues or problems, without allowing any one participant to dominate the process. The method was developed at the RAND Corporation.

DEMAND (FOR HEALTH SERVICES) Willingness and/or ability to seek, use, and in some settings, pay for services. Sometimes further subdivided into *expressed demand* (equated with use) and *potential demand* or *need*.

DEMOGRAPHIC TRANSITION The evolution from high to low fertility and mortality rates in a country. Formerly thought to be related to technological change and industrialization but probably more directly caused by improvements in female literacy and the status of women. It is accompanied by a change in the age composition of the population as birthrates and death rates decline; usually infant and child mortality rates decline as well. As a result there is a decrease in the proportion of children and young adults and an increase in the proportion of older persons in the population, i.e., an AGING OF THE POPULATION. See also ECOLOGICAL TRANSITION; "EPIDEMIOLOGICAL TRANSITION" THEORY.

DEMOGRAPHIC ENTRAPMENT A community may be said to be demographically trapped if (1) it exceeds the CARRYING CAPACITY of its local ecosystem; (2) there is no other land to which it can migrate; and (3) it has too few exports to exchange for food and other essentials. Common outcomes include poverty, stunting, starvation, and violence. There may be a warning stage, during which starvation or violence can be expected (e.g., because population is increasing rapidly).

DEMOGRAPHY The study of populations, especially with reference to size and density, fertility, mortality, growth, age distribution, migration, and VITAL STATISTICS, and the interaction of all these with social and economic conditions.

DEMONSTRATION MODEL An experimental health care facility, program, or system with built-in provision for measuring aspects such as costs per unit of service, rates of use by patients or clients, and outcomes of encounters between providers and users. The aim usually is to determine the feasibility, efficacy, effectiveness, and/or efficiency of the model service.

DENOMINATOR The lower portion of a fraction, used to calculate a rate or ratio. The population (or population experience, as in person-years, passenger-miles, etc.) at risk in the calculation of a rate or ratio. Valid information on denominators is essential in clinical and epidemiological research and also in many public health activities. See also NUMERATOR.

DENSITY CASE-CONTROL STUDY A variant of the case-control design in which the controls are drawn in such a way that they represent the person-time experience that generated the cases, usually by DENSITY SAMPLING. This design provides an estimate of the rate ratio with no RARE DISEASE ASSUMPTION. A type of CASE-BASE STUDY. See also CASE-COHORT STUDY.

DENSITY-EQUALIZING MAP See ISODEMOGRAPHIC MAP.

DENSITY OF POPULATION Demographic term meaning numbers of persons in relation to available space.

DENSITY SAMPLING A method of selecting controls in a CASE-CONTROL STUDY in which cases are sampled only from incident cases over a specific time period and controls are sampled and interviewed throughout that period (rather than simply at one point in time, such as the end of the period). This method can reduce bias due to changing exposure patterns in the source population and allows estimation of the rate ratio without any rare-disease assumption.

DEONTOLOGICAL A duty-based theoretical approach to ETHICS. Right actions stem from freely embraced obligations to universal moral imperatives, such as the obligation to respect persons as ends and not as means.[36]

DEPENDENCY RATIO Ratio of children and old people in a population in comparison to all others (i.e., the proportion of economically inactive to economically active); "children" are usually defined those below 15 years of age and "old people" as those 65 years of age and above.

DEPENDENT VARIABLE

1. A variable the value of which is dependent on the effect of other variable(s)—independent variable(s)—in the relationship under study. A manifestation or outcome whose variation we seek to explain or account for by the influence of independent variables.

2. In REGRESSION ANALYSIS, the variable whose average value is being studied in relation to regressors (covariates or "independent" variables).[20] See also INDEPENDENT VARIABLE; REGRESSAND; REGRESSOR.

DESCRIPTIVE EPIDEMIOLOGY Epidemiological studies and activities (e.g., SURVEILLANCE) whose descriptive components are much stronger than their analytic components or that clearly fall within the descriptive area of the descriptive-analytic spectrum. Descriptive study of the occurrence of disease and other health-related characteristics in human populations. General descriptions concerning the relationship of disease to basic characteristics such as age, gender, race, occupation, social class, and geographic location; even such general descriptions may have analytic dimensions. The major characteristics in descriptive epidemiology can be classified under the headings *persons, place*, and *time*. Descriptive epidemiology is always observational, never experimental; hence observational epidemiological studies may be descriptive; nevertheless, EPIDEMIOLOGICAL RESEARCH studies are often analytic. See also ANALYTIC STUDY; CASE REPORTS; ETIOLOGICAL STUDY; OBSERVATIONAL STUDY.

DESCRIPTIVE STUDY A study concerned with and designed only to describe the existing distribution of variables without much regard to causal relationships or other hypotheses. An example is a community health survey used to determine the health status of the people in a community. In a descriptive study, a parameter of disease occurrence is related to a determinant without concern for a causal interpretation of the relation.[5] Descriptive studies (e.g., analyses of population registries) can be used to measure risks or trends in health indicators, generate hypotheses, monitor public health policies, etc. Contrast ANALYTIC STUDY; ETIOLOGICAL STUDY.

DESIGN See RESEARCH DESIGN.

DESIGN BIAS The difference between a true value and that obtained as a result of faulty design of a study. Examples include uncontrolled studies where the effects of two or more processes cannot be separated for lack of measurement of key causes of the exposure or outcome (confounding); also studies done on poorly defined populations or with unsuitable control groups.

DESIGN EFFECT A BIAS in study findings attributable to the study design. A specific form is bias attributable to intraclass correlation in CLUSTER SAMPLING. The design effect for a cluster design is the ratio of the variance for that design to the variance calculated from a simple random sample of the same size.

DESIGN VARIABLE

1. A study variable whose distribution in the subjects is determined by the investigator.
2. In statistics, a variable taking on the value 1 to indicate membership in a particular category and 0 or –1 to indicate nonmembership in the category. Used primarily in ANALYSIS OF VARIANCE. See also INDICATOR VARIABLE.

DESMOTERIC MEDICINE The practice of medicine in a prison. Derived from the Greek *desmoterion*, prison.

DETECTABLE PRECLINICAL PERIOD The period between the time when a disease is capable of yielding a positive screening test and the appearance of clinical symptoms and/or signs. See also LEAD TIME.

DETECTION BIAS Bias due to systematic differences between the study groups in ascertainment, assessment, diagnosis, or verification of outcomes. As with other biases, there are many mechanisms and forms of detection bias.[10,12,14,31] An example is verification of diagnosis by laboratory tests in hospital cases but failure to apply the same tests to cases outside the hospital.

DETERMINANT Any factor that brings about change in a health condition or other defined characteristic. Single specified causes. A determinant makes a difference to a given outcome. Does not imply a DETERMINISTIC philosophy of health. See also CAUSALITY; DISEASES OF COMPLEX ETIOLOGY; MATHEMATICAL MODEL.

DETERMINANT, DISTAL (DISTANT) (Syn: upstream determinant) A causal factor that is remote or far apart in position or time to the outcome of concern, making it more difficult to discern or trace within the causal pathway than other causal factors that are less far away from the outcome.[71,72] An example is atmospheric contamination with ozone-destroying substances that increase the risk of skin cancer.[111] In infectious diseases, the microbial agent is more proximal to the disease than social factors such as poverty, which are more distant or upstream but no less influential on the individual risk of developing the disease. See also STRATEGY, "POPULATION."

DETERMINANT, PROXIMAL (PROXIMATE) (Syn: downstream determinant) An established or postulated RISK FACTOR that is nearer in time or distance before an outcome of concern. The causal pathway is clearly enough defined to allow confident assertion of linkage between the determinant and the outcome. See also STRATEGY, "HIGH-RISK."

DETERMINISM, GENETIC A view of genetics according to which genetic inheritance not only influences but strongly constrains human development, health, and behavior. It disregards environmental influences on GENE EXPRESSION and social influences on health states. See also EPIGENETIC INHERITANCE; GENETIC PENETRANCE; MONOGENIC DISEASES; POLYGENIC DISEASES.

DETERMINISTIC METHOD A method that predicts outcomes perfectly, without allowance for statistical (chance) variation.

DETERMINISTIC MODEL A representation of a system, process, or relationship in mathematical form in which relationships are fixed (i.e., they take no account of probability and CHANCE), so that any given input invariably yields the same result.[6,10–12] See also MATHEMATICAL MODEL.

DETERMINANT OF FERTILITY, PROXIMATE Factor having a direct influence on fertility, such as contraceptive use, age at marriage, age at first sexual intercourse, breastfeeding, or abortion.

DEVELOPMENTAL AND LIFE-COURSE EPIDEMIOLOGY The study of long-term effects on later health or disease risk of physical or social exposures during gestation, childhood, adolescence, young adulthood, and later adult life. The premise is that various biological and social factors throughout life independently, cumulatively, and interactively influence health and disease in adult life. The aim is to elucidate biological, behavioral, and psychosocial processes that operate across an individual's life course or across generations to influence disease risk.[16,112,113]

DEVELOPMENTAL ORIGINS HYPOTHESIS The hypothesis that cardiovascular disease and type 2 diabetes originate through developmental PLASTICITY in response to undernutrition. A hypothesis proposed in 1990 by the British epidemiologist David Barker (b. 1939) that intrauterine growth retardation, low birth weight, and premature birth have a causal relationship to the origins of hypertension, coronary heart disease, and non–insulin dependent diabetes in middle age.[114,115] As growth during infancy and early childhood is also linked to later disease, *developmental origins hypothesis* is preferred to *fetal origins hypothesis*.[45] The hypothesis is evolving to include evidence that exposure to environmental factors early in development involves EPIGENETIC modifications, such as DNA methylation, which influence adult disease susceptibility;[116,117] e.g., in utero or neonatal exposure to bisphenol A (BPA), a high-production-volume chemical used in the manufacture of polycarbonate plastic, may be associated with higher body weight, increased risk of breast and prostate cancer, and altered reproductive function.[118] See also THRIFTY PHENOTYPE.

DIAGNOSIS The process of determining health status and the factors responsible for producing it; may be applied to an individual, family, group, or community. The term is applied both to the process of determination and to its findings. See also DISEASE LABEL; SEMIOLOGY.

DIAGNOSIS-RELATED GROUP (DRG) Classification of hospital patients according to diagnosis and intensity of care required, used by insurance carriers to set reimbursement scales.

DIAGNOSTIC AND STATISTICAL MANUAL OF MENTAL DISORDERS (DSM) A manual that aims to systematize and standardize the definitions of mental disorders developed by the American Psychiatric Association. It contains a listing of psychiatric disorders and their corresponding diagnostic codes; each disorder is accompanied by a set of diagnostic criteria and text containing information about the disorder (associated features; prevalence; familial patterns; age-, culture-, and gender-specific features; and differential diagnosis). No information about treatment or presumed etiology is included. It is used by mental health professionals from a variety of disciplines for clinical, research, administrative, and educational purposes. DSM-IV is the fourth edition, published in 1994. The DSM-V is currently in preparation.

DIAGNOSTIC INDEX A system for recording diagnoses, diseases, or problems of patients or clients in a medical practice or service, usually including identifying information (name, birthdate, sex) and dates of encounters.

DIAGNOSTIC SUSPICION BIAS A bias that may occur when knowledge of the subject's prior exposure to a putative cause (ethnicity, drug intake, a second disorder, an environmental exposure) influences both the intensity and the outcome of the diagnostic process.[14,63]

DICHOTOMOUS SCALE See MEASUREMENT SCALE.

DIFFERENTIAL The difference(s) shown in tabulation of health and vital statistics according to age, sex, or some other factor; age differentials are the differences revealed in the tabulations of rates in age groups, sex differentials are the differences in rates between males and females, income differentials are differences between designated income categories, etc.

DIFFUSION THEORY

1. The concept that infectious pathogens and ideas diffuse through a population.[119]
2. Theories explaining the dissemination of ideas and customs to other populations.
3. The "innovation-diffusion theory" explains how innovative ideas spread through segments of society, including the role of opinion leaders and the media.

DIGIT PREFERENCE A preference for certain numbers that leads to rounding off measurements. Rounding off may be to the nearest whole number, even number, multiple of 5 or 10, or (when time units like a week are involved) 7, 14, etc. This can be a form of OBSERVER VARIATION or an attribute of respondent(s) in a survey.

DIMENSIONALITY The number of dimensions (i.e., scalar quantities) needed for accurate description of an element of a vector space. See also DEGREES OF FREEDOM.

DIRECT ADJUSTMENT, DIRECT STANDARDIZATION See STANDARDIZATION.

DIRECTED ACYCLIC GRAPH (DAG) See CAUSAL DIAGRAM.

DIRECTION Blalock's[120] synonym for David Hume's CONNECTION.[71] It indicates a linkage from cause to effect that is repeatedly demonstrable, hence predictable.

DIRECTIONALITY

1. The direction of inference of a study.[12,31,121] It may be retrospective (backward-looking) or prospective (forward-looking).
2. The sign of a relationship between variables. Correlation coefficients are directional measures of association because the sign changes if one of the variables is reversed.

DIRECTIVES See GUIDELINES.

DIRECT OBSTETRICAL DEATH See MATERNAL MORTALITY.

DISABILITY Temporary or long-term reduction of a person's capacity to function. See also INTERNATIONAL CLASSIFICATION OF IMPAIRMENTS, DISABILITIES, AND HANDICAPS for the official WHO definition.

DISABILITY-ADJUSTED LIFE YEARS (DALYs) A DALY lost is a measure of the BURDEN OF DISEASE on a defined population. It is hence an indicator of POPULATION HEALTH. DALYs are advocated as an alternative to QUALITY-ADJUSTED LIFE YEARS (QALYs). They are based on adjustment of LIFE EXPECTANCY to allow for long-term disability as estimated from official statistics; the necessary data to do so may not be available in some areas. The concept postulates a continuum from disease to disability to death that is not universally accepted, particularly by the community of persons with disabilities. DALYs are calculated using a "disability weight" (a proportion less than 1) multiplied by chronological age to reflect the burden of the disability. DALYs can thus produce estimates that accord greater value to fit than to disabled persons and to the middle years of life rather than to youth or old age.[122] See also DISABILITY-FREE LIFE EXPECTANCY.

DISABILITY-FREE LIFE EXPECTANCY (Syn: active life expectancy) The average number of years an individual is expected to live free of disability if current patterns of mortality and disability continue to apply.[123] A statistical abstraction based on existing age-specific death rates and either age-specific disability prevalences or age-specific disability transition rates.

DISASTER EPIDEMIOLOGY The application of epidemiological principles and tools to managing emergency public health programs (e.g., to reduce morbidity and mortality among displaced populations).

DISCLOSURE OF INTERESTS

1. In health sciences research and other professional activities (e.g., lecturing, consulting), the action of making researchers' interests on a given issue known. Following requirements of the International Committee of Medical Journal Editors (www.icmje.org), all participants in the peer review and publication process must disclose all relationships that could be viewed as presenting a potential conflict of interest. Editors may use information disclosed in conflict-of-interest and financial interest statements as a basis for editorial decisions. Editors should publish this information if they believe it is important in judging the manuscript. Editors should also publish regular disclosure statements about potential conflicts of interest related to the commitments of journal staff. A similar rationale is applied by governments that receive expert advice from health scientists. See also CONFLICT OF INTEREST.
2. In certain types of law, the obligation that each party has to the other parties to reveal or make known all facts relevant to the subject matter of the contract.

The provision of financial and other types of information concerning a company to those with an interest in the economic activities of the company.

DISCORDANT A term used in TWIN STUDIES to describe a twin pair in which one twin exhibits a certain trait and the other does not. Also used in matched-pair case-control studies to describe a pair whose members had different exposures to the risk factor under study. Under conventional analytical methods, only the discordant pairs are informative about the association between exposure and disease.

DISCOUNT RATE A measure of costs, benefits, and outcomes in relation to time that allows for the fact that money (and health) have greater value in the present than at some future time. A term used mainly in economics and in CLINICAL DECISION ANALYSIS.

DISCRETE DATA Data that can be arranged into naturally occurring or arbitrarily selected groups or sets of values as opposed to data in which there are no naturally occurring breaks in continuity (i.e., CONTINUOUS DATA). An example is number of decayed, missing, and filled teeth (DMF).

DISCRIMINANT FUNCTION ANALYSIS A statistical analytical technique used with discrete dependent variables; it is concerned with separating sets of observed values and allocating new values and can sometimes be used instead of logistic regression analysis. Kendall and Buckland[98] refer to this as "discriminatory analysis" and describe it as a rule for allocating individuals or values from two or more discrete populations to the correct population with minimal probability of misclassification.

DISEASE

1. Literally, *dis-ease*, the opposite of *ease*, when something is wrong with a bodily function.
2. The words *disease, illness*, and *sickness* are sometimes used as if they were loosely interchangeable, but they are better regarded as not synonymous:[22,124–126]
   i. DISEASE is the biological dimension of nonhealth, an essentially physiological dysfunction.
   ii. ILLNESS is a subjective or psychological state of the person who feels aware of not being well; the experience of a person with a disease; a social construct fashioned out of transactions between healers and patients in the context of their common culture.
   iii. SICKNESS is a state of social dysfunction of a person with a disease; the role that the individual assumes when ill; a result of being defined by others as "unhealthy."

In the real world, lay concepts of illness and medical concepts of disease interact and shape each other. Neither disease nor illness is infinitely malleable: both are constrained by biology and by culture.[127,128] See also DISORDER; EMBODIMENT; SEMIOLOGY; SICKNESS "CAREER."

DISEASE, PRECLINICAL Disease with no signs or symptoms because these have not yet developed. See also INAPPARENT INFECTION.

DISEASE, SUBCLINICAL A condition in which disease is detectable by special tests but does not reveal itself by signs or symptoms.

DISEASE FREQUENCY SURVEY See CROSS-SECTIONAL STUDY; morbidity survey.

DISEASE INTENSITY See FORCE OF MORBIDITY.

DISEASE LABEL The identity of the condition from which a patient suffers. It may be the name of a precisely defined disorder identified by a battery of tests, a probability statement based on consideration of what is most likely among several possibilities, or an opinion based on pattern recognition. Use of the word *label* can convey stigma. See also DIAGNOSIS; SEMIOLOGY; SICKNESS "CAREER."

DISEASE MAPPING A method for displaying spatial distribution of cases of disease, most often used in veterinary epidemiology. Disease maps may display raw numbers or rates (i.e., CHOROPLETHIC MAPS). See also GEOGRAPHIC INFORMATION SYSTEM; MEDICAL GEOGRAPHY.

DISEASE MODEL Quantitative simulation of the natural history of a disease (incidence, progression, prognosis, etc.) based on epidemiological data. A *public health model* is population-based and is used in planning and evaluating health services, whereas a *clinical model* is used in individual patient care.[129]

DISEASE ODDS RATIO See ODDS RATIO.

DISEASE PROGRESSION BIAS

1. In studies on the clinical accuracy and validity of diagnostic tests, a bias that occurs if results of the diagnostic test under study and of the reference standard test are not collected on the same patients at the same time, and if spontaneous recovery or progression to a more advanced stage of disease takes place. See also QUADAS.
2. In etiologic studies, biases that occur when disease progression entails metabolic and other pathophysiologic changes that alter the characteristics or concentrations (e.g., in blood, adipose tissue, target organs, peritumoral tissue) of the study exposure biomarkers. Biomarkers of exposure collected during subclinical or overt disease will then not reflect exposures of etiologic significance that took place in more distant time windows. For instance, during the progression of some cancers, blood concentrations of lipophilic substances of putative etiologic interest (e.g., lipophilic vitamins, organochlorine compounds) may be increased or decreased due to pathophysiologic changes associated with cancer-induced weight loss, cholestasis or lipid mobilization.

DISEASE REGISTRY See REGISTER, REGISTRY.

DISEASE TAXONOMY See TAXONOMY OF DISEASE.

DISEASES OF COMPLEX ETIOLOGY Diseases that result from complex causal pathways (e.g., from interactions between sociocultural, environmental, clinical, genetic, and epigenetic processes) often over long periods of life. Common diseases with late-onset phenotypes often result from interactions between the EPIGENOME, the GENOME, and the environment.[43,116] See also POLYGENIC DISEASES; WEB OF CAUSATION.

DISENTRAPMENT Some form of escape from DEMOGRAPHIC ENTRAPMENT.

DISINFECTION Killing of infectious agents outside the body by direct exposure to chemical or physical agents.

Concurrent disinfection is the application of disinfective measures as soon as possible after the discharge of infectious material from the body of an infected person or after the soiling of articles with such infectious discharges, all personal contact with such discharges or articles being minimized prior to such disinfection.

Terminal disinfection is the application of disinfective measures after the patient has been removed by death or to a hospital, or has ceased to be a source of infection, or after other hospital isolation practices have been discontinued. Terminal disinfection is rarely practiced; terminal cleaning generally suffices, along with airing and sunning of rooms, furniture, and bedding. Disinfection is necessary only for diseases spread by indirect contact; steam sterilization or incineration of bedding and other items is desirable after a disease such as plague or anthrax.[52]

DISINFESTATION Any physical or chemical process serving to destroy or remove undesired small animal forms, particularly arthropods or rodents, present upon the person, the clothing, or in the environment of an individual or on domestic animals. Disinfestation includes delousing for infestation with *Pediculus humanus humanus*, the body louse. Synonyms include the terms *disinsection* and *disinsectization* when insects only are involved.

DISMOD A model designed to help disease experts arrive at internally consistent estimates of incidence, duration, and case fatality rates of BURDEN OF DISEASE. It uses a life-table approach in following an initially disease-free cohort over time while applying the risks (incidence, remission, case fatality rate) associated with a disease and the competing risk of all other diseases as represented by general mortality. Using a competing risk approach, it calculates the relative proportions of each cohort that will develop, recover from, or die from the disease, die from other causes of mortality, or continue to live disease-free. To the extent that it takes into account other competing risk factors of mortality, this approach may be more realistic than one that simply assumes that Prevalence = incidence x duration. Differences between the two approaches seem most marked in chronic diseases with low rates of remission and cause-specific mortality.[46]

DISORDER, DISEASE, SYNDROME A *disorder* is a disturbance or departure—for example, of an organ or body system—from normal healthy function; i.e., an IMPAIRMENT. A *disease* is a disorder that can be assigned to a diagnostic category; it usually has a distinct clinical course and often a distinct etiology. A *syndrome* is a group of symptoms and signs that tend to appear together and collectively characterize a disorder.

DISTAL DETERMINANT See DETERMINANT, DISTAL (DISTANT).

DISTRIBUTION

1. (Syn: frequency distribution) The complete summary of the frequencies of the values or categories of a measurement made on a group of persons. The distribution tells either how many or what proportion of the group was found to have each value (or each range of values) out of all the possible values that the measurement can have.
2. In statistics, a DISTRIBUTION FUNCTION.

DISTRIBUTION-FREE METHOD (Syn: nonparametric method) A method that does not depend upon the form of the underlying distribution. Like all statistical methods, however, it depends on assumptions of randomness (in sampling or in allocation to exposure) and thus may be subject to BIAS.

DISTRIBUTION FUNCTION (Syn: probability distribution) A mathematical function that gives the relative frequency or probability with which a random variable falls at or below each of a series of values. Examples include the normal distribution, log-normal distribution, chi-square distribution, *t* distribution, *F* distribution, logistic distribution, binomial distribution, Poisson distribution, and multinomial distribution, all of which have applications in epidemiology.

DMF Decayed, missing, and filled teeth. Lowercase letters (i.e., dmf) are used for deciduous dentition, uppercase for permanent teeth. The DMF number is widely used in dental epidemiology.

DOMINANCE A concept from biological and urban ecology describing how one group or species has more influence or control than the others. In an urban community, dominance may be related to competition over land value, strategic geographical location, or a healthier environment.[18]

DOMINANT In genetics, alleles that fully manifest their phenotype when present in the heterozygous state. Contrast RECESSIVE.

DOSE The amount of a substance available for interaction with metabolic processes or biologically significant receptors after crossing the relevant boundary (epidermis, gut, respiratory tract); the absorbed dose is the amount crossing a specific absorption barrier. In lay usage, the amount of a medication to be taken at one time.[130]

DOSE-RESPONSE RELATIONSHIP (Syn: dose-effect relationship) An association between a given dose or set of doses (i.e., amount, duration, concentration) of an agent and the magnitude of a graded effect in an individual or a population.The relationship of observed outcomes (responses) in a population to varying levels of a protective or harmful agent such as a drug or an environmental contaminant. Commonly displayed as a graph, sometimes as a histogram. Important aspects include the rate at zero dose (baseline, or control), the presence or absence of a THRESHOLD DOSE, the presence or absence of MONOTONICITY, and the form of the mathematical expression that better fits the relationship between the dose and the response (linear, logarithmic, etc.). Other relevant features include the time element (e.g., How soon after the dose is the response observed? Is there a latent period?) and the range of individual variation (What proportion of those exposed experience no response, and a slight, moderate, or severe response?).

DOT CHART, DOT PLOT A display (plot) of the individual values of a set of numbers. The x axis represents categories of a noncontinuous variable and the y axis represents the values displayed by the observations.

DOUBLE-BLIND TRIAL A procedure of blind assignment to study and control groups and blind assessment of outcome, designed to ensure that ascertainment of outcome is not biased by knowledge of the group to which an individual was assigned. *Double* refers to both parties—the observer(s) in contact with the subjects and the subjects

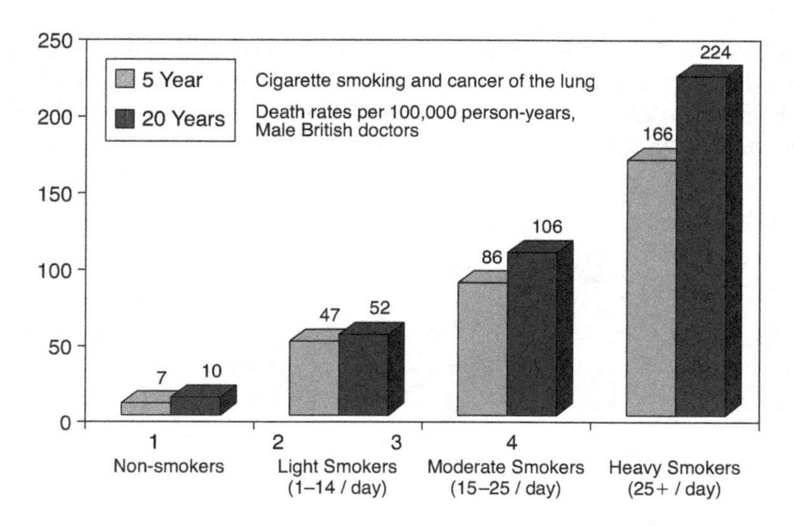

Dose-response relationship. Data from Doll R, Hill AB. Lung cancer and other causes of death in relation to smoking; a second report on the mortality of British doctors. *Br Med J* 1956, 2:1071–1082; Doll R, Peto R. Mortality in relation to smoking; 20 years' observations on male British doctors. *Br Med J* 1976, 2:1525–1536. With permission.

in the study and control groups. See also BLIND(ED) STUDY; RANDOMIZED CONTROLLED TRIAL.

DOUBLING TIME The average time taken for a population to double in numbers.

DRIFT See GENETIC DRIFT; SOCIAL DRIFT.

DROPLET NUCLEI A type of particle implicated in the spread of airborne infection. Droplet nuclei are tiny particles (1–10 μm diameter) that represent the dried residue of droplets. They may be formed by (1) evaporation of droplets coughed or sneezed into the air or (2) aerosolization of infective materials. See also TRANSMISSION OF INFECTION.

DROPOUT A person enrolled in a study who becomes inaccessible or ineligible for follow-up (e.g., because of inability or unwillingness to remain enrolled in the study). The occurrence of dropouts can lead to biases in study results. See also ATTRITION BIAS.

DRUG RESISTANCE The ability of an organism to develop strains that are impervious to specific threats to their existence.[131]

DRUG RESISTANCE, MULTIPLE (MDR) Simultaneous resistances to several structurally and functionally distinct drugs.

DRUG-RESISTANT TUBERCULOSIS, MULTIPLE (MDR tuberculosis) A form of tuberculosis that is resistant to two or more of the primary drugs used for the treatment of tuberculosis (at least isoniazid and rifampin). It occurs when bacteria develop the ability to withstand antibiotic attack and relay that ability to newly produced bacteria. It can spread from one person to another. On an individual basis, improper use of the antituberculosis medications remains an important cause of drug-resistant tuberculosis.[132] Treatment of MDR tuberculosis requires second-line drugs (SLDs) that are less effective, more toxic, and costlier than first-line isoniazid- and rifampin-based regimens.

DRUG-RESISTANT TUBERCULOSIS, EXTENSIVELY (XDR) A form of tuberculosis caused by a strain of *Mycobacterium tuberculosis* resistant to isoniazid and rifampin, to any fluoroquinolone, and to at least one of the three following injectable drugs: capreomycin, kanamycin, and amikacin.[133]

DUMMY VARIABLE See INDICATOR VARIABLE.

DYNAMIC POPULATION A population that gains and loses members; all natural populations are dynamic—a fact recognized by the term *population dynamics*, which is used by demographers to denote changing composition. See also POPULATION DYNAMICS; STABLE POPULATION; FIXED COHORT.

e Symbol for the base of natural or Napierian logarithms. It may be defined mathematically as the sum of the exponential series

$$e^x = 1 + x + x^2/2! + x^3/3! + \ldots x^n/n!$$

where $x = 1$ and n approaches infinity, i.e.,

$$e = 1 + 1 + 1/2 + 1/6 + 1/24 + \ldots = 2.71828\ldots$$

EARLY DETECTION OF DISEASE Identification of a specific disease at an early stage in the NATURAL HISTORY OF THE DISEASE. Detection before the usual clinical diagnosis does not guarantee diagnosis at an early stage, nor does it assure a more effective treatment. Often an ambiguous and misleading expression because of the term *detection*, which implies that the disease would otherwise be diagnosed "late," and because sometimes no disease is diagnosed, just a putatively precursor lesion (perhaps, naturally reversible) or a genetic or biochemical alteration (the actual risk of disease conferred by the latter may not have been demonstrated by longitudinal studies).[62,63,134] Since *detection* is not a synonym of *diagnosis*, confirmation of the suspected diagnosis will require additional tests, properly diagnostic. By definition, early detection of disease does not prevent disease occurrence. It may do so only if early detection of a precursor lesion leads to complete and definitive removal of all such lesions; otherwise long-term medical surveillance of precursor lesions or other alterations (and, as usual, of overt disease) will be required, and no gain will exist over diagnosis of disease through customary clinical paths.

Early detection may be accomplished both by EARLY CLINICAL DETECTION and by population-based SCREENING programs. It includes both symptomatic and asymptomatic individuals. It may be a form of SECONDARY PREVENTION; in certain diseases it may contribute to TERTIARY PREVENTION. Early detection of disease will usually appear to improve survival, even when it is ineffective (e.g., because treatment is not administered earlier, treatment is not more effective when administered earlier, or no effective treatment is available). Early detection (of disease, of precursor lesions, of genetic factors putatively conferring disease susceptibility, and even of classic RISK FACTORS) is not an aim in itself: it is justified only if it improves outcomes meaningful to individuals or communities. SEE ALSO CASE-FINDING; LEAD TIME BIAS; SCREENING.

EARLY CLINICAL DETECTION Early detection of disease in a clinical setting among persons presenting to a clinician or using medical services (by contrast with early detection of disease through a population-based screening program). In principle the term includes both symptomatic and asymptomatic individuals, but in practice most individuals who undergo early clinical etection show signs and symptoms of the diease to be detected or have precursor lesions (i.e., alterations that have conclusively been demonstrated to increase risk of the target disease). See also CASE FINDING.

EARLY-WARNING SYSTEM In disease surveillance, a specific procedure to detect as early as possible any departure from usual or normally observed frequency of phenomena. For example, the routine MONITORING of numbers of deaths from pneumonia and influenza in large American cities has been used as an early warning system for the identification of influenza epidemics. In developing countries, a change in children's average weights is an early warning signal of nutritional deficiency. See also CASE REPORT.

EBM See EVIDENCE-BASED MEDICINE.

E-BOOK A method of recording encounters in primary medical care: encounters are arranged by problem or diagnostic category, thus making it possible to count the number of persons seen (and the number of times each was seen) according to problem or diagnostic category in a given period of time.[135] It was used in epidemiological studies of primary medical care. See also AGE-SEX REGISTER; DIAGNOSTIC INDEX.

EBPH See EVIDENCE-BASED PUBLIC HEALTH.

EC European Community or European Commission.

ECDC European Centre for Disease Prevention and Control (www.ecdc.eu.int).

ECLOSION Emergence of imago (adult) from pupal case, hatching of larva from egg; a term descriptive of life stages of insect vectors.

ECOEPIDEMIOLOGY In the early 1980s this term was applied to the study of ecological influences on human health, whether related to environmental chemical agents or biological interactions such as life cycles of parasites. Mervyn Susser[136] (b. 1921) used the term within a conceptual approach that unifies molecular, clinical, and SOCIAL EPIDEMIOLOGY in a multilevel application of methods aimed at identifying causes, categorizing risks, and controlling public health problems. A perspective that balances traditional biomedical concepts of risk with the broader social and environmental context.[18]

ECOLOGICAL CASE-REFERENT DESIGN A study design suitable for use in the evaluation of communitywide interventions and characterized by measurement of the exposure on a ecological scale and of the outcome on a individual scale.

ECOLOGICAL ANALYSIS Analysis based on aggregated or grouped data; errors in inference may result because associations may be artifactually created or masked by the aggregation process.[107] See AGGREGATIVE FALLACY; ECOLOGICAL FALLACY; ATOMISTIC FALLACY.

ECOLOGICAL BIAS See AGGREGATIVE FALLACY; ATOMISTIC FALLACY; CROSS-LEVEL BIAS; ECOLOGICAL FALLACY.

ECOLOGICAL CORRELATION A correlation in which the units studied are populations or groups rather than individuals. Correlations found in this manner may not hold true for the individual members of the same populations. See also ECOLOGICAL FALLACY.

ECOLOGICAL DEPTH A criterion used for assessing the impact or penetration of an intervention into the local system; it includes the intervention scope (number of levels) and the duration of effect. An epidemiological program with high ecological depth yields an effect at multiple levels (individual, environmental) that endures over time.[18]

ECOLOGICAL FALLACY (Syn: aggregation bias, ecological bias)

1. An erronous inference that may occur because an association observed between variables on an aggregate level does not necessarily represent or reflect the association that exists at an individual level; a causal relationship that exists on a group level or among groups may not exist among the group individuals.[18,31,107]
2. An error in inference due to failure to distinguish between different levels of organization. A correlation between variables based on group (ecological) characteristics is not necessarily reproduced between variables based on individual characteristics; an association at one level may disappear at another or even be reversed. Example: At the ecological level, a correlation has been found in several studies between the quality of drinking water and mortality rates from heart disease; it would be an ecological fallacy to infer from this alone that exposure to water of a particular level of hardness necessarily influences the individual's chances of dying from heart disease. Policies, decisions, and actions at a given level (individual, municipal, regional, etc.) must be based on evidence—on causal relationships at that level. See also AGGREGATIVE FALLACY, ATOMISTIC FALLACY, CROSS-LEVEL BIAS.

ECOLOGICAL FOOTPRINT The dimensions and composition of the ecosystem required to sustain the actions or goods of a population, such as a hospital, a factory, a holiday resort, an aircraft. An estimate of the impact of an individual, group, or organization on the environment based on consumption and pollution. The term is applied mainly to the required input of resources and output of waste products. Ecological footprint analysis compares human demand and consumption of natural resources with the system's ecological capacity to regenerate them.

ECOLOGICAL STUDY In epidemiology, a study in which the units of analysis are populations or groups of people rather than individuals. An example is the study of the relationship between the distribution of income and mortality rates in states or provinces. Conclusions of ecological studies may not apply to individuals; thus caution is needed to avoid the ECOLOGICAL FALLACY. Ecological studies can reach valid causal inferences on causal relationships at the ecological level—i.e., on causal processes that occur at the group level or among groups.[107] Ecological studies are necessary for decisions that affect entire groups (e.g., for public and private policies that are developed across an entire state, country, or region). See also AGGREGATIVE FALLACY, ATOMISTIC FALLACY, CROSS-LEVEL BIAS.

ECOLOGICAL TRANSITION Within a framework of human development, ecological transitions are shifts in roles or settings that occur across the LIFE COURSE (e.g., arrival of a new sibling, entering school, finding a job, getting married, moving one's household, retiring). These transitions usually entail a change in a person's role or behavioral expectations.[18]

ECOLOGY The study of the relationships among living organisms and their environment. The comprehensive science of the relation of the organism to the environment. See also HUMAN ECOLOGY.

ECOSOCIAL THEORY OF DISEASE DISTRIBUTION One of the multilevel epidemiological frameworks that seek to integrate social and biological reasoning and a historical and ecological perspective so as to develop new insights into determinants of population distributions of disease and social inequalities in health. The central question for the theory is: "Who and what is responsible for population patterns of health, disease, and well-being as manifested in social inequalities in health?"[137]

ECOSYSTEM Plant and animal life systems considered in relation to the environmental factors and processes that influence them. The fundamental unit in ecology, comprising the living organisms and the nonliving elements that interact in a defined region. This region may be any size, from a drop of pond water to the entire biosphere. A comparatively stable and enduring arrangement of a population with mutual dependencies, including all living and nonliving (e.g., water, climate) elements within an area. The population operates collectively as a unit in ways that maintain a viable relationship with the environment. Edges of ecosystems are seldom clearly defined.[18,138]

EFFECT The result of a cause. In epidemiology, frequently a synonym for EFFECT MEASURE.

EFFECTIVENESS In the usage made common among epidemiologists by Archibald L. Cochrane (1909–1988)[139] and others, it is a measure of the extent to which a specific intervention, procedure, regimen, or service, when deployed in the field in the usual circumstances, does what it is intended to do for a specified population.[140] A measure of the extent to which a health care intervention fulfills its objectives in practice. To be distinguished from EFFICACY and EFFICIENCY. See also INTENTION-TO-TREAT ANALYSIS; PRAGMATIC STUDY.

EFFECTIVE POPULATION SIZE The average number of individuals in a population that contribute genes to the next generation.

EFFECTIVE SAMPLE SIZE Sample size after dropouts, deaths, and other specified exclusions from an original sample.

EFFECT MEASURE A quantity that measures the effect of a factor on the frequency or risk of a health outcome. Three such measures are ATTRIBUTABLE FRACTIONS, which measure the fraction of cases due to a factor; risk and rate differences, which measure the amount a factor adds to the risk or rate of a disease; and risk and rate ratios, which measure the amount by which a factor multiplies the risk or rate of disease.

EFFECT MODIFICATION (Syn: effect-measure modification) Variation in the selected effect measure for the factor under study across levels of another factor.[12,24] See also INTERACTION.

EFFECT MODIFIER (Syn: modifying factor)

1. A factor that modifies the measure of effect of a putative causal factor under study. There is effect modification when the selected effect measure for the factor under study varies across levels of another factor. An effect modifier may modify different measures in different directions and may modify one measure but not another.
2. A factor that biologically, clinically, socially, or otherwise alters the effects of a causal factor under study. For example, age-related decline in liver function can lead to stronger effects of toxins in the elderly; immunization reduces or eliminates the adverse consequences of exposure to pathogenic organisms. As another example, age is an effect modifier for many conditions, and immunization status is an effect modifier for the consequences of exposure to pathogenic organisms. See also CAUSALITY; INTERACTION.

EFFICACY The extent to which a specific intervention, procedure, regimen, or service produces a beneficial result under ideal conditions; the benefit or UTILITY to the individual or the population of the service, treatment regimen, or intervention. Ideally, the determination of efficacy is based on the results of a RANDOMIZED CONTROLLED TRIAL.

EFFICIENCY

1. The effects or end results achieved in relation to the effort expended in terms of money, resources, and time. The extent to which the resources used to provide a specific intervention, procedure, regimen, or service of known efficacy and effectiveness are minimized. A measure of the economy (or cost in resources) with

which a procedure of known efficacy and effectiveness is carried out. The process of making the best use of scare resources.

2. In statistics, the relative PRECISION with which a particular study design or estimator will estimate a parameter of interest.
3. Health economists identify several types of efficiency:[141]

TECHNICAL EFFICIENCY refers to the relationship between resources (capital and labor) and health outcomes.

PRODUCTIVE EFFICIENCY refers to maximizing health outcomes for a given cost or minimizing cost for a given outcome.

ALLOCATIVE EFFICIENCY is maximizing community health at given levels of technical and productive efficiency.

4. Other types of efficiency include:

STATISTICAL EFFICIENCY is the extent to which a study design maximizes the precision of effect estimates obtained from a given number of subjects or given amount of person-time.

STUDY EFFICIENCY is the value of information obtained from a study in relation to the number of subjects (or person-time) and/or to the monetary and other costs of the study.

EGG COUNT See WORM COUNT.

EIS See EPIDEMIC INTELLIGENCE SERVICE.

ELECTROPHILIC Having an affinity for negative charge. Molecules that behave as electron acceptors are electrophilic. Only sufficiently reactive, electrophilic compounds are capable of directly interacting with cellular proteins and DNA. See also NUCLEOPHILIC; CARCINOGEN; PROCARCINOGEN.

ELIGIBILITY CRITERIA An explicit statement of the conditions under which persons are admitted to an epidemiological study, such as a case-control study or a randomized controlled trial.

ELIMINATION Reduction of case transmission to a predetermined very low level; e.g., elimination of tuberculosis as a public health problem was defined by the WHO (1991) as reduction of prevalence to a level below one case per million population. Compare ERADICATION (OF DISEASE).

ELISA Enzyme-linked immunosorbent assay.

EMBODIMENT

1. Processes through which extrinsic factors experienced at different life stages are inscribed into an individual's body functions or structures, and the result of such processes.[16] How humans biologically *incorporate* the world in which we live, including aspects of the societal and ecological CONTEXT. Recognizing that humans are simultaneously social beings and biological organisms, the concept aims to highlight that (1) bodies tell stories about—and cannot be studied divorced from—the conditions of human existence; (2) bodies tell stories that often match people's stated accounts; and (3) bodies tell stories that people cannot or will not tell. A multilevel phenomenon, integrating soma, psyche, and society within historical and ecological context; hence an antonym to disembodied genes, minds, and behaviors. Pathophysiological responses and clinical expressions of social inequalities result from and reflect how people literally embody and express their experiences of inequality.[125–128,137,142–144]
2. A tangible or visible form of an idea, quality, or feeling. The representation or expression of something in such a form.[76] A key concept for some schools of phenomenology. The subjective experience of one's own body is different from the objective or scientific picture of a body in physiological terms. The specific ways in

which we experience ourselves as embodied thus become prime data for analyses about knowledge and experience.[77,127] See also DISEASE.

EMBRYO Biologically, in the human, the stage of the conceptus from uterine implantation (about 7 days after fertilization) to completion of organ development (about 54–60 days); conventionally, 8 weeks after conception, 10 weeks after the last menstrual period. The distinction between an embryo and a FETUS can be important in law and in perinatal epidemiology.

EMERGING INFECTIONS (Syn: emerging pathogens) Infectious diseases that have recently been identified and taxonomically classified. Many of them are capable of causing dangerous epidemics. They include human immunodeficiency virus (HIV) infection, Ebola virus disease, hantavirus pulmonary syndrome and other viral hemorrhagic fevers, *Campylobacter* infection, transmissable spongiform encephalopathies, Legionnaires' disease, and Lyme disease. Some appear to be new diseases of humans (e.g., HIV infection). Others, such as the viral hemorrhagic fevers, may have existed for many centuries and have been recognized only recently, because ecological or other environmental and demographic changes have increased the risk of human infection. *Reemerging infections* are certain "old" diseases, such as tuberculosis and syphilis, that have experienced a resurgence because of changed host-agent-environment conditions.

EMPIRICAL Based directly on experience (e.g., observation or experiment) rather than on reasoning or theory alone.

EMPIRICAL-BAYES METHODS Statistical methods that have the mathematical form of BAYESIAN STATISTICS but that estimate the prior distributions from the data being analyzed instead of deriving them from external data or expert judgment. Such methods are especially useful for addressing MULTIPLE COMPARISONS PROBLEMS, as they arise, for example, in genomewide "scans." See also SHRINKAGE ESTIMATION.

EMPORIATRICS The specialty of travel medicine.[145] From the Greek *emporion* (trade).

ENABLING FACTORS See CAUSATION OF DISEASE, FACTORS IN.

ENCOUNTER A face-to-face transaction between a personal health worker and a patient or client. Not limited to health care settings.

ENDEMIC DISEASE The constant presence of a disease or infectious agent within a given geographic area or population group; may also refer to the usual prevalence of a given disease within such an area or group. See also HOLOENDEMIC DISEASE; HYPERENDEMIC DISEASE; PREVALENCE.

ENDOBIOTIC An endogenous substance that produces a toxic metabolite when it is metabolized. A substance or organisms that grows within a living organism. Contrast XENOBIOTIC.

END RESULTS See OUTCOMES.

ENEE European Network for Education in Epidemiology.

ENTROPY In thermodynamics, entropy is a measure of the disorder in a system. In statistics, entropy means the same; it is a measure of disorder, uncertainty, or chaos or, more loosely, randomness.[146]

ENVIRONMENT All that which is external to the individual human host. Can be divided into physical, biological, social, cultural, etc., any or all of which can influence the health status of populations.[9,72,130,138] "The environment provides the food people eat, the water they drink, the air they breathe, the energy they command, the plagues and pests they combat and the mountains, seas, lakes, streams, plants and animals that they enjoy and depend upon."[147]

ENVIRONMENTAL EPIDEMIOLOGY A branch or subspecialty of EPIDEMIOLOGY that uses epidemiological principles, reasoning, and methods to study the health effects on populations of exposure to physical, chemical, and biological agents external to the human body and of immediate and remote social, economic, and cultural factors (e.g., urbanization, agricultural development, energy production/combustion) related to these physical, chemical, and biological agents. By studying populations in different exposure circumstances, environmental epidemiologists aim to clarify relationships between exogenous agents and/or factors and health. Recognition of health hazards posed by large-scale environmental changes and by ecological disruption, often via indirect pathways, has added an extra dimension to this field of inquiry.

ENVIRONMENTAL HEALTH CRITERIA DOCUMENT Official publication containing a review of existing knowledge about chemicals, radiation, etc., and their identifiable immediate and long-term effects on health. Environmental health criteria documents are produced by the WHO, the International Agency for Research on Cancer (IARC), and many national agencies, such as the National Institute for Occupational Safety and Health (NIOSH) in the United States.

ENVIRONMENTAL HEALTH IMPACT ASSESSMENT A statement of the beneficial or adverse health effects or risks due to an environmental exposure or likely to follow an environmental change. Such statements may contain or refer to results of epidemiological and/or toxicological studies of environmental health hazards.

ENVIRONMENTAL HYPERSENSITIVITY An ill-defined concept that refers to a set of poorly understood conditions and syndromes that some authors deem potentially related to exposure to low concentrations of chemical, physical, or other environmental agents. Related conditions might include the sick building syndrome, the chronic fatigue syndrome, and multiple chemical sensitivity.

ENVIRONMENTAL TOBACCO SMOKE (ETS) A specific form of air pollution due to burning tobacco, especially SIDESTREAM SMOKE. ETS is carcinogenic to humans; e.g., it is classified in group 1 by the International Agency for Research on Cancer (IARC). Closely related terms are INVOLUNTARY SMOKING or *passive smoking* and *secondhand smoke*.

EPA Environmental Protection Agency (United States).

EPI Expanded Programme on Immunization (WHO/UNICEF).

EPIDEMIC [from the Greek *epi* (upon), *dēmos* (people)] The occurrence in a community or region of cases of an illness, specific health-related behavior, or other health-related events clearly in excess of normal expectancy.

The community or region and the period in which the cases occur must be specified precisely. The number of cases indicating the presence of an epidemic varies according to the agent, size, and type of population exposed; previous experience or lack of exposure to the disease; and time and place of occurrence. Epidemicity is thus relative to usual frequency of the disease in the same area, among the specified population, at the same season of the year.

A single case of a communicable disease long absent from a population or first invasion by a disease not previously recognized in that area requires immediate reporting and full field investigation; two cases of such a disease associated in time and place may be sufficient evidence to be considered an epidemic. Classic epidemics initially identified following the occurrence of small numbers of cases include the epidemic of vaginal cancer in daughters of women who took diethylstilbestrol during pregnancy[148] and the pandemic of AIDS, which was heralded by a report[149] of cases of *Pneumocystis carinii* pneumonia among gay men in Los Angeles in 1981.

The purpose of surveillance systems such as the EPIDEMIC INTELLIGENCE SERVICE is to identify epidemics as early as possible so that effective control measures can be put in place. This remains a most important use of epidemiology.

The word may be used also to describe outbreaks of disease in animal or plant populations. See also EPIZOOTIC; EPORNITHIC.

EPIDEMIC, COMMON SOURCE (Syn: common vehicle epidemic, holomiantic disease) Outbreak due to exposure of a group of persons to a noxious influence that is common to the individuals in the group. When the exposure is brief and essentially simultaneous, the resultant cases all develop within one incubation period of the disease (a "point" or "point source" epidemic). The term *holomiantic disease* was used by Stallybrass (1931) to describe outbreaks of this type, but as with several other terms created from Greek or Latin roots, transmission to epidemiologists who lacked a classical education did not take place.

EPIDEMIC, MATHEMATICAL MODEL OF See MATHEMATICAL MODEL.

EPIDEMIC, POINT SOURCE See EPIDEMIC, COMMON SOURCE.

EPIDEMIC CURVE A graphic plotting of the distribution of cases by time of onset.

EPIDEMIC INTELLIGENCE (Syn: epidemiological intelligence) The process of detecting, verifying, analyzing, assessing, and investigating signals that may represent a threat to public health.[150] Activities aimed at managing epidemiological crises, biochemical threats, radiological risks, natural disasters, or the public health impact of terrorist attacks and wars. A government body engaged in collecting secret or sensitive information related to epidemic outbreaks. The Global Public Health Intelligence Network (GPHIN) of the World Health Organization is an Internet-based multilingual early-warning tool that continuously searches news wires and websites to identify information about disease outbreaks and other events of potential international public health concern. To ensure a comprehensive picture of the epidemic threat to global health security, WHO also gathers epidemic intelligence from informal sources. With the advent of modern communication technologies, many initial outbreak reports now originate in the electronic media and electronic discussion groups.[151]

EPIDEMIC INTELLIGENCE SERVICE (EIS) A postgraduate training program in epidemiology of the U.S. Centers for Disease Control and Prevention (CDC). Established in 1951 owing to biological warfare concerns arising from the Korean War. EIS officers have been decisive in the investigation of many epidemics, including AIDS, anthrax, hantavirus, and West Nile virus in the United States and Ebola in Uganda and Zaire.

EPIDEMICS, HISTORY OF The effect of diseases on the course of history fascinates epidemiologists and historians alike.[10,152] It has preoccupied scholars since the biblical plagues, Hippocrates, and the epidemic, described by Thucydides, that struck the Athenians at the end of the first year of the Peloponnesian War (429 B.C.). Measles and smallpox brought by Europeans defeated the Aztecs and Incas, who, in return, gave tobacco and perhaps syphilis to Europeans. There are innumerable scholarly and popular works on the subject. Early treatises include those of Hecker[153] and Creighton[154]; a modern work by a historian is *Plagues and Peoples*.[155] Perhaps the nearest to a comprehensive monograph by an epidemiologist is Thomas McKeown's *The Origins of Human Disease*.[156] Partial accounts include histories of the impact on societies and civilizations of syphilis,[157] tuberculosis,[158] poliomyelitis,[159] typhus,[160] and many other conditions.[125,161]

EPIDEMIC THRESHOLD The number or density of susceptibles required for an epidemic to occur. According to the MASS ACTION PRINCIPLE, the epidemic threshold is the reciprocal of the INFECTION TRANSMISSION PARAMETER.

EPIDEMIOLOGICAL CASE DEFINITION See CASE DEFINITION.

EPIDEMIOLOGICAL METHODS, HISTORY OF A domain of history that deals specifically with the evolution of epidemiological methods and concepts.[5–11,81]

EPIDEMIOLOGICAL RESEARCH Occurrence research—i.e., research among people into the frequency of occurrence of phenomena of public health, clinical, social, or biological RELEVANCE, with measures of frequency and causal assessments related to the DETERMINANTS of such phenomena.[5] See also CREATIVITY; INTEGRATIVE RESEARCH.

"EPIDEMIOLOGICAL TRANSITION" THEORY Traditionally,[162] the mortality component of the DEMOGRAPHIC TRANSITION was considered to have three phases: (1) The "age of pestilence and famine"; (2) the "age of receding pandemics"; (3) the "age of degenerative and man-made diseases." According to Omran,[162] the shift from the first to third phases took about 100 years in the Western industrial nations, but it occurred more rapidly in Japan and eastern Europe; many developing countries have yet to undergo the shift. Mackenbach[163] shows that the transition from first to third phase took considerably longer in Western industrial nations and asserts that "degenerative and man-made diseases" is a misleading term for conditions such as cancer and cardiovascular disease, which have complex etiologies.

EPIDEMIOLOGIST A professional who strives to study and control the factors that influence the occurrence of disease or other health-related conditions and events in defined populations and societies, has an expertise in POPULATION THINKING and epidemiological methods, and is knowledgeable about public health and causal inferences in health. The control of disease in populations is often considered to be a core task for the epidemiologist involved in the provision of public health services. Epidemiologists may study disease in populations of animals and plants as well as among human populations.

EPIDEMIOLOGY The study of the occurrence and distribution of health-related states or events in specified populations, including the study of the DETERMINANTS influencing such states, and the application of this knowledge to control the health problems.

Study includes surveillance, observation, hypothesis testing, analytic research, and experiments. *Distribution* refers to analysis by time, place, and classes or subgroups of persons affected in a population or in a society. *Determinants* are all the physical, biological, social, cultural, economic and behavioral factors that influence health. *Health-related states and events* include diseases, causes of death, behaviors, reactions to preventive programs, and provision and use of health services. *Specified populations* are those with common identifiable characteristics. Application to control... makes explicit the aim of epidemiology—to promote, protect, and restore health.

The primary "knowledge object" of epidemiology as a scientific discipline are causes of health-related events in populations. In the past 70 years, the definition has broadened from concern with communicable disease epidemics to take in all processes and phenomena related to health in populations.[4,5,9,11,152,164] Therefore epidemiology is much more than a branch of medicine treating of epidemics. There was a London Epidemiological Society in the 1850s. *Epidemiología* appears in the title of a Spanish history of epidemics, *Epidemiología española* (Madrid, 1802). The term *epidemic* is much older; for instance, it appears in Johnson's *Dictionary* (1775), and the *Oxford English Dictionary* gives a citation dated 1603. The word was, of course, used by Hippocrates. See also POPULATION THINKING; GROUP COMPARISON.

EPIDEMIOLOGY, DEMARCATION OF Marking or fixing the boundaries or limits of epidemiology as a scientific discipline; assessing epidemiology's methodologies, objects of research, legitimate uses and applications (e.g., in public health policy, in clinical practice, in basic research); examining its distinctiveness, similarities, or relationships with other scientific disciplines. Defense of scientific identity and solidarity, disciplinary autonomy, and EPISTEMIC authority of epidemiology are additional important elements of boundary work. These forms of scientific discourse are important components of the process by which various sciences establish their scientific and intellectual nature, moral order, social status, and mission.[4] Epidemiology benefits from a rich plurality of scientific cultures and practices; consequently, it enjoys diverse demarcation discourses.[4–12,111,136,164–170] Demarcation of many scientific disciplines evolved historically as their intellectual, institutional, and professional environments evolved.[4]

EPIDEMIOLOGY, ANALYTIC See ANALYTIC STUDY.

EPIDEMIOLOGY, APPLIED See APPLIED EPIDEMIOLOGY.

EPIDEMIOLOGY, BLACK-BOX See "BLACK-BOX EPIDEMIOLOGY."

EPIDEMIOLOGY, CANCER See CANCER EPIDEMIOLOGY.

EPIDEMIOLOGY, CARDIOVASCULAR See CARDIOVASCULAR EPIDEMIOLOGY.

EPIDEMIOLOGY, DESCRIPTIVE See DESCRIPTIVE EPIDEMIOLOGY.

EPIDEMIOLOGY, DEVELOPMENTAL See DEVELOPMENTAL AND LIFE-COURSE EPIDEMIOLOGY.

EPIDEMIOLOGY, DISASTER See DISASTER EPIDEMIOLOGY.

EPIDEMIOLOGY, ENVIRONMENTAL See ENVIRONMENTAL EPIDEMIOLOGY.

EPIDEMIOLOGY, EXPERIMENTAL See EXPERIMENTAL EPIDEMIOLOGY.

EPIDEMIOLOGY, FIELD See FIELD EPIDEMIOLOGY.

EPIDEMIOLOGY, FORENSIC See FORENSIC EPIDEMIOLOGY.

EPIDEMIOLOGY, HEALTHCARE See HOSPITAL EPIDEMIOLOGY.

EPIDEMIOLOGY, HOSPITAL See HOSPITAL EPIDEMIOLOGY.

EPIDEMIOLOGY, LIFE COURSE See DEVELOPMENTAL AND LIFE-COURSE EPIDEMIOLOGY.

EPIDEMIOLOGY, MECHANISTIC See MECHANISTIC EPIDEMIOLOGY.

EPIDEMIOLOGY, OBSERVATIONAL See OBSERVATIONAL EPIDEMIOLOGY.

EPIDEMIOLOGY, OCCUPATIONAL See OCCUPATIONAL EPIDEMIOLOGY.

EPIDEMIOLOGY, PRIMARY CARE See PRIMARY CARE EPIDEMIOLOGY.

EPIDEMIOLOGY, PSYCHOSOCIAL See SOCIAL EPIDEMIOLOGY.

EPIDEMIOLOGY, SOCIAL See SOCIAL EPIDEMIOLOGY.

EPIDEMIOLOGY, SOCIOLOGY OF. See SOCIOLOGY OF EPIDEMIOLOGY.

EPIDEMIOLOGY, THEORETICAL See THEORETICAL EPIDEMIOLOGY.

EPIGENETIC INHERITANCE A set of reversible heritable changes in gene function or other cell phenotype that occur without a change in the genotype. Such changes may be spontaneous, in response to environmental factors, or in response to other genetic events. Several types of epigenetic inheritance systems exist.[171] Epigenetic processes include PARAMUTATION, BOOKMARKING, IMPRINTING, GENE SILENCING, X CHROMOSOME INACTIVATION, POSITION EFFECT, REPROGRAMMING, or TRANSVECTION.

EPIGENETICS The study of heritable changes that are not the result of changes in the DNA sequence. Information heritable during cell division other than the DNA sequence itself. Changes in GENE EXPRESSION that are not regulated by the DNA nucleotide sequence (e.g., GENE SILENCING by promoter HYPERMETHYLATION or HISTONE MODIFICATION). Amazingly, given that they are not coded in the DNA, some epigenetic changes are heritable across several generations. Changes in gene-expression patterns caused by epigenetic alterations have been observed in biological systems exposed to nickel, cadmium, or arsenic. Complex diseases like cancer arise from the stepwise accumulation of genetic and epigenetic alterations that confer upon an incipient neoplastic cell (a "clone") the properties of unlimited, self-sufficient growth and resistance to normal homeostatic regulatory mechanisms.[116,172–176]

EPIGENOME The overall epigenetic state of a cell. At the intersection between environment and genetic variation, the epigenome is an important target of environmental factors. According to the COMMON DISEASE GENETIC AND EPIGENETIC (CDGE) HYPOTHESIS, the epigenome may modulate the effect of genetic variation either by affecting the gene's expression through the action of chromatin proteins or DNA methylation or by modulating protein folding of the gene product. The epigenome may, in turn, be affected by sequence variation in the genes encoding chromatin or chaperone proteins. Environmental factors (e.g., toxins, growth factors, dietary methyl donors, and hormones) can affect the GENOME and the epigenome. Although the epigenome is particularly susceptible to dysregulation during gestation, neonatal development, puberty, and old age, it is most vulnerable to environmental exposures during embryogenesis, because the elaborate DNA methylation and chromatin patterning required for normal tissue development is programmed during early development. Many XENOBIOTICS have the potential to modify the epigenome.[118] One key component of the cancer epigenome, for example, is an altered DNA methylation pattern composed of global demethylation and promoter localized hypermethylation; these changes fundamentally participate in an altered structure and function of DNA (e.g., unwanted transcription of repeat elements, abnormal activation of oncogenes, genomic instability, aberrant silencing of genes important to the initiation and progression of tumors).[177] See also DEVELOPMENTAL ORIGINS HYPOTHESIS.

EPI INFO Free software developed by the CDC for epidemiologists and other health professionals. Supports development of a questionnaire or form, the data entry process, and data analysis, inluding epidemiological measures, tables, graphs, and maps (www.cdc.gov/epiinfo).

EPISODE Period in which a health problem or illness exists, from its onset to its resolution. See also ENCOUNTER.

EPISTASIS Gene interaction; particularly interaction between different alleles at different genes (e.g., the suppression by a gene of the effect of another gene).

EPISTEMIC Relating to knowledge or to the degree of its validation.

EPISTEMIC COMMUNITIES

1. Transnational networks of scientists and of other knowledge-based professionals. Scientific associations have features of epistemic communities; subgroups within them may act as epistemic communities.[7]
2. Networks of experts who define for policy makers what the problems they face are and what they should do about them.
3. A group of people who do not have any specific history together but share ideas. Those who accept one version of a story that is particularly meaningful for their communities.

EPISTEMIC CULTURES Sets of practices, arrangements, and mechanisms bound together by necessity, affinity, interest, and historical coincidence that, in a given scientific field or area of professional expertise, make up how we know what we know.[178] Cultures of pursuing and warranting knowledge; they are pursued by specialists separated off from other specialists by long training periods, stringent division of labor, distinctive technological tools and methodologies, financing sources, scientific associations, journals, and dictionaries ... Interiorized processes of knowledge creation. They build the epistemic subject and referents, the meaning of *empirical*, methods of consensus formation, or forms of engagement with the social world.[4] They draw on different background knowledges, which become merged in knowledge work. They are forms of life and agree on acceptable forms of life (e.g., what it is to be a "postdoc" in epidemiology). See also KNOWLEDGE CONSTRUCTION; SOCIOLOGY OF SCIENTIFIC KNOWLEDGE.

EPISTEMOLOGY

1. The theory of knowledge. Epistemological questions include the origin of knowledge; the place of experience and reason in generating knowledge; the relationship between knowledge and certainty and between knowledge and the impossibility of error; the changing forms of knowledge as societies change. These issues are linked with others, such as the nature of truth and the nature of experience and meaning.[77]
2. The study of the relation between the knower (or would-be knower) and what can be known. Answers to these questions are constrained by answers to ontological questions.[179]

In epidemiology and other health sciences, debates have benefited from clarifying the methodological, epistemological, and ontological nature of the issues under analysis[4,5,10,180–182] For instance, the proposition that methods used in an epidemiological study must be coherent with the "knowledge object"[181] of the study does not primarily address a methodological issue but an epistemological one; also of an essentially epistemological nature are criticisms of studies that suffer from a hypertrophy or a dissonance of the methodological apparatus vis-à-vis the study hypotheses, of studies based on a poor conception of the hypotheses, or of statistical analyses unguided by knowledge available on the study subject.[5,68,93] See also ONTOLOGY.

EPIZOOTIC An outbreak (epidemic) of disease in an animal population; often with the implication that it may also affect human populations.

EPORNITHIC An outbreak (epidemic) of disease in a bird population.

EPR Epidemic and Pandemic (Alert and) Response. See also EPIDEMIOLOGICAL INTELLIGENCE.

EQUIPOISE A state of genuine uncertainty about the benefits or harms that may result from different exposures or interventions. A state of equipoise is an indication for a RANDOMIZED CONTROLLED TRIAL, because there are no ethical concerns about one regimen being better for a particular patient.

EQUITY Fairness, impartiality. An important concept in bioethics, especially in relation to human rights. See also HEALTH EQUITY.

EQUIVALENCE TESTS Significance tests in which the NULL HYPOTHESIS is that samples differ to a prescribed degree. A significant result of an equivalence test comparing the effects of two treatments would support the alternative hypothesis, i.e., that the effects are equivalent. The size of the differences tested is generally the upper limit of dissimilarity that is considered trivial or not clinically significant.

ERADICATION (OF DISEASE) Termination of all transmission of infection by extermination of the infectious agent through surveillance and containment. Eradication, as in the instance of smallpox, is based on the joint activities of control and surveillance. Regional eradication has been successful with poliomyelitis and in some countries appears close to succeeding for measles. The term ELIMINATION is sometimes used to describe eradication of diseases such as measles from a large geographic region or political jurisdiction. In 1992, the WHO put it this way: "Eradication is defined as achievement of a status whereby no further cases of a disease occur anywhere, and continued control measures are unnecessary." Smallpox was eradicated in 1977, based on joint control and surveillance activities.

ERROR A false or mistaken result of a measurement. Any other false or mistaken result obtained in a study or experiment. Two broad kinds of error can occur in studies in the health, life, and social sciences:

1. Random error: the portion of variation in a measurement that has no apparent connection to any other measurement or variable, generally regarded as due to CHANCE.
2. Systematic error: error that is consistently wrong in a particular direction; it often has a recognizable source (e.g., a faulty measuring instrument). See BIAS.

ERROR, TYPE I (Syn: alpha error) The error of wrongly rejecting a NULL HYPOTHESIS, i.e., declaring that a difference exists when it does not. See also MULTIPLE COMPARISON PROBLEM; *P* VALUE; SIGNIFICANCE, STATISTICAL; STATISTICAL TEST.

ERROR, TYPE II (Syn: beta error) The error of failing to reject a false null hypothesis, i.e., declaring that a difference does not exist when in fact it does. See also POWER; STATISTICAL TEST.

ERROR, TYPE III Wrongly assessing the causes of interindividual variation within a population when the research question requires an analysis of causes of differences between populations or time periods. When the objects of the study are risk differences between groups or periods, the study must examine multiple groups or periods; otherwise a type III error can result. Risk differences between individuals within a particular population may not have the same causes as differences in the average risk between two different populations.[183] See also ATOMISTIC FALLACY; EPISTEMOLOGY; ONTOLOGY; STRATEGY, "POPULATION."

ERROR BAR A graphical display of the statistical uncertainty of an estimate, displayed as lines having the length of one or more standard deviations, standard errors, or confidence intervals for the estimate that extend out from the plotted estimated value.

ESTIMATE A measurement or a statement about the value of some quantity is said to be an estimate if it is known, believed, or suspected to incorporate some degree of error.

ESTIMATOR In statistics, a function (formula) for computing estimates of a parameter from observed data (e.g., the MANTEL-HAENSZEL ODDS RATIO).

ETHICS The branch of philosophy that deals with distinctions between right and wrong—with the moral consequences of human actions. Ethical principles govern the conduct of epidemiology, as they do all human activities.[36,85–87] The ethical issues that arise in epidemiological practice and research include informed consent, confidentiality, respect for human rights, and scientific integrity. Epidemiologists and others have developed guidelines for the ethical conduct of epidemiological studies.[184–187] See also INFORMED CONSENT.

ETHICS (ETHICAL) REVIEW COMMITTEE See INSTITUTIONAL REVIEW BOARD.

ETHNIC GROUP, ETHNICITY

1. A social group characterized by a distinctive social and cultural tradition maintained within the group from generation to generation, a common history and origin, and a sense of identification with the group. Members of the group have distinctive features in their way of life, shared experiences, and often a common genetic heritage. These features may be reflected in their health and disease experience.
2. The social group a person belongs to and either identifies with or is identified with by others as a result of a mix of cultural and other factors, including language,

diet, religion, ancestry, and physical features traditionally associated with RACE. Increasingly, the concept is being used synonymously with race, but the trend is pragmatic rather than scientific.[108,188]

ETHNOEPIDEMIOLOGY Epidemiological study of causal factors for health and disease among different ethnic groups, with development of intervention strategies that take culture into account.[189]

ETIOLOGICAL FRACTION (EXPOSED)

1. A synonym for the ATTRIBUTABLE FRACTION (EXPOSED).
2. The fraction of exposed cases for which exposure played a role in the development of their disease. See probability of causation.

ETIOLOGICAL FRACTION (POPULATION)

1. A synonym for the ATTRIBUTABLE FRACTION (POPULATION).
2. The fraction of all cases for which exposure played a role in the development of their disease. See probability of causation.

ETIOLOGICAL STUDY A study that aims to unveil causal relationships. Although most ANALYTICAL STUDIES may be considered to have such an aim, the term may be useful to the extent that it emphasizes that the purpose is not just to analyze relationships but to interpret relationships in causal terms. The etiological study is paradigmal to the intervention study, not vice versa.[5] See also CAUSAL INFERENCE.

ETIOLOGY Literally, the science of causes, causality; in common usage, cause. See also CAUSALITY; PATHOGENESIS.

EU European Union.

EUPHA European Public Health Association.

EVALUATION A process that attempts to determine as systematically and objectively as possible the relevance, effectiveness, and impact of activities in the light of their objectives. Several varieties of evaluation can be distinguished (e.g., evaluation of structure, process, and outcome). See also CLINICAL TRIAL; EFFECTIVENESS; EFFICACY; EFFICIENCY; HEALTH SERVICES RESEARCH; PROGRAM EVALUATION AND REVIEW TECHNIQUES; QUALITY OF CARE.

EVANS'S POSTULATES Expanding biomedical knowledge has led to revision of the HENLE-KOCH POSTULATES.[10] Alfred Evans[190] developed those that follow, partly based on the Henle-Koch model:

1. Prevalence of the disease should be significantly higher in those exposed to the hypothesized cause than in controls not so exposed.
2. Exposure to the hypothesized cause should be more frequent among those with the disease than in controls without the disease—when all other RISK FACTORS are held constant.
3. Incidence of the disease should be significantly higher in those exposed to the hypothesized cause than in those not so exposed, as shown by prospective studies.
4. The disease should follow exposure to the hypothesized causative agent with a normal or log-normal distribution of incubation periods.
5. A spectrum of host responses should follow exposure to the hypothesized agent along a logical biological gradient from mild to severe.
6. A measurable host response following exposure to the hypothesized cause should have a high probability of appearing in those lacking this before exposure (e.g., antibody, cancer cells) or should increase in magnitude if present before exposure. This response pattern should occur infrequently in persons not so exposed.

7. Experimental reproduction of the disease should occur more frequently in animals or humans appropriately exposed to the hypothesized cause than in those not so exposed; this exposure may be deliberate in volunteers, experimentally induced in the laboratory, or may represent a regulation of natural exposure.
8. Elimination or modification of the hypothesized cause should decrease the incidence of the disease (e.g., attenuation of a virus, removal of tar from cigarettes).
9. Prevention or modification of the host's response on exposure to the hypothesized cause should decrease or eliminate the disease (e.g., immunization, drugs to lower cholesterol, specific lymphocyte transfer factor in cancer).
10. All of the relationships and findings should make biological and epidemiological sense.

See also CAUSALITY; HILL'S CRITERIA OF CAUSATION; MILL'S CANONS.

EVENT RATE The number of people experiencing an event as a proportion of the number of people in the population or relative to the PERSON-TIME experience of the population.

EVIDENCE Scientific knowledge. Results of research used to support decision making.

EVIDENCE-BASED MEDICINE (EBM) The consistent use of knowledge derived from biological, clinical, and EPIDEMIOLOGICAL RESEARCH in the management of patients, with particular attention to the balance of benefits, risks, and costs of diagnostic tests, screening programs, and treatment regimens, taking account of each patient's circumstances, including baseline risk, comorbid conditions, culture, and personal preferences.[14,62,63,191] There are no major intellectual reasons either against evidence-based (EB) nursing, EB health care planning, EB proteomics,[192,193] or, for that matter, EB justice and EB economics.

EVIDENCE-BASED PUBLIC HEALTH (EBPH) Application of the best available evidence (i.e., the most valid, precise, and relevant scientific knowledge) in setting public health policies and practices. The evidence may be derived from epidemiological, statistical, medical, economic, demographic, sociological, and several other scientific disciplines. Sources of evidence should preferably be published, peer-reviewed, and critically appraised articles and reports. Implementation of public health policies, programs, and practices requires good evidence on FEASIBILITY, EFFICACY, EFFECTIVENESS, EFFICIENCY, COST, acceptability to the target population, and careful analysis of ethical and political implications.[194–197] Evidence on acceptability and ethical and cultural implications may also be obtained from FOCUS GROUPS. Another definition is: The development, implementation, and evaluation of effective programs and policies in public health through application of the principles of scientific reasoning, including systematic uses of data and information systems and appropriate use of behavioral and social science theory and program planning models. In EBPH, public health activities are explicitly linked with the underlying scientific evidence that suggests relevance and purpose and which demonstrates effectiveness.[70,104,194]

EXACT METHOD A statistical method based on the actual (i.e., "exact") probability distribution of the study data rather than on an approximation, such as a normal or a chi-square distribution (e.g., Fisher's exact test).

EXACT TEST A statistical test based on the actual null probability distribution of the study data rather than, say, a normal approximation. The most used exact test is the Fisher-Irwin test for fourfold tables (or Fisher's exact test).

EXCEPTION FLAGGING (REPORTING) SYSTEM An automated system of data analysis that calculates thresholds for unusual events. Used in SURVEILLANCE.

EXCESS RATE AMONG EXPOSED See RATE DIFFERENCE.

EXCESS RISK A term sometimes used to refer to the POPULATION EXCESS RISK and sometimes to the RISK DIFFERENCE or ABSOLUTE RISK REDUCTION.

EXPANDED PROGRAMME ON IMMUNIZATION (EPI) A program of immunizing against diphtheria, tetanus, measles, pertussis, poliomyelitis, and tuberculosis conducted especially in developing countries. Part of the effort to achieve "Health for All by the Year 2000" under the auspices of WHO, UNICEF, and other agencies.

EXPANSION OF MORBIDITY As life expectancy increases, the prevalence of long-term disease, especially among older persons, increases. Mental disorders such as dementia may be an example.[198] Thus this is the opposite of COMPRESSION OF MORBIDITY. Both phenomena may coexist in the same population, some disorders becoming less prevalent, others more so.

EXPECTATION OF LIFE (Syn: life expectancy or expectation) The average number of years an individual of a given age is expected to live if current mortality rates continue to apply. A statistical abstraction based on existing age-specific death rates.

Life expectancy at birth ($\mathring{e}_0$): Average number of years a newborn baby can be expected to live if current mortality trends continue. Corresponds to the total number of years a given BIRTH COHORT can be expected to live divided by the number of children in the cohort. Life expectancy at birth is partly dependent on mortality in the first year of life; therefore it is lower in poor than in rich countries because of the higher infant and child mortality rates in the former.

Life expectancy at a given age, age x ($\mathring{e}_x$): The average number of additional years a person of age x will live, based on the age-specific death rates for a given year, if current mortality trends continue to apply.

Life expectancy is a hypothetical measure and indicator of current health and mortality conditions. It is not a rate.

EXPECTED YEARS OF LIFE LOST A measure of the impact of a disease on society as a result of early death. The expected years of life lost due to a particular cause is the sum, over all persons dying from that cause, of the years these persons would have lived had they experienced normal life expectancy. Life expectancies are usually taken from the population concerned, but another population can be used (e.g., the one with the highest life expectancy), which yields the *standard expected years of life lost*.[199] See also BURDEN OF DISEASE; POTENTIAL YEARS OF LIFE LOST.

EXPERIMENT The core of an experimental study. Manipulation of one or more independent variables and control of potential confounders by the investigator in order to test a specific hypothesis involving the causal effect of the independent variables on an outcome.

EXPERIMENT, NATURAL See NATURAL EXPERIMENT.

EXPERIMENTAL STUDY A study in which the investigator intentionally alters one or more factors and controls the other study conditions in order to analyze the effects of so doing. A study in which conditions are under the direct control of the investigator.

EXPERIMENTAL EPIDEMIOLOGICAL STUDY An epidemiological study with a clear experimental component; usually, a large phase III or a phase IV RANDOMIZED CONTROLLED TRIAL or a COMMUNITY TRIAL. In community trials (e.g., of fluoridation of drinking water), whole communities are (nonrandomly) allocated to experimental and control groups. See also OBSERVATIONAL STUDY; RANDOM ALLOCATION.

EXPERIMENTAL EPIDEMIOLOGY

1. The application of epidemiological reasoning, knowledge, and methods to experiments, particularly to phase III and phase IV RANDOMIZED CONTROLLED TRIALS and to community trials. If the word *experiment* is qualified by the adjective *epidemiological*, it usually refers to a RANDOMIZED CONTROLLED TRIAL or to a COMMUNITY TRIAL. Clinical or community-based studies merit the term *experiment* or *quasi-experiment* only if it is possible to modify conditions during the period of study. See also NATURAL EXPERIMENT.
2. To epidemiologists in the 1920s, it meant the study of epidemics among colonies of experimental animals such as rats and mice. See also ANIMAL MODEL; MECHANISTIC EPIDEMIOLOGY; OBSERVATIONAL STUDY.

EXPLANATORY STUDY, EXPLANATORY TRIAL A study (including randomized clinical trials) whose main objective is to explain, rather than merely describe, a situation by isolating the effects of specific variables and understanding the mechanisms of action.[14] Contrast with PRAGMATIC STUDY.

EXPLANATORY VARIABLE

1. A variable that causally explains the association or outcome under study.
2. In statistics, a synonym for INDEPENDENT VARIABLE.

EXPLORATORY STUDY A study whose main objective is to examine or ascertain some preliminary facts or to familiarize researchers with a problem or technology, often without clear or precise hypotheses; or, sometimes, to screen several hypotheses at once in a preliminary fashion. It may be even more preliminary than a PILOT INVESTIGATION. See also DATA DREDGING; DATA MINING; FISHING EXPEDITION.

EXPOSED In epidemiology, the exposed group (or simply, *the exposed*) is often used to connote a group whose members have been exposed to a supposed cause of a disease or health state of interest or possess a characteristic that is a determinant of the health outcome of interest.

EXPOSED CASES IMPACT NUMBER See IMPACT NUMBERS

EXPOSURE

1. The variable whose causal effect is to be estimated. Examples of exposures assessed by epidemiological studies are environmental and lifestyle factors, socioeconomic and working conditions, medical treatments, and genetic traits. Exposures may be harmful or beneficial—or even both (e.g., if an immunizable disease is circulating, exposure to immunizing agents helps most recipients but may harm those with adverse reactions to the vaccine).
2. Proximity and/or contact with a source of a disease agent in such a manner that effective transmission of the agent or harmful effects of the agent may occur.
3. The amount of a factor to which a group or individual was exposed; sometimes contrasted with dose, the amount that enters or interacts with the organism.
4. The process by which an agent comes into contact with a person or animal in such a way that the person or animal may develop the relevant outcome, such as a disease.

EXPOSURE ASSESSMENT Process of estimating concentration or intensity, duration, and frequency of exposure to an agent that can affect health.[200]

EXPOSURE CONTROL See RISK MANAGEMENT.

EXPOSURE IMPACT NUMBER See IMPACT NUMBERS.

EXPOSURE LIMIT General term defining the regulated level of exposure that should not be exceeded.[200]

EXPOSURE-ODDS RATIO See ODDS RATIO.

EXPOSURE RATIO The ratio of rates at which persons in the case and control groups of a CASE-CONTROL STUDY are exposed to the RISK FACTOR (or to the protective factor) of interest.

EXPRESSION, GENE See GENE EXPRESSION.

EXPRESSIVITY In genetics, the extent to which a gene is expressed, i.e., demonstrated in the phenotype.

EXTENDED TRIAL A study using additional data collected from the same patients after completion of a formal phase III randomized controlled trial. Analysis of such data allows researchers to collect additional information on toleration and efficacy. See also CLINICAL TRIAL.

EXTENSIVELY DRUG-RESISTANT TUBERCULOSIS (XDR) See DRUG-RESISTANT TUBERCULOSIS, EXTENSIVELY.

EXTERNAL VALIDITY See VALIDITY, STUDY.

EXTERNALITIES Social benefits and costs that are not included in the market price of an economic good. Examples include benefits to others of treating a case of infectious disease, adverse health effects of industrial air pollution not included in the price of the industrial product, and impact on national economy of natural resource depletion not included in calculation of national income.

EXTRAPOLATE, EXTRAPOLATION To predict the value of a variate outside the range of observations; the resulting prediction. See also INTERPOLATE.

EXTREMAL QUOTIENT The ratio of the rate in the geographic region with the highest rate of interventions, such as surgical procedures, to the rate in the region with the lowest rate.[201]

EXTRINSIC INCUBATION PERIOD Time required for development of a disease agent in a vector from the time of uptake of the agent to the time when the vector is infective. See also INCUBATION PERIOD; VECTOR-BORNE INFECTION.

F_1 ("F one") Term used in genetics to describe first-generation progeny of a mating.

F TEST Most commonly, a test used to test that several groups come from populations with the same variance.

FACE VALIDITY The extent to which a measurement or a measurement instrument appears reasonable on superficial inspection. See also VALIDITY and VALIDITY, MEASUREMENT.

FACTOR

1. An event, characteristic, or other definable entity that leads to a change in a health condition or other defined outcome. See also CAUSALITY; CAUSATION OF DISEASE, FACTORS IN.
2. A synonym for *(categorical) independent variable*, or, more precisely, an independent variable used to identify, with numerical codes, membership of qualitatively different groups. A causal role may be implied, as in "overcrowding is a factor in disease transmission," where overcrowding represents the highest level of the factor "crowding."

FACTOR ANALYSIS A set of statistical methods for analyzing the correlations among several variables in order to estimate the number of fundamental dimensions that underlie the observed data and to describe and measure those dimensions. Used frequently in the development of scoring systems for rating scales and questionnaires.

FACTORIAL DESIGN A method of setting up an experiment or study to ensure that all levels of each intervention or classificatory factor occur with all levels of the others.

FALSE NEGATIVE Negative test result in a person who possesses the attribute for which the test is conducted. The labeling of a diseased person as healthy when screening in the detection of disease. See also SCREENING; SENSITIVITY.

FALSE POSITIVE Positive test result in a person who does not possess the attribute for which the test is conducted. The labeling of a healthy person as diseased when screening in the detection of disease. See also SCREENING; SPECIFICITY.

FAMILIAL AGGREGATION A tendency of some diseases to cluster in families, which may be the result of a genetic mechanism, an environmental factor or process common to family members (e.g., diet), or a combination of both. ASCERTAINMENT BIAS should be seriously considered.

FAMILIAL DISEASE Disease that exhibits a tendency toward familial occurrence or aggregation. Familial occurrence of disease may be due to genetic transmission, intrafamilial transmission of infection or culture, interaction within the family, or the family's shared experience, including its exposure to common environmental factors.[23,134]

FAMILY A group of two or more persons united by blood, adoptive or marital ties, or the common-law equivalent; the family may include members who do not share the household but are united to other members by blood, adoptive or marital ties, or equivalent ties. Epidemiological studies may be concerned with family members or with those who share the same household or dwelling unit.

FAMILY, EXTENDED A group of persons comprising members of several generations united by blood, adoptive and marital ties, or equivalent ties. See also FAMILY, NUCLEAR.

FAMILY, NUCLEAR A group of persons comprising members of a single or at most two generations, usually husband-wife-children, united by blood, adoptive or marital ties, or equivalent ties.

FAMILY CONTACT DISEASE Disease that occurs among members of the family of a worker who is exposed to a toxic substance such as asbestos dust and carries this home on his or her person or clothing, causing exposure to other family members.

FAMILY OF CLASSIFICATIONS The Conference for the Tenth Revision of the International Statistical Classification of Diseases and Related Health Problems recommended adopting the concept of the family of disease and health-related classifications.[202] This "family" comprises ICD-10 (the ICD three-character core classification), its short tabulation lists, and the ICD four-character classification; lay reporting and other community-based information schemes in health; specialty-based adaptations for oncology, psychiatry, etc.; other health-related classifications (ICIDH, procedures, reasons for encounter); and the International Nomenclature of Diseases (IND).

FAMILY STUDY An epidemiological study of a family or a group of families. The term has been used to describe surveillance of family groups (e.g., for tuberculosis). In genetics, investigation of families showing an unusual characteristic in order to determine whether the characteristic clusters in certain families, and if so, why.

FARR'S LAWS OF EPIDEMICS William Farr (1807–1883), who was the first Compiler of Abstracts in the General Register Office of England and Wales, enunciated several "laws" of epidemics.[203] He observed that epidemics appear to be generated in unhealthy places, go through a regular course, and decline. In his Second Annual Report (1840), he demonstrated mathematically that the decline in mortality of a waning epidemic occurs at a uniformly accelerating rate. He constructed mathematical models to explain the natural history of epidemic diseases, often correctly and elegantly.

FATALITY RATE The death rate observed in a designated series of persons affected by a simultaneous event (e.g., victims of a disaster). A term to be avoided, because it can be confused with CASE FATALITY RATE.

F DISTRIBUTION (Syn: variance ratio distribution) The distribution of the ratio of two independent quantities each of which is distributed like a variance in normally distributed samples. So named in honor of R. A. Fisher (1890–1962), who first described this distribution.

FEASIBILITY (of a study, program, intervention) The viability, practicability, or workability of the study, program or intervention. How possible or practicable it is to carry it out. The feasibility of clinical and epidemiological research studies is strongly influenced by clinical, cultural, logistic, economic, and ethical factors. In assessing the weaknesses of a study in terms of internal and external validity and statistical precision, the feasibility of the theoretically better alternatives must be considered.

Family of disease and health-related classifications

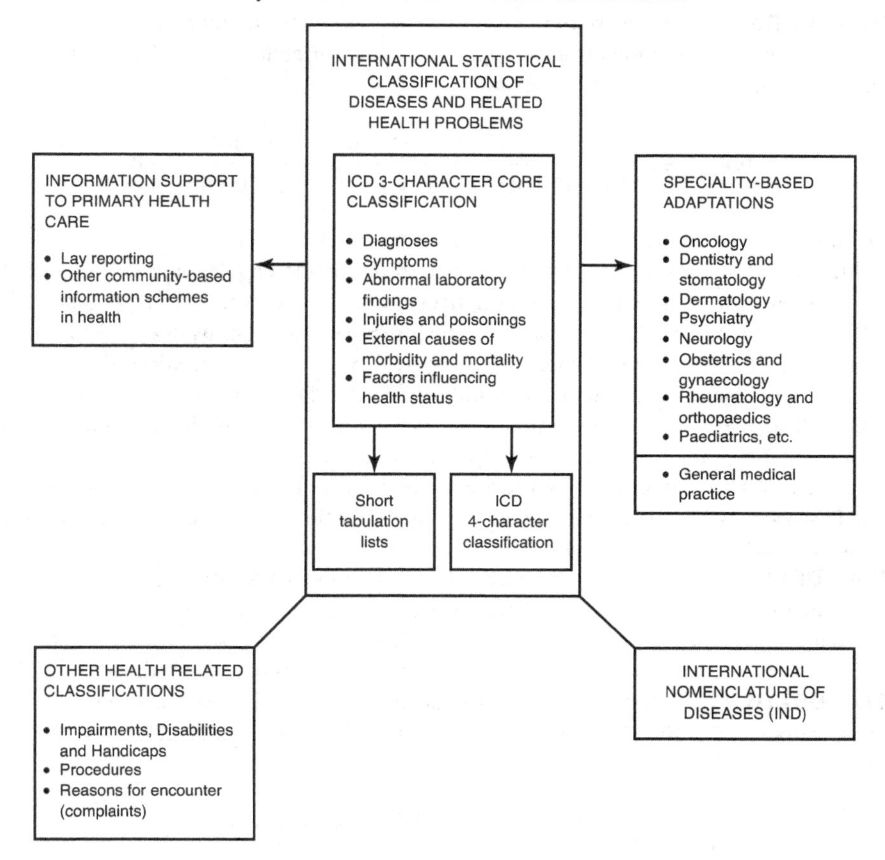

INTERNATIONAL STATISTICAL CLASSIFICATION OF DISEASES AND RELATED HEALTH PROBLEMS
INFORMATION SUPPORT TO PRIMARY HEALTH CARE
• Lay reporting
• Other community-based information schemes in health
ICD 3-CHARACTER CORE CLASSIFICATION
• Diagnoses
• Symptoms
• Abnormal laboratory findings
• Injuries and poisonings
• External causes of morbidity and mortality
• Factors influencing health status
SPECIALITY-BASED ADAPTATIONS
• Oncology
• Dentistry and stomatology
• Dermatology
• Psychiatry
• Neurology
• Obstetrics and gynaecology
• Rheumatology and orthopaedics
• Paediatrics, etc.
• General medical practice
Short tabulation lists
ICD 4-character classification
OTHER HEALTH RELATED CLASSIFICATIONS
• Impairments, Disabilities and Handicaps
• Procedures
• Reasons for encounter (complaints)
INTERNATIONAL NOMENCLATURE OF DISEASES (IND)

Family of disease and health-related classifications. The WHO family of classifications. From *International Statistical Classification of Diseases and Related Health Problems*, 10th rev. (ICD-10), vol. 1. Geneva: World Health Organization, 1991. With permission.

FEASIBILITY STUDY Preliminary study to determine the practicability of a proposed health program or procedure or of a larger study and to appraise the factors that may influence its practicability. See also PILOT INVESTIGATION, STUDY.

FECUNDITY The ability to produce live offspring. Fecundity is difficult to measure, since it refers to the theoretical ability of a woman to conceive and carry a fetus to term. If a woman produces a live birth, it is known that she and her consort were fecund during some time in the past.

FEMALE-MALE GAP A set of national, regional, or other estimates—for example, of health status or literacy—in which all the figures for females are expressed as a percentage of the corresponding figures for males, which are indexed to 100. In some countries, a useful indicator of selective female abortion and infanticide.

FERTILITY The actual production of live offspring. Stillbirths, fetal deaths, and abortions are not included in the measurement of fertility in a population. See also GRAVIDITY; PARITY.

FERTILITY RATE See GENERAL FERTILITY RATE.

FERTILITY RATIO A measure of the fertility of the population that restricts the denominator to the female population of appropriate age for childbearing. The fertility ratio is defined as

$$\text{Fertility ratio} = \frac{\text{number of girls under 15 years of age}}{\text{number of women in the 15–49 age group}} \times 1000$$

It should not be confused with GENERAL FERTILITY RATE.

FETAL DEATH (Syn: stillbirth) Death prior to the complete expulsion or extraction from its mother of a product of conception, irrespective of the duration of pregnancy. The death is indicated by the fact that, after such separation, the fetus does not breathe or show any other evidence of life, such as beating of the heart, pulsation of the umbilical cord, or definite movement of voluntary muscles. Defined variously as death after the 20th or 28th week of gestation. (The definition of the length of gestation varies between different jurisdictions, making this event difficult to compare internationally.) The WHO Conference for the Tenth Revision of the International Classification of Diseases (ICD-10) recommended that the definition of fetal death should remain unchanged. See also LIVE BIRTH.

FETAL DEATH CERTIFICATE (Syn: certificate of stillbirth) A vital record registering a fetal death, or stillbirth. Some health jurisdictions require the use of a fetal death certificate for all products of conception, whereas others require its use only in cases in which gestation has reached a particular duration, usually the 20th or the 28th week.

FETAL DEATH RATE (Syn: stillbirth rate) The number of fetal deaths in a year expressed as a proportion of the total number of births (live births plus fetal deaths) in the same year.

$$\text{Fetal death rate} = \frac{\text{number of fetal deaths in a year}}{\text{number of fetal deaths plus live births in the same year}} \times 1000$$

Note that the denominator is larger than for the FETAL DEATH RATIO and that the fetal death rate is therefore lower than the fetal death ratio, which is used in some jurisdictions. International comparisons of stillbirth or fetal death statistics will be flawed if the distinction is not appreciated.

FETAL DEATH RATIO A measure of fetal wastage, related to the number of live births. Defined as

$$\text{Fetal death ratio} = \frac{\text{number of fetal deaths in a year}}{\text{number of live births in the same year}}$$

(Can be expressed as a rate per 1000.)

FETAL ORIGINS HYPOTHESIS See DEVELOPMENTAL ORIGINS HYPOTHESIS.

FETUS Biologically, the stage of the conceptus after organ development is complete; in humans, 8 weeks after conception, 10 weeks after the last menstrual period. Vital statistical and medicolegal usage is less precise. Sometimes it means any stage of the conceptus between fertilization and expulsion; more often it means a gestational age less than 26 weeks from conception, 28 weeks from the last menstrual period. Recently it has come to mean less than 18 or 20 weeks, respectively, reflecting the current capability of perinatology to enhance survival prospects for a very immature developing conceptus.

FIELD EPIDEMIOLOGY The practice of epidemiology in the field—in the community—commonly in a public health service (i.e., a unit of government or a closely allied institution). Field epidemiology is how epidemics and outbreaks are investigated, and it is a tool for implementing measures to protect and improve the health of the public. Field epidemiologists must deal with unexpected, sometimes urgent problems that demand immediate solution. Its methods are designed to answer specific epidemiological questions in order to plan, implement, and/or evaluate public health interventions. These studies must consider the needs of those who will use the results. The task of a field epidemiologist is not complete until results of a study have been clearly communicated in a timely manner to those who need to know and an intervention has been made to improve the health of the people.[204] See also APPLIED EPIDEMIOLOGY.

FIELD SURVEY The planned collection of data in "the field," usually among noninstitutionalized persons in the GENERAL POPULATION.[27] A method of establishing a relationship between two or more variables in a population in numerical terms by eliciting and collating information from existing sources (not only records but people who can say how they feel or what happened). See also CROSS-SECTIONAL STUDY.

FIELD TRIALS Clinical trials or other types of CLINICAL STUDIES (e.g., on vaccines, drugs, bed nets, exercise programs) conducted outside the laboratory, in the general population, in primary care; often, as opposed to studies in academic, tertiary care settings. See also PRAGMATIC STUDY.

FISHER'S EXACT TEST The test for association in a two-by-two table that is based upon the exact hypergeometric distribution of the frequencies within the table.

FISHING EXPEDITION Exploratory study to find clues and leads for further study. Although the term is sometimes used pejoratively, such "expeditions" may be done for worthwhile causes (e.g., to seek clues to the cause of a major life-threatening outbreak). See also DATA DREDGING.

FITNESS This word has specific meanings in several fields related to epidemiology.

1. In population genetics, a measure of the relative survival and reproductive success of a given phenotype or population subgroup.
2. In HEALTH PROMOTION and health risk appraisal, physical fitness is a set of attributes that people have or achieve that relate to their ability to perform physical activity. Intellectual and emotional fitness can also be described and to some extent measured.

FIXED COHORT A cohort in which no additional membership is allowed—that is, it is fixed by being present at some defining event ("zero time"); an example is the cohort comprising survivors of the atomic bomb exploded at Hiroshima. See also DYNAMIC POPULATION.

FLOW CHART See FLOW DIAGRAM.

FLOW DIAGRAM (Syn: logic model, flow chart) A diagram comprising blocks connected by arrows representing steps in a process. An ALGORITHM used in decision analysis. Flow diagrams have many uses (e.g., to show eligibility, recruitment, and losses in design and execution of a study or to show how a program is intended to work).

FOCUS GROUP A small convenience sample of people brought together to discuss a topic or issue with the aim of ascertaining the range and intensity of their views rather than arriving at a consensus. This sociological method is used by epidemiologists to, for example, appraise perceptions of health problems, assess acceptability of a field study, or refine the questions to be used in a field study. The distinction between a focus group and a DELPHI survey is that the latter does aim to reach a consensus, is more formal, is usually made up of experts, generally functions by mail or telephone, and the identities of members preferably are unknown to one another. In a focus group, persons meet face to face, although it is possible for their identities to remain unknown to one another.

FOCUS OF INFECTION A defined and circumscribed locality containing the epidemiological factors needed for transmission: a human community, a source of infection, a vector population, and appropriate environmental conditions.

FOLLOW-UP Observation over a period of time of an individual, group, or an initially defined population whose appropriate characteristics have been assessed in order to observe changes in health status or health-related variables. See also ATTRITION BIAS; COHORT.

FOLLOW-UP STUDY

1. A study in which individuals or populations—selected on the basis of whether they have been exposed to risk, received a specified preventive or therapeutic procedure, or possess a certain characteristic—are followed to assess the outcome of exposure, the procedure, or effect of the characteristic (e.g., occurrence of disease).
2. Synonym for COHORT STUDY.

FOMITES (singular, fomes) Articles that convey infection to others because they have been contaminated by pathogenic organisms. Examples include a handkerchief, drinking glass, door handle, clothing, and toys.

FORCE OF MORBIDITY (Syn: hazard rate, instantaneous incidence rate, person-time incidence rate) A theoretical measure of the number of new cases that occur per unit of population-time (e.g., person-years at risk). This is a measure of the occurrence of disease at a point in time, t, defined mathematically as the limit, as Δt approaches zero, of

$$\frac{\text{Probability that a person well at time } t \text{ will develop the disease in the interval } t + \Delta t}{\Delta t}$$

The average value of this quantity over the interval t to $(t + \Delta t)$ can be estimated as

$$\frac{\text{Incident cases observed from } t \text{ to } (t + \Delta t)}{\text{Number of person-time units of experience observed from } t \text{ to } (t + \Delta t)}$$

FORCE OF MORTALITY [Syn: actuarial (death) rate] The hazard rate of the occurrence of death at a point in time t—the limit as Δt approaches zero—of the probability that an individual alive at time t will die by time $t + \Delta t$, divided by Δt. Distinct from cumulative death rate.

FORECASTING A method of estimating what may happen in the future that relies on extrapolation of existing trends (demographic, epidemiological, etc.). It may be less useful than SCENARIO BUILDING, which has greater flexibility. For example, extrapolation of mortality trends for coronary heart disease in the early 1960s in the United States suggested that the mortality rates would continue to rise, whereas in fact the rates began to fall soon after that time.

FORENSIC EPIDEMIOLOGY The use of epidemiological reasoning, knowledge, and methods in the investigation of public health problems that may have been caused by or associated with intentional and/or criminal acts.[205] As mentioned above, EPIDEMIOLOGY is applied in many populations, professional specialties, and health care settings; hence this dictionary includes just some examples of definitions for a few specialty-based branches of epidemiology.

FOREST PLOT A plot that summarizes results of studies included in a META-ANALYSIS. The name was introduced at a time when the graph had vertical lines representing the studies.

FORTUITOUS RELATIONSHIP See ASSOCIATION, FORTUITOUS.

FORWARD SURVIVAL ESTIMATE A procedure for estimating the age distribution at some later date by projecting forward an observed age distribution. The procedure uses survival ratios, often obtained from model life tables.

FOURFOLD TABLE See CONTINGENCY TABLE.

"FOURTH WORLD" The environmental and socioeconomic situation of decayed urban neighborhoods in affluent nations, resembling the conditions encountered in the poorest developing countries. It includes homeless people, who are among an underclass (often disenfranchised) found in urban communities in rich countries. This term should not be used without explanation in scientific writing.

FRACTALS Mathematical patterns in which smaller parts have the same shape as larger parts, indefinitely down to ever finer levels of magnification. Blood vessels and the bronchial tree behave according to fractal theory. An application of fractals occurs in studies of the way human and other populations grow and spread. The same rules may apply to the spread of some infections and neoplasms.

FRAGILE DATA Data derived from a well-designed study that do not quite reach a level of statistical significance but arrive at unexpected and/or important conclusions. Alternatively, data that reach or imply important conclusions from a poorly designed study. Hence an ambiguous and potentially misleading term.

FRAMINGHAM STUDY Probably the best-known cohort study of heart disease. Since 1949, samples of residents of Framingham, Massachusetts, have been subjects of investigations of risk factors in relation to the occurrence of heart disease and later, other outcomes.

FREQUENCY See OCCURRENCE.

FREQUENCY DISTRIBUTION See DISTRIBUTION.

FREQUENCY MATCHING See MATCHING.

FREQUENCY POLYGON A graphic illustration of a distribution, made by joining a set of points, for each of which the abscissa is the midpoint of the class and the ordinate, or height, is the frequency.

FUNCTION A quality, trait, or fact that is so related to another as to be dependent upon and to vary with this other.

FUNDING BIAS Bias in characterizing an association (usually between an exposure and a set of outcomes) owing to the absence or withdrawal of financial and other types of support. Lack of support obstructs or discourages the conduct of research. It may lead to PUBLICATION BIAS. See also CONFLICT OF INTEREST.

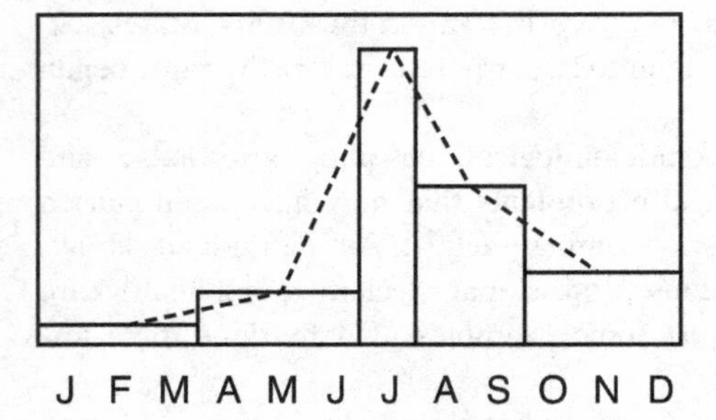

Frequency polygon. Numbers of notified cases in specified months. From Abramson JH. *Making Sense of Data*, 2nd ed. 1994 .

FUNNEL PLOT A plotting device used in META-ANALYSIS to detect PUBLICATION BIAS. The estimate of risk is plotted against sample size. If there is no publication bias, the plot is funnel-shaped; but if studies showing positive results are more likely to be published than NULL STUDIES, there is a "hole in the lower left corner" of the funnel.[106, 206]

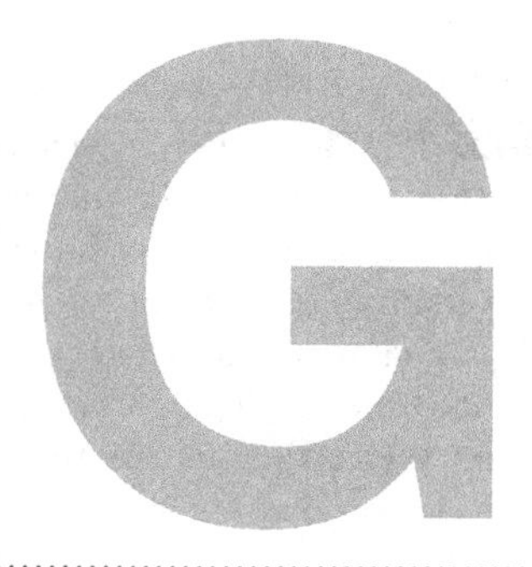

GAMBLER'S FALLACY (Syn: Monte-Carlo fallacy) The notion that the probability of an event occurring increases with the length of time since the event previously occurred when no such relation exists (e.g., as with properly randomized games of chance).

GAME THEORY A branch of mathematical logic concerned with the range of possible reactions to a particular strategy; each reaction can be assigned a probability, and each reaction can lead to further action by the "adversary" in the game. Used in systems analysis. It has occasional applications in disease surveillance and control. It is one of the underlying theories used in CLINICAL DECISION ANALYSIS and in determining utilities (e.g., in calculating QALYs).

GAMETE A mature sex cell: the ovum of the female or the spermatozoon of the male. Gametes are haploid, containing half the normal number of chromosomes of a somatic cell, and fusing with its counterpart at fertilization to produce a zygote, which has the normal number of diploid chromosomes and develops into an embryo.

GAMETOCYTE

1. A cell that is in the process of developing into a GAMETE by undergoing gametogenesis.
2. The sexual stage of malaria parasites. Male gametocytes (microgametocytes) and female gametocytes (macrogametocytes) are inside red blood cells in the bloodstream. If they are ingested by a female *Anopheles* mosquito, they undergo sexual reproduction, which starts the extrinsic (sporogonic) cycle of the parasite in the mosquito.

GATEKEEPER A person or system that selectively regulates or controls access to a HEALTH CARE service.

GAUSSIAN DISTRIBUTION See NORMAL DISTRIBUTION.

GCP (GOOD CLINICAL PRACTICE) An international set of ethical and scientific quality standards for designing, conducting, recording, and reporting trials that involve participation of human subjects. It originates from the International Conference for Harmonization (ICH) (www.ich.org) and derives from the Helsinki Declaration of the World Medical Association on Ethical Principles for Medical Research Involving Human Subjects (www.wma.net/e/policy/b3.htm). The GCP standards are implemented, among others, by the European Medicines Agency (www.emea.europa.eu/Inspections/GCP-general.html), and the U.S. Food and Drug Administration (FDA) (www.fda.gov/oc/gcp/default.htm).

GDP Gross domestic product.

G-ESTIMATION A method to estimate the parameters of structural nested models (SNMs). The method requires the assumption of no unmeasured confounding, or the slightly weaker assumption of known magnitude of the unmeasured confounding. The general version of G-estimation was proposed by Robins.[393,394] The standard instrumental variable estimator is a particular case of g-estimator. A method for estimation of the causal effect of a time-varying treatment in the presence of time-varying confounders. Other methods for such estimation are the parametric G-computation algorithm formula estimator, the iterative conditional expectations (ICE) estimator, and inverse-probability-of-treatment weighted (IPTW) estimation of MARGINAL STRUCTURAL MODELS (MSMs). When MSMs cannot be used, G-estimation of structural nested models (SNMs) can be used instead (e.g., to estimate the effect of an exposure on mortality in occupational cohort studies). Logistic SNMs cannot be fit by G-estimation. An advantage of using MSMs over G-estimation to control for time-dependent confounding is their resemblance to standard modeling techniques. See also INVERSE PROBABILITY WEIGHTING.

GENDER

1. In grammar, the term to designate a noun (person, animal, or object) as masculine, feminine, or neuter.
2. The totality of culturally constructed awareness, attitudes, beliefs, and behaviors about males and females and sometimes their sexual orientation. A social construct regarding culture-bound conventions, roles, and behaviors for, as well as relationships between and among, women and men and boys and girls.[128,137]

GENE A sequence of DNA that codes for a particular protein product or that regulates other genes. A DNA segment that is transcribed into messenger RNA and translated into a protein. Traditionally, genes have been deemed to comprise the exons that are actually translated plus the intervening introns.[23] Today, the nature of genes is in the midst of a profound reanalysis by genetics and other branches of science. They are no longer what they used to be in number and in essence.[43,134,207–209]

GENE EXPRESSION The amount and timing of appearance of the functional product of a gene. The process by which the DNA sequence of a gene is converted into functional proteins. Non–proteincoding genes (e.g., rRNA genes, tRNA genes) are not translated into protein. Gene expression is a multistep process that begins with the transcription of DNA (of which genes are made) into messenger RNA. It is then followed by posttranscriptional modification and translation into a gene product, followed by folding, posttranslational modification, and targeting. The amount of protein that a cell expresses depends on the tissue, the developmental stage of the organism, and the physiologic state of the cell. The expression of many genes is known to be regulated after transcription; thus, an increase in the concentration of mRNA may not increase expression. See also EPIGENETICS.

GENE POOL The total of all genes possessed by reproductive members of a population.

GENERAL FERTILITY RATE A more refined measure of fertility than the crude birthrate. The denominator is restricted to the number of women of childbearing age (i.e., 15–44 or 15–49. Defined as

$$\text{General fertility rate} = \frac{\text{number of live births in an area during a year}}{\text{midyear female population age 15–44 in same area in same year}} \times 1000$$

The upper age limit for this rate is 44—sometimes 49—years in most jurisdictions.

GENERALIZABILITY The degree to which results of a study may apply, be relevant, or be generalized to populations or groups that did not participate in the study. In etiological research, such inferences to an external population are not merely statistical in nature but must be based on theory, judgment, and evidence external to the study (e.g., on available knowledge on biological, clinical, or social mechanisms linking a given exposure to the risk of developing the disease). See VALIDITY, STUDY.

GENERAL POPULATION All members of a human population, defined essentially on the basis of geographical location, as in a country, region, city, etc. All inhabitants of some given area. Everyone in the POPULATION being studied, irrespective of race, ethnicity, or professional status.[188] Individuals admitted to hospitals, other health care facilities, and prisons are usually excluded from the concept (i.e., considered not to be part of the general population). The term is often used to underline the different results that studies tend to obtain in the general population and in specific populations, subgroups, or settings (e.g., in the professionally active or working population, the hospitalized population).

GENERATION EFFECT (Syn: cohort effect) Variation in health status that arises from the different causal factors to which each BIRTH COHORT in the population is exposed as the environment and society change. Each consecutive birth cohort is exposed to a unique environment that coincides with its life span.

GENERATION TIME The interval between receipt of infection by the host and the latter's maximal infectivity. This applies to both clinical cases and inapparent infections. With person-to-person transmission of infection, the interval between cases is determined by the generation time. See SERIAL INTERVAL. See also INCUBATION PERIOD.

GENE SILENCING One of several EPIGENETIC processes that regulate GENE EXPRESSION. A term commonly used to describe that instead of being expressed ("turned on"), a gene is "switched off" by an epigenetic mechanism. Transcriptional gene silencing is the result of histone modifications, creating an environment of heterochromatin around a gene that makes it inaccessible to transcriptional machinery (RNA polymerase, transcription factors). Posttranscriptional gene silencing results when the mRNA of a particular gene has been destroyed, thus preventing its translation to form an active gene product (e.g., a protein). See also EPIGENETIC INHERITANCE.

GENETIC DIVERSITY The variety of different types of genes in a species or population. A form of BIODIVERSITY.

GENETIC DRIFT Random variation in gene frequency from generation to generation, most often observed in small populations. The process of evolution through random statistical fluctuation of genetic composition of populations.

GENETIC ENGINEERING Manipulation of the genome of a living organism.

GENETIC EPIDEMIOLOGY The specialty that deals with the etiology, distribution, and control of disease in groups of people (e.g., relatives), and with genetic and epigenetic inheritance of disease in populations. The study of the role of genetic factors and their interaction with environmental factors in the occurrence of disease in human populations.[23,134,210–212] In recent years it has experienced a certain convergence with MOLECULAR EPIDEMIOLOGY.

GENETIC LINKAGE The phenomenon whereby phenotypes and alleles at one or more marker alleles tend to be inherited together. Particular genes occupy specific sites in chromosomes, one member of each pair of chromosomes coming from each parent.

When two genes are fairly close to each other in the same chromosome pair, they tend to be inherited together. Such genes are said to be linked, and the phenomenon is called genetic linkage. See also LINKAGE DISEQUILIBRIUM.

GENETIC PENETRANCE The penetrance of a genetic variant is the frequency with which the characteristic that the variant controls (the phenotype) is seen in people who carry the variant. The extent to which a genetically determined condition is expressed in an individual. The proportion of individuals with a given GENOTYPE that show the PHENOTYPE under specific environmental conditions. When all individuals carrying a dominant mutation show the mutant phenotype, the gene is said to show complete penetrance. The relation between the frequency of a variant and its penetrance is often inverse: the more penetrant (e.g., deleterious) a variant, the less frequent it is in the population. Only highly penetrant mutations may act with no INTERACTION with external factors. Gene-environment interactions are intrinsic to the mode of action of low-penetrant genes. Current knowledge suggests that low-penetrant genetic traits cause a smaller fraction of the BURDEN OF DISEASE than certain environmental agents (e.g., smoking, air pollution, chemical carcinogens).[213–215] See also EPIGENETICS; MONOGENIC DISEASES; POLYGENIC DISEASES.

GENETIC POLYMORPHISM See POLYMORPHISM, GENETIC.

GENETICS The branch of biology dealing with genetic heredity and variation of individual members of a species. Its branches include population genetics, which partly overlaps with genetic and molecular epidemiology; therefore pertinent genetic terms are part of this dictionary.

GENETIC SCREENING The use of genetic, clinical and epidemiological knowledge, reasoning, and techniques to detect genetic variants that have been demonstrated to place an individual at increased risk of a given disease. Ethical problems may arise in genetic screening (e.g., regarding the provision of information to persons of their putative increased risk when there is no effective treatment, and potential loss of eligibility for employment and insurance benefits).[134, 213] See also NUMBER NEEDED TO SCREEN (NNS).

GENETIZATION The process by which issues traditionally considered to be medical but not necessarily genetic become defined as problems with a strong or a single genetic component or as having a genetic cause and, sometimes, also a genetic treatment. The expansion of genetics into the life and health sciences and professions (e.g., the genetization of prenatal medicine, oncology, primary care). More generally, the attribution of physiological, pathological, behavioral, or social conditions and problems to genetic causes, often at the expense of clinical, environmental, cultural, economic, or social explanations. The expansion of genetics into the domains of everyday existence. In genetization processes *genetic* is often considered to be synonymous with *inherited*, and vice versa, thus neglecting somatic (acquired) genetic alterations and cultural inheritance.[108, 142–144, 207, 216, 217] See also INTEGRATION; MEDICALIZATION; REDUCTIONISM.

GENOME The array of genes carried by an individual. The total genetic material of an organism. The whole set of the DNA of a species. See also EPIGENOME.

GENOTOXIC A substance, setting or process that is toxic or harmful to the genetic material. An agent or process that interacts with cellular DNA, either directly or after metabolic biotransformation, resulting in alteration of DNA structure. DNA-adduct formation is one type of genotoxicity.[218] See also CARCINOGEN.

GENOTOXIC CARCINOGENS Chemical carcinogens capable of causing damage to DNA. They can be MUTAGENIC, CLASTOGENIC, or ANEUGENIC. Inside the cell, carcinogens or their metabolic products can either directly or indirectly affect the regulation and expression of genes involved in cell-cycle control, DNA repair, cell differentiation, or apoptosis. Some carcinogens act by genotoxic mechanisms, such as forming DNA adducts or inducing chromosome breakage, fusion, deletion, missegregation and nondisjunction; for example, carcinogenic ions or compounds of nickel, arsenic, and cadmium can induce structural and numerical chromosomal aberrations. DNA binding and induction of mutations in cancer-related genes, such as *TP53* and K-*ras*, are important genotoxic mechanisms of tumor initiation. Also important in causing diseases of complex etiology, such as cancer, is the accompanying ability of many compounds to promote the outgrowth of transformed cell clones through NONGENOTOXIC mechanisms.[219]

GENOTYPE The genetic constitution inherited by an organism or a person, as distinct from the physical characteristics and appearance that emerge with development (i.e., the PHENOTYPE). The genetic constitution of an organism; modulated by the environment, it is then expressed as a phenotype.

GEOGRAPHICAL INFORMATION SYSTEM (GIS) An information system that incorporates digitally constructed maps and uses sophisticated modeling techniques to analyze and display information patterns. Satellite imaging and remote sensing have greatly expanded the scope of GISs (e.g., trends in specific diseases are suggested after analyzing the composition of vegetation and the amounts of precipitation in tropical regions, which relate to changes in the distribution and abundance of predators and insect vectors). Another application is digitally prepared spot maps of disease clusters using postal codes and notified cases.[220] An important application is in GEOMATICS.

GEOGRAPHICAL PATHOLOGY (Syn: medical geography) The comparative study of countries or of regions within them with regard to variations in morbidity/mortality. The (implied) aim of such study is usually to demonstrate that the variations are caused by or related to differences in the geographical environment.

GEOMATICS The collection, processing, storage, and analysis of geographical information. An important application is sequentially generated computer maps to show regional and temporal trends and variations in various sectors of society, including the health sector. Its uses include the assessment of time trends in the geographical distribution of diseases such as malaria.

GEOMETRIC MEAN See MEAN, GEOMETRIC.

GESTATIONAL AGE Strictly speaking, the gestational age of a fetus is the elapsed time since conception. However, as the moment when conception occurred is rarely known precisely, the duration of gestation is measured from the first day of the last normal menstrual period. Gestational age is expressed in completed days or completed weeks (e.g., events occurring 280–286 days after the onset of the last normal menstrual period are considered to have occurred at 40 weeks of gestation).

Measurements of fetal growth, as they represent continuous variables, are expressed in relation to a specific week of gestational age (e.g., the mean birth weight for 40 weeks is that obtained at 280–286 days of gestation on a weight-for-gestational-age curve). Some specified variations of gestational age are *preterm*, less than 37 completed weeks (less than 259 days); *term*, from 37 to less than 42 completed weeks (259–293 days); *postterm*, 42 completed weeks or more (294 days or more).

GESTATION LENGTH An ambiguous term for the duration of pregnancy because it can be calculated in different ways:

1. Biologically, as used by embryologists and teratologists, the time from fertilization (conception) to expulsion of the fetus; in humans the mean is 266 days (38 weeks).
2. In obstetrics and often in epidemiology, gestation is dated from the last menstrual period, on average 2 weeks earlier than the time of fertilization, i.e., mean 280 days (40 weeks).

GINI COEFFICIENT A measure of dispersion in a set of values. Devised by Corrado Gini (1884–1965), Italian demographer and economist. A common measure of income inequality derived from the Lorenz curve; the curve shows the percentage of total income earned by the cumulative percentage of the population. In a "perfectly equal society," the poorest 15% of the population would earn 15% of the total income, the poorest 65% of the population would earn 65% of the total income, and the Lorenz curve would equal the 45-degree "theoretical line of perfect equality." As inequality increases in a community, the Lorenz curve deviates from the line of equality. The Gini coefficient is the size of the area between the line of equality and the Lorenz curve (area A in the figure) divided by the total area under the line of equality (A+B). Thus, the more the Lorenz curve departs from the theoretical line, the higher the Gini coefficient is. The coefficient can take a value between 0 and 1: a 0 would be obtained in a society where all income was equally shared, and a 1 (or 100%) in a totally unequal society. Assumptions and properties of the Lorenz curve and the Gini coefficient must be assessed before comparing values across different groups.[221]

GLOBAL BURDEN OF DISEASE See BURDEN OF DISEASE.

GLOVER PHENOMENON An old term referring to the wide variation in rates at which many common medical procedures are conducted in seemingly comparable communities with similar morbidity rates—a phenomenon analyzed by J.A. Glover[221] and many others.

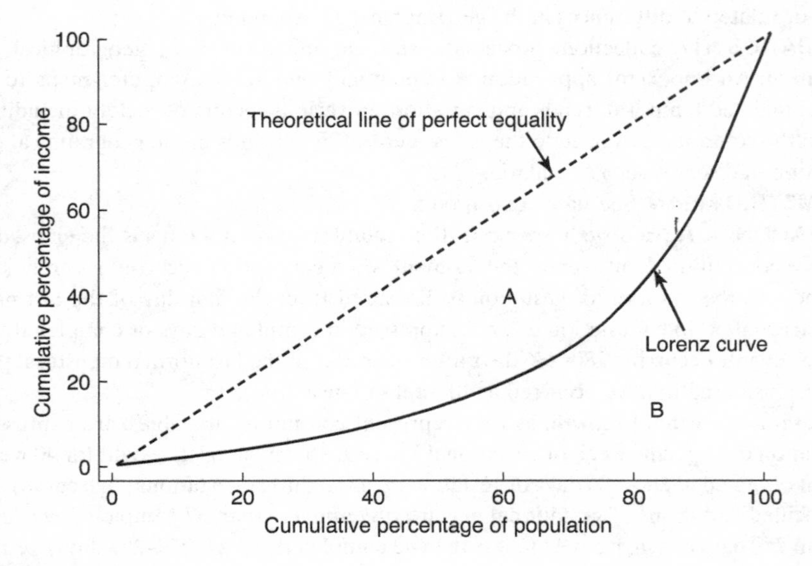

Gini coefficient.

GOAL A desired state to be achieved within a specified time. See also TARGET.

"GOLD STANDARD" A method, procedure, or measurement that is widely accepted as being the best available. Often used to compare with new methods of unknown effectiveness (e.g., a potential new diagnostic test is assessed against the best available diagnostic test).

GOMPERTZ-MAKEHAM FORMULA A formula describing the relationship of mortality rate to age. There is an age-independent component and a component that increases exponentially with age. Benjamin Gompertz, a nineteenth-century demographer, first identified the proportionate relationship of mortality to age. This was refined by W. M. Makeham in 1867 to provide a better model of the age-specific pattern of the instantaneous death rate. If q_x is the probability of dying at age x and A, B, and C are constants, $q_x = A + BC^x$. For ages beyond childhood, the Gompertz-Makeham formula closely fits observed patterns.

GONADOTROPHIC CYCLE One complete round of ovarian development in the mosquito (or other insect vector) from the time when the blood meal is taken to the time when the fully developed eggs are laid.

GOBI/FFF Growth monitoring, oral rehydration, breast-feeding, immunization/family planning, food production, female education (WHO/UNICEF/World Bank).

GOODNESS OF FIT Degree of agreement between an empirically observed distribution and a mathematical or theoretical distribution.

GOODNESS-OF-FIT TEST A statistical test of the hypothesis that data have been randomly sampled or generated from a population that follows a particular theoretical distribution or model. Perhaps the most common such tests are chi-square tests.

GPA Global Programme on AIDS (WHO); superseded by UNAIDS.

GPHIN Global Public Health Intelligence Network of the World Health Organization. See also EPIDEMIOLOGICAL INTELLIGENCE.

GRAB SAMPLE See SAMPLE.

GRADIENT OF INFECTION The variety of host responses to infection ranging from inapparent infection to fatal illness.

GRAPH A general term for visual display of the relationship between variables; for example, the values of one set of variables are plotted along the horizontal, or *x*, axis, of a second variable, along the vertical, or *y*, axis. Three-dimensional graphs of relationships between three variables can be represented and comprehended visually in two dimensions. The relationship between *x* and *y* may be linear, exponential, logarithmic, etc. See also AXIS; ABSCISSA, ORDINATE. "Graph" is also a descriptive term for histograms, bar charts, etc.

GRAVIDITY The number of pregnancies (completed or incomplete) experienced by a woman. See also PARITY.

"GRAY LITERATURE" (Syn: fugitive literature) Technical reports, studies, and essays that are not specifically aimed for conventional publication, have restricted distribution, and are hence seldom included in the bibliographic retrieval systems commonly available to scholars, officers, and the public. They may be commissioned, sponsored, or owned by companies, academic units, financial institutions, or government agencies, including local or regional health departments. This literature used to include many unpublished masters' or doctoral dissertations, but these and many other papers are nowadays enjoying wider access in digital formats. Scientific articles published in journals using languages other than English do not per se have the features mentioned above (e.g., they have wide circulations among scholars and health professionals).

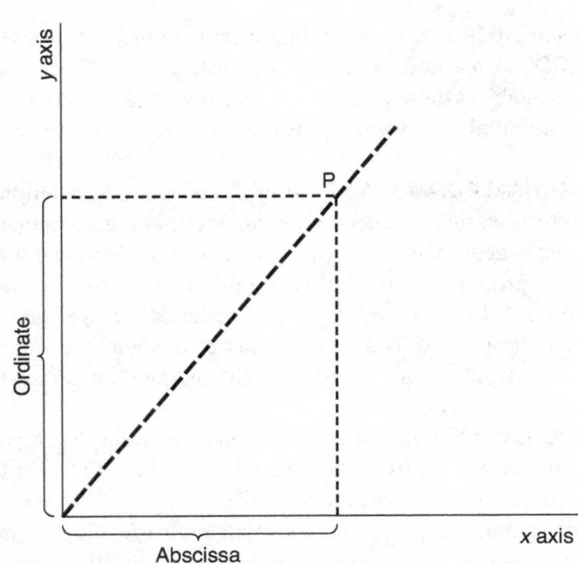

Graph showing abscissa, ordinate, and locus of a point, P, in relation to x and y axis.

Gray literature, including epidemiological studies, may not be peer reviewed. Nonetheless, such literature may contain highly valid and relevant scientific findings, including information useful in META-ANALYSIS and in PUBLIC HEALTH IMPACT ASSESSMENT.

GROSS REPRODUCTION RATE (Syn: raw coefficient of reproduction) The average number of female children a woman would have if she survived to the end of her childbearing years and if, throughout that period, she were subject to a given set of age-specific fertility rates and a given sex ratio at birth. It provides a measure of REPLACEMENT-LEVEL FERTILITY (or of the *replacement of the generations*) in the absence of mortality. In a hypothetical generation, it is equal to the number of girls born to a woman until the end of the reproduction period at a given (current year) age-specific fertility. See also NET REPRODUCTION RATE.

GROUP COMPARISONS Comparisons that consist in contrasting what is observed in a group of people in the presence of exposure to what would have occurred had the group of interest not been exposed to the postulated cause. Differences in frequency of disease occurrence between groups can logically be interpreted as being caused by the exposure. This is the main mode of knowledge acquisition in epidemiology.[10] See also POPULATION THINKING.

GROWTH RATE OF POPULATION A measure of population growth (in the absence of migration) comprising addition of newborns to the population and subtraction of deaths. The result, known as *natural rate of increase*, is calculated as

$$\frac{\text{Live births during the year — deaths during the year}}{\text{Midyear population}} \times 1000$$

Alternatively, it is the difference between crude birthrate and crude death rate.

GUIDELINES A formal statement about a defined task or function. Examples include clinical practice guidelines, guidelines for application of preventive screening procedures, and guidelines for ethical conduct of epidemiological practice and research.[184–187,222] Contrast CODE OF CONDUCT, in which the rules are intended to be strictly adhered to and may include penalties for violation. In the terminology developed by the European Community, *directives* are stronger than *recommendations*, which are stronger than *guidelines*. In North America, *guidelines* is normal usage also for recommendations.

GUTTMAN SCALE A measurement scale that ranks response categories to a question, with each unit representing an increasingly strong expression of an attribute, such as pain or disability, or an attitude.

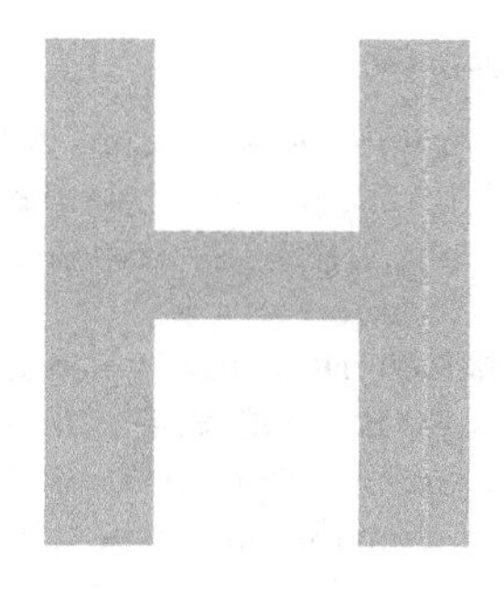

HACKETT SPLEEN CLASSIFICATION A numerical means of recording the size of an enlarged spleen, especially in malaria. This is a six-point scale of 0 (no enlargement) to 5 (enlarged to umbilicus or larger).

HALF-LIFE Time in which the concentration of a substance (especially if radioactive) is reduced by 50%.

HALO EFFECT

1. The influence upon an observation of the observer's perception of the characteristics of the individual observed (other than the characteristic under study). The influence of the observer's recollection or knowledge of findings on a previous occasion.
2. The effect (usually beneficial) that the manner, attention, and caring of a provider have on a patient during a medical encounter regardless of what medical procedures or services the encounter involves. See also PLACEBO EFFECT.

HANDICAP Reduction in a person's capacity to fulfill a social role as a consequence of an IMPAIRMENT or disability, inadequate training for the role, or other circumstances. Applied to children, the term usually refers to the presence of an impairment or other circumstance that is likely to interfere with normal growth and development or with the capacity to learn. See also INTERNATIONAL CLASSIFICATION OF IMPAIRMENTS, DISABILITIES, AND HANDICAPS for the official WHO definition.

HANDICAP-FREE LIFE EXPECTANCY The average number of years an individual is expected to live free of handicap if current patterns of mortality and handicap continue to apply.[123] See also DISABILITY-FREE LIFE EXPECTANCY; HEALTH EXPECTANCY.

HAPHAZARD SAMPLE Selection of a group for study without thought as to whether they are representative of the population. The word *haphazard* here implies selection based on a mixture of criteria such as convenience, accessibility, turning up at the time an investigation or study is in progress, belonging to some existing list or registry, etc. Because they have an unknown chance of being unrepresentative of the population, haphazard samples are unsatisfactory for generalization.

HARDY-WEINBERG EQUILIBRIUM State in which the allele and genotype frequencies do not change from one generation to the next in a population.[23,210] Although conditions for Hardy-Weinberg equilibrium are seldom strictly met, genotype frequencies are often consistent with the Hardy-Weinberg law. Several software packages exist to test whether a set of genotypic frequencies are in Hardy-Weinberg equilibrium.

HARDY-WEINBERG LAW The principle that both gene and genotype frequencies will remain in equilibrium in an infinitely large population in the absence of mutation, migration, selection, and nonrandom mating. If p is the frequency of one allele and q is the frequency of another and $p + q = 1$, then p^2 is the frequency of homozygotes for the allele, q^2 is the frequency of homozygotes for the other allele, and $2\,pq$ is the frequency of heterozygotes.

HARMONIC MEAN See MEAN, HARMONIC.

HAWTHORNE EFFECT The effect (usually positive or beneficial) of being under study upon the persons being studied; their knowledge of the study often influences their behavior. The name derives from work studies by Whitehead, Dickson, Roethlisberger, and others, in the Western Electric Plant, Hawthorne, Illinois, reported by Elton Mayo in *The Social Problems of an Industrial Civilization* (London: Routledge, 1949).

HAZARD

1. Inherent capability of an agent or a situation to have an adverse effect. A factor or exposure that may adversely affect health. Loosely, in lay speech a synonym for RISK; in epidemiology, a similar concept to RISK FACTOR.
2. (Syn: force of morbidity, instantaneous incidence rate) A theoretical measure of the probability of occurrence of an event per unit time at risk; e.g., death or new disease, at a point in time, t, defined mathematically as the limit, as Δt approaches zero, of the probability that an individual well at time t will experience the event by $t + \Delta t$, divided by Δt.

HAZARD IDENTIFICATION See RISK ASSESSMENT.

HEALTH

1. The World Health Organization (WHO) described it in 1948, in the preamble to its constitution, as: "A state of complete physical, mental, and social well-being and not merely the absence of disease or infirmity."
2. In 1984, a WHO health promotion initiative led to expansion of the original WHO description, which can be abbreviated to: "The extent to which an individual or a group is able to realize aspirations and satisfy needs, and to change or cope with the environment. Health is a resource for everyday life, not the objective of living; it is a positive concept, emphasizing social and personal resources as well as physical capabilities."[223]
3. A state characterized by anatomical, physiological, and psychological integrity; ability to perform personally valued family, work, and community roles; ability to deal with physical, biological, psychological, and social stress; a feeling of well-being; and freedom from the risk of disease and untimely death.[224]
4. A state of equilibrium between humans and the physical, biological, and social environment compatible with full functional activity.[225] A sustainable state in which humans and other living creatures with which they interact can coexist indefinitely in equilibrium. *Health* is derived from the Old English *hal*, meaning whole, sound in wind and limb. See also SUSTAINABILITY.

HEALTH-ADJUSTED LIFE EXPECTANCY Life expectancy expressed in quality-adjusted life years. See HEALTH EXPECTANCY.

HEALTH BEHAVIOR The combination of knowledge, practices, and attitudes that together contribute to motivate the actions we take regarding health. Health behavior may promote and preserve good health or, if the behavior is harmful (e.g., tobacco smoking), may be a determinant of disease. This combination of knowledge, practices, and attitudes has been described and discussed by several writers.[226] See also DISEASE; ILLNESS BEHAVIOR; SICKNESS "CAREER."

HEALTH CARE Services provided to individuals or communities by agents of the health services or professions to promote, maintain, monitor, or restore health. Health care is not limited to medical care, which implies action by or under the supervision of a physician. The term is sometimes extended to include health-related self-care.

HEALTHCARE EPIDEMIOLOGY See HOSPITAL EPIDEMIOLOGY.

HEALTH DETERMINANT See DETERMINANT.

HEALTH DEVELOPMENT A collective effort to improve health and well-being in all individuals and communities of a society, taking into account prevailing political, cultural, social, and economic features.

HEALTH EDUCATION Learning resources and teaching programs concerned with health—its protection and promotion. It often begins in the family and continues through primary and secondary education, with emphasis on exercise, diet, care of teeth, avoidance of sexually transmitted disease, sexuality, social relationships, smoking, alcohol, and other drugs, accidents, violence, etc. Health education may be provided by school teachers and nurses as well as by specially trained educators or physicians. It is also conducted in the community and with subsets of the population, including pregnant women, workers, people about to retire, or the elderly. See also ACQUAINTANCE NETWORK; CONTEXT; PREVENTION.

HEALTH EQUITY Fairnes and impartiality in any health-related determinant (e.g., exposure, policy) or outcome. Equity in epidemiologic risk management aims to ensure that communities near sites hazardous to health (e.g., polluting industrial facilities) are not more exposed to such environmental health risks than are more affluent communities removed from the source of pollution. Achieving equity of access to health care services regardless of social, ethnic, and cultural status has become a high-priority health policy issue in many countries.[85–87,137,138,221]

HEALTH EXPECTANCY A general term for several health indicators in which life expectancy is weighted for health status. The term refers to the average amount of time (years, months, weeks, days) a person is expected to live in a given health state if current patterns of mortality and health states continue to apply; the patterns are derived from epidemiological and vital statistics data. Health expectancy is therefore a statistical abstraction, based on existing age-specific death rates and age-specific prevalences for health states or on age-specific transition rates between health states.[227] Specific health expectancies are based on health states defined by the International Classification of Impairments, Disabilities and Handicaps (ICIDH) concepts of impairment, disability, and handicap. Examples include DISABILITY-FREE LIFE EXPECTANCY and HANDICAP-FREE LIFE EXPECTANCY. *Health expectancy* – also called *life expectancy in good health* or *healthy life expectancy* and *disability-free life expectancy* – considers only the time spent in good health. *Health-adjusted life expectancy* and *disability-adjusted life expectancy* assign values to ranges of health states.

HEALTH FOR ALL The cultural, social, and political objective of health policy, enshrined in the WHO Alma-Ata Declaration (1978). It was interpreted as a goal to be achieved by the year 2000, as a slogan, and as an aspiration that might be realized by implementing primary health care for all citizens of a country.

HEALTH GAP General term for a group of health indicators in which lost life expectancy is weighted by health status. They may be distinguished on the basis of a specified or implied health target or norm for a population, definition and weighting of health states, and inclusion or exclusion of values other than health. Unlike health expectancies,

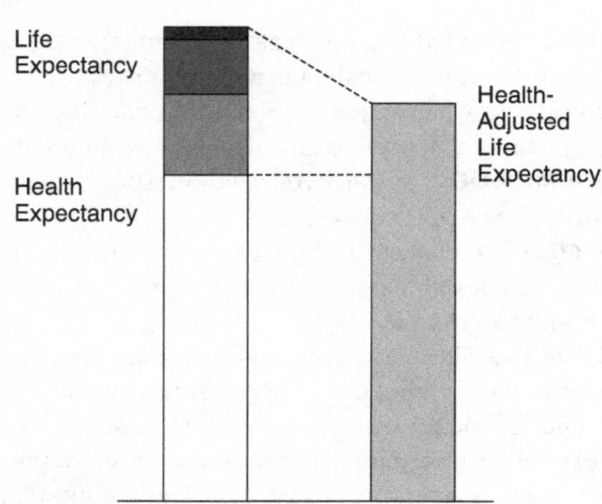

Relationships between life expectancy, health expectancy, and health-adjusted life expectancy. The shaded areas in the left bar indicate varying degrees of illness or disability. The right bar is a weighted average of all the components of the left bar and is necessarily greater than health expectancy but less than life expectancy. From Spasoff, 1999. With permission.

they can be computed for specific causes of mortality and morbidity. POTENTIAL YEARS OF LIFE LOST and EXPECTED YEARS OF LIFE LOST use a target selected arbitrarily or drawn from a life table and give all remaining years of life equal weight; DISABILITY-ADJUSTED LIFE YEARS (DALYs) assign weights to years of life remaining.

HEALTH IMPACT ASSESSMENT (HIA) See PUBLIC HEALTH IMPACT ASSESSMENT.

HEALTH IN ALL POLICIES (HIAP) A theme or slogan for INTERSECTORAL ACTION, horizontal health policies and HEALTHY PUBLIC POLICIES. The main health theme of the Finnish European Union Presidency in 2006 (www.stm.fi). A strategy to help strengthen links between health and other policies. HiAP addresses the effects on health across all policies (such as agriculture, education, the environment, fiscal policies, housing, and transport). It seeks to improve health and at the same time contribute to the well-being and the wealth of the nations through structures, mechanisms, and actions planned and managed mainly by sectors other than health. An approach that promotes coordination mechanisms to ensure that the health dimension is integrated into activities of all government agencies and services. While the health sector has gradually increased its cooperation with other government sectors, industry, and nongovernmental organizations in the past four decades, other sectors have increasingly taken health and the well-being of citizens into account in their policies. The key factor enabling such a development has been that health and well-being are shared values across societal sectors. HiAP is a political result of the growing recognition of the importance of health for the overall objectives of a society: health is a key foundation stone of strategies of growth, competitiveness, and sustainable development. The HiAP approach uses an integrated approach to HEALTH IMPACT ASSESSMENT (HIA).

HEALTH INDEX A numerical indication of the health of a given population derived from a specified composite formula. The components of the formula may be INFANT MORTALITY RATES, INCIDENCE RATE for particular disease, or other HEALTH INDICATOR.

HEALTH INDICATOR A variable, susceptible to direct measurement, that reflects the state of health of persons in a community. Examples include infant mortality rates, incidence rates based on notified cases of disease, disability days, etc. These measurements may be used as components in the calculation of a HEALTH INDEX.

HEALTH PROMOTION The process of enabling people to increase control over their health and improve it. It involves the population as a whole in the CONTEXT of their everyday lives rather than focusing on people at risk for specific diseases and is directed toward action on the determinants or causes of health.[228] See also PREVENTION; PREVENTIVE MEDICINE.

HEALTH RISK APPRAISAL (HRA) [(Syn: health hazard appraisal (HHA)] A generic term applied to methods for describing an individual's chances of becoming ill or dying from selected causes. The many versions available share several common features: Starting from the average risk of death for the individual's age and sex, a consideration of various lifestyle and physical factors indicates whether the individual is at greater or less than average risk of death from the commonest causes of death for his or her age and sex. All methods also indicate what reduction in risk could be achieved by altering any of the causal factors (such as cigarette smoking) that the individual could modify. The premise underlying such methods is that information on the extent to which an individual's characteristics, habits, and health practices are influencing his or her future risk of dying will assist health care workers in counseling their patients.

HEALTH SECTOR The sector of society that is concerned with and deals with all issues and services related to health, sickness, and the provision of health care to the population. See also DETERMINANT.

HEALTH SERVICES Services performed by health professionals or by others under their direction for the purpose of promoting, maintaining, or restoring health. In addition to personal health care, health services include measures for health protection, health promotion, and disease prevention.

HEALTH SERVICES RESEARCH The integration of knowledge from clinical, epidemiological, sociological, economic, management, and other sciences in the study of the organization, functioning, and performance of health services. Health services research is usually concerned with relationships between NEEDS, DEMAND, supply, use, and OUTCOMES of health services. The aim of health services research is evaluation; several components of evaluative health services research are distinguished, namely:

1. Evaluation of *structure*, concerned with resources, facilities, and manpower.
2. Evaluation of *process*, concerned with matters such as where, by whom, and how health care is provided.
3. Evaluation of *output*, concerned with the amount and nature of health services provided.
4. Evaluation of *outcome*, concerned with the results—i.e., whether persons using health services experience measurable benefits, such as improved survival or reduced disability.

HEALTH STATISTICS Aggregated data describing and enumerating attributes, events, behaviors, services, resources, outcomes, or costs related to health, disease, and health services. The data may be derived from survey instruments, medical records, and administrative documents. VITAL STATISTICS are a subset of health statistics.

HEALTH STATUS The degree to which a person is able to function physically, emotionally, and socially with or without aid from the health care system. Compare QUALITY OF LIFE.

HEALTH STATUS INDEX A set of measurements designed to detect short-term fluctuations in the health of members of a population; these measurements include physical function, emotional well-being, activities of daily living, feelings, etc. Most indexes require the use of carefully composed questions designed with reference to matters of fact rather than shades of opinion. The results are usually expressed by a numerical score that gives a profile of the well-being of the individual.

HEALTH SURVEY A survey designed to provide information on the health status of a population. It may be descriptive, exploratory, or explanatory. See also MORBIDITY SURVEY; CROSS-SECTIONAL STUDY.

HEALTH SYSTEMS RESEARCH (Syn: health research) The multidisciplinary study of health systems, including HEALTH SERVICES RESEARCH, supported by data on DETERMINANTS of health and accurate health statistics. A term popularized by the WHO.

HEALTH TECHNOLOGY ASSESSMENT (HTA) The formal evaluation of technologies used in health care, including medicine, and in public health. It explicitly involves not only EFFICACY but also COST-EFFECTIVENESS, COST-UTILITY, and all other aspects of technology that may be important for society. HTA supports evidence-based decision making in health care policy and practice.

HEALTHY PUBLIC POLICIES Policies that improve the conditions under which people live: such as secure, safe, adequate, and sustainable livelihoods, lifestyles, and environments, including housing, education, nutrition, access to information, child care, transportation, and necessary community and personal social and health services.[229] POLICY adequacy may be measured by its impact on POPULATION HEALTH.[70,196] See also HEALTH IN ALL POLICIES; PREVENTION.

HEALTHY WORKER EFFECT A phenomenon observed initially in studies of occupational diseases: workers often exhibit lower overall death rates than the GENERAL POPULATION, because persons who are severely ill and chronically disabled are ordinarily excluded from employment or leave employment early.[230] Death rates in the general population may be inappropriate for comparison if this effect is not taken into account. Similar effects are known for military personnel, migrants, and other groups.

HEALTHY YEARS EQUIVALENTS (HYEs) A measure of health-related quality of life that incorporates two sets of preferences; one set reflects individuals' preferences for life years or duration of life, and the other reflects preferences for states of health.[231]

HEALY (healthy life years) A composite indicator that incorporates mortality and morbidity in a single number.[232] See also BURDEN OF DISEASE; DISABILITY-ADJUSTED LIFE YEARS (DALYs); DISABILITY-FREE LIFE EXPECTANCY; LIFE EXPECTANCY FREE FROM DISABILITY (LEFD); QUALITY-ADJUSTED LIFE YEARS (QALY).

HEBDOMADAL MORTALITY RATE The mortality rate in the first week of life; the denominator is the number of live births in a year.

HENLE–KOCH POSTULATES A set of CAUSAL CRITERIA for making judgments about microorganisms as causes of infectious diseases. They were first formulated by F. G. Jacob Henle and adapted by Robert Koch in 1877 and 1882. Koch stated that these postulates should be met before a causal relationship can be accepted between a particular bacterial parasite or disease agent and the disease in question:

1. The agent must be shown to be present in every case of the disease by isolation in pure culture.
2. The agent must not be found in cases of other disease.
3. Once isolated, the agent must be capable of reproducing the disease in experimental animals.
4. The agent must be recovered from the experimental disease produced.

Postulates 1 and 2 require complete specificity in a unique and unconfounded bacterial cause; 3 demands biological coherence; and 4 requires performance as predicted in experimental tests. Insistence on the invariable presence of the organism (postulate 1) conforms with Galileo's original notion of necessary and sufficient cause. For the more recently recognized viruses and prions, which lack independent life and often specificity also, the generalizations of the postulates do not hold. Nor do they hold for DISEASES OF COMPLEX ETIOLOGY, which cause most of the BURDEN OF DISEASE in many areas of the world.[10,66,67,169,190] See also CAUSAL CRITERIA.

HERD IMMUNITY The immunity of a group or community. The resistance of a group to invasion and spread of an infectious agent, based on the resistance to infection of a high proportion of individual members of the group. The resistance is a product of the number susceptible and the probability that those who are susceptible will come into contact with an infected person. Resistance of a population to invasion and spread of an infectious agent, based on the agent-specific immunity of a high proportion of the population. The proportion of the population required to be immune varies according to the agent, its transmission characteristics, the distribution of immunes and susceptibles, and other (e.g., environmental) factors.

HERD IMMUNITY THRESHOLD The proportion of immunes in a population, above which the incidence of the infection decreases.[233] This can be mathematically expressed as

$$H = 1 - 1/R_0 = (R_0 - 1)/R_0 = (rT - 1)/rT$$

where H is the herd immunity threshold, R_0 is the BASIC REPRODUCTIVE RATE, r is the TRANSMISSION PARAMETER, and T is the total population.

HEREDITY The passing on of biological (including genetic) characteristics from one generation to the next. Nonbiological traits and attributes may also be passed on from parents to offspring (e.g., religious and health beliefs). The transmission of characters and dispositions in the process of organic reproduction. Introduced in the biomedical sciences from the legal sphere, where it was used synonymous with INHERITANCE and *succession*.[234,235]

HERITABILITY The degree to which a trait is genetically determined, calculated by regression-correlation analyses among close relatives.

HETEROSCEDASTICITY Nonconstancy of the variance of a measure over the levels of the factors under study.

HEURISTIC METHOD A method of reasoning that relies on a combination of empirical observations and unproven theories to produce a solution that may be correct and defensible but cannot be proven sound under the given conditions of application. The word, not always perfectly understood by users or audience, sounds more impressive than the method. In common parlance, rule of thumb.

HIBERNATION Survival of organisms (including arthropod vectors) during cold periods by reducing the metabolic rate.

HIERARCHICAL ANALYSIS See MULTILEVEL ANALYSIS.

HIERARCHICAL MODEL See MULTILEVEL MODEL.

HIERARCHY OF EVIDENCE The quality of epidemiological evidence was appraised by the Canadian Task Force on the Periodic Health Examination[236] and the U.S. Preventive Services Task Force[237] as an essential prerequisite to their recommendations about

SCREENING and preventive interventions. The classes of evidence that these groups used are as follows:

I: Evidence from at least one properly designed randomized controlled trial.
II-1: Evidence from well-designed controlled trials without RANDOM ALLOCATION.
II-2: Evidence from well-designed cohort or case-control analytic studies, preferably from more than one center or research group.
II-3: Evidence obtained from multiple time series, with or without the intervention; dramatic results in uncontrolled experiments (e.g., first use of penicillin in the 1940s) also are in this category.
III: Opinions of respected authorities, based on clinical experience, descriptive studies, reports of expert committees, consensus conferences, etc.

It is not always possible to achieve complete scientific rigor; for example, randomized controlled trials or cohort studies may be unethical or not feasible.

"HIGH-RISK" PREVENTIVE STRATEGY See STRATEGY, "HIGH-RISK."

HILL'S CRITERIA OF CAUSATION or **HILL'S CONSIDERATIONS FOR CAUSAL INFERENCE** A series of logical, empirical, and theoretical checks that causal relations may or may not satisfy, described by Austin Bradford Hill (1897–1991)[238] and elaborated by others, including Mervyn Susser.[67] The considerations are often called "criteria," even though Hill did not use the latter term. They are:

Consistency: The association is consistent when results are replicated in studies in different settings using different methods. Replicability and survivability.

Strength: This is defined by the size of the risk as measured by appropriate statistical estimates. The stronger, the more likely to be causal, although weak relationships may also be causal.[43] See also ABSOLUTE RISK DIFFERENCE; RELATIVE RISK; RISK DIFFERENCE.

Specificity: Present when a putative cause produces a specific effect, as hypothesized or predicted by background theory (e.g., exogenous estrogen usage is expected to show a relation to hormone-sensitive conditions but not to seat-belt use). The particularity with which one variable predicts the occurrence of another.

Dose-response relationship: An increasing level of exposure (in amount and/or time) increases the risk. More generally, the relation of exposure to risk follows the expected theoretical pattern (e.g., morbidity and mortality follow a U-shaped relation to some vitamins).

Temporal relationship: Exposure always precedes the outcome. This is the only absolutely essential or necessary criterion of causality. See also TIME ORDER.

Biological plausibility: The association is coherent with firmly established knowledge on pathobiological processes. Exceptional caution is needed in this consideration: when the understanding of biological mechanisms is incomplete, implausible and speculative biological explanations will seem plausible and even coherent. See also PLAUSIBILITY.

Coherence: The association should be compatible with existing theory and knowledge. It may be theoretical and factual; biological, clinical, epidemiological, social, statistical, etc. See also COHERENCE, EPIDEMIOLOGICAL.

Experiment: The caused condition can be altered (e.g., prevented or ameliorated) by an appropriate experimental regimen that changes the putative effect.

See also ASSOCIATION; CAUSAL CRITERIA; CAUSALITY; CAUSATION OF DISEASE, FACTORS IN; COHERENCE; DISEASES OF COMPLEX ETIOLOGY; EVANS'S POSTULATES; HENLE-KOCH POSTULATES; MILL'S CANONS; NECESSARY CAUSE; PROBABILITY OF CAUSATION.

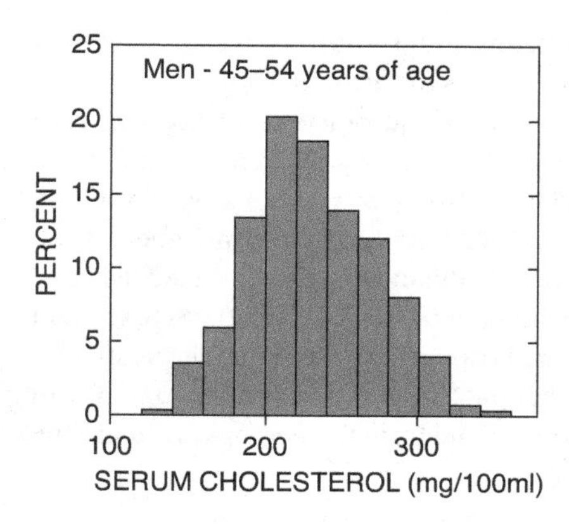

Histogram. Distribution of serum cholesterol levels in men aged 45–54 years.

HISTOGRAM A graphic representation of the frequency distribution of a variable. Rectangles are drawn in such a way that their bases lie on a linear scale representing different intervals, and their areas are proportional to the frequencies of the values within each of the intervals. See also BAR CHART.

HISTORICAL COHORT STUDY See COHORT STUDY, HISTORICAL.

HISTORICAL CONTROL Control subject(s) for whom data were collected at a time preceding that at which the data are gathered on the group being studied. Because of differences in exposure, etc., use of historical controls can lead to bias in analysis.

HISTORY OF EPIDEMIOLOGICAL METHODS See EPIDEMIOLOGICAL METHODS, HISTORY OF.

HIV SEROCONCORDANT/-DISCORDANT Sexual partners having/not having the same HIV serological status.

HOGBEN NUMBER A unique personal identifying number constructed by using a sequence of digits for birth date, sex, birthplace, and other identifiers. Suggested by the English mathematician Lancelot Hogben. Used in PRIMARY CARE EPIDEMIOLOGY in some countries and usable in RECORD LINKAGE. See also IDENTIFICATION NUMBER; SOUNDEX CODE.

HOLLERITH CARDS See PUNCH CARD.

HOLOENDEMIC DISEASE A disease for which a high prevalent level of infection begins early in life and affects most of the child population, leading to a state of equilibrium such that the adult population shows evidence of the disease much less commonly than do the children. Malaria in many communities is a holoendemic disease.

HOLOMIANTIC INFECTION See COMMON SOURCE EPIDEMIC.

HOMOSCEDASTICITY Constancy of the variance of a measure over the levels of the factors under study.

HOSPITAL-ACQUIRED INFECTION See NOSOCOMIAL INFECTION.

HOSPITAL DISCHARGE ABSTRACT SYSTEM Abstraction of MINIMUM DATA SET from hospital charts for the purpose of producing summary statistics about hospitalized patients. Examples include the HOSPITAL INPATIENT ENQUIRY (HIPE) and Professional Activity Study (PAS). The statistical tabulations commonly include length of stay by final diagnosis, surgical operations, specified hospital service (i.e., medical, surgical, gynecological, etc.) and also give outcomes such as "death" and "discharged alive from hospital." This system cannot generally be used for epidemiological purposes as it is not possible to infer representativeness or to generalize; this is because the data usually lack a defined denominator and the same person may be counted more than once in the event of two or more HOSPITAL SEPARATIONS in the period of study. However, such data can be a fruitful source of cases for case-control studies of rare conditions.

The systematic use of summary statistics on the process and outcome of hospital care began in the nineteenth century, pioneered in England by Florence Nightingale (1820–1910) and in Vienna by Ignaz Semmelweis (1818–1865). Nightingale was the founder of modern nursing care and an accomplished statistician—a member of the Royal Statistical Society. She was also a confrere of William Farr, Edwin Chadwick, and other great nineteenth-century reformers. Her *Notes on Hospitals* (1859) discussed and illustrated the importance of statistical analysis of hospital activity. Semmelweis studied the outcome of obstetric care, demonstrating that puerperal sepsis was associated with attendance on women in labor by doctors who had come from the necropsy room to the labor room without washing their hands.

HOSPITAL EPIDEMIOLOGY The application of epidemiological reasoning, knowledge, and methods in hospitals (and, by extension, in other health care settings), in order to address a wide range of preventive issues and in particular to enhance the quality of patient care and the safety of health professionals. Intense efforts are always devoted to infection prevention and control and to the prevention of other adverse outcomes. As mentioned before, EPIDEMIOLOGY is applied in many settings; for space reasons, this dictionary includes only a few illustrative examples of specialties. See also FIELD EPIDEMIOLOGY; NOSOCOMIAL INFECTION; PRIMARY CARE EPIDEMIOLOGY.

HOSPITAL INPATIENT ENQUIRY (HIPE) Statistical tables of a 10% sample of hospital patients in England and Wales, showing class of hospital, diagnosis, length of stay, outcomes, etc.

HOSPITAL SEPARATION A term used in commentaries on hospital statistics to describe the departure of a patient from hospital without distinguishing whether the patient departed alive or dead. The distinction is unimportant insofar as the statistics of hospital activity, such as bed occupancy, are concerned.

HOST

1. A person or other living animal, including birds and arthropods, that affords subsistence or lodgment to an infectious agent under natural conditions. Some protozoa and helminths pass successive stages in alternate hosts of different species. Hosts in which the parasite attains maturity or passes its sexual stage are primary or definitive hosts; those in which the parasite is in a larval or asexual state are secondary or intermediate hosts. A transport host is a carrier in which the organism remains alive but does not undergo development.[52]
2. In an epidemiological context, the host may also be the population or group; biological, social, and behavioral characteristics of this group relevant to health are called "host factors."

HOST, DEFINITIVE In parasitology, the host in which sexual maturation occurs. In malaria, the mosquito (invertebrate host).

HOST, INTERMEDIATE In parasitology, the host in which asexual forms of the parasite develop. In malaria, this is a human or other vertebrate mammal or bird (vertebrate host).

HOUSEHOLD One or more persons who occupy a dwelling (i.e., a place that provides shelter, cooking, washing, and sleeping facilities); this may or may not be a family. The term is also used to describe the dwelling unit in which the persons live.

HOUSEHOLD SAMPLE SURVEY A survey of persons in a sample of households. This, in many variations, is a favored method of gathering data for health-related and many other purposes. The households may be sampled in any of several ways—e.g., by cluster or use of random numbers in relation to numbered dwelling units. The survey may be conducted by interview, telephone survey, or self-completed responses to presented questions. The method is used in developing nations as well as in the industrial world.

HUMAN BLOOD INDEX Proportion of insect vectors found to contain human blood.

HUMAN DEVELOPMENT The process by which individuals, social groups, and populations achieve their potential level of health and well-being. Human development includes physical, biological, mental, emotional, educational, economic, social, and cultural components; some of these are expressed in the HUMAN DEVELOPMENT INDEX (HDI).

HUMAN DEVELOPMENT INDEX (HDI) A composite index combining indicators representing three dimensions—longevity (life expectancy at birth); knowledge (adult literacy rate and mean years of schooling); and income (real GDP per capita in purchasing-power-parity dollars) (source: World Bank). The validity of the HDI has been questioned because it attempts to express multiple complex variables on a unidimensional scale.

HUMAN ECOLOGY The study of human groups as influenced by environmental factors, including social and behavioral factors. A macrolevel, holistic approach to the study of human organization. See also ECOLOGY.

HUMAN GENOME EPIDEMIOLOGY NETWORK (HUGENET) A collaboration committed to assess the impact of human genome variation on population health and how genetic information can be used to improve health and prevent disease, including assessment of the role and quality of genetic tests for screening (www.cdc.gov/genomics/hugenet). See also GENETIC EPIDEMIOLOGY; MOLECULAR EPIDEMIOLOGY.

HUMAN IMMUNODEFICIENCY VIRUS (HIV) The pathogenic organism responsible for the acquired immunodeficiency syndrome (AIDS). Formerly known as the lymphadenopathy virus (LAV), the name given by Montagnier et al., the original French discoverers, in 1983; it was also known as the human T-cell lymphotropic virus, type III (HTLV-III), the name given by Gallo et al. to the virus they reported in 1984. The retrovirus responsible for HIV disease, it is transmissible in blood, serum, semen, breastfeeding, body tissues, and other body fluids. The are two types: HIV-1 (responsible of the AIDS pandemic) and HIV-2; they compromise immune responses to organisms that are destroyed by a healthy immune system. The virus is immunologically unstable, but it produces antibodies that can be detected by Western blot and ELISA tests of blood, serum, semen, saliva, etc.

HUMAN IMMUNODEFICIENCY VIRUS (HIV) INFECTION The surveillance case definition for HIV infection uses either laboratory, clinical, or other criteria. The laboratory criteria include positive screening test for HIV antibody and other laboratory evidence of HIV infection. Additional criteria of the presence and absence of HIV infection are defined for infants.

HYGIENE The principles and laws governing the preservation of health and their practical application. Practices conducive to good health. The sum of the procedures and techniques that promote human development and harmonious adaptation to the individual's milieu.

HYPERENDEMIC DISEASE A disease that is constantly present at a high incidence and/or prevalence and affects most or all age groups equally.

HYPERGEOMETRIC DISTRIBUTION The exact probability distribution of the frequencies in a two-by-two contingency table, conditional on the marginal frequencies being fixed at their observed levels.

HYPNOZOITE Dormant form of malaria parasites found in liver cells. After sporozoites (inoculated by the mosquito) invade liver cells, some sporozoites develop into dormant forms (the hypnozoites), which do not cause symptoms. Hypnozoites can become activated months or years after the initial infection, producing a RELAPSE.

HYPOTHESIS

1. A supposition, arrived at from observation or reflection, that leads to refutable predictions.
2. Any conjecture cast in a form that will allow it to be tested and refuted. See also NULL HYPOTHESIS.

HYPOTHETICO-DEDUCTIVE METHOD Karl Popper's language (following Hume) for DEDUCTIVE LOGIC as applied to scientific research. For Popper, science is that which is testable.[239] Therefore a hypothesis must be stated a priori in order to test its *survivability* by efforts to reject it. Popper's underlying assumption is that no hypothesis can be truly verified and proved; at best, it can be *corroborated*. Many scientists reject Popper's assumption of *nonverifiability*. In order to verify ideas and hypotheses, scientists are often obliged to argue by induction. But that does not preclude resort to the hypothetico-deductive method as a testing procedure.[71] See also INDUCTIVE LOGIC; LOGIC.

I

IARC International Agency for Research on Cancer. A WHO agency (www.iarc.fr).

IATROGENESIS Literally, "doctor-generated"; often broadly used to refer to adverse effects of preventive, diagnostic, therapeutic, surgical, and other medical, sanitary and health procedures, interventions, or programs. The entire process through which a professional health activity generates an adverse health effect. There is a natural plurality of views on what constitutes iatrogenesis and its scope (e.g., clinical, social, and cultural iatrogenesis). Medicine and public health are obviously not the only professions that cause adverse effects: others are also part of some excessive professionalizing and bureaucratization of contemporary societies.[78,240] See also PREVENTION, QUATERNARY.

IATROGENIC EFFECT An adverse effect on health resulting from the activity of a health professional (e.g., a physician, a nurse, a professional of health promotion).

ICD See INTERNATIONAL CLASSIFICATION OF DISEASE.

ICEBERG PHENOMENON That portion of disease which remains unrecorded or undetected despite physicians' diagnostic endeavors and community disease surveillance procedures is referred to as the "submerged portion of the iceberg." Detected or diagnosed disease is the "tip of the iceberg." The submerged portion comprises disease not medically attended, medically attended but not accurately diagnosed, and diagnosed but not reported.[241] Other terms have been proposed to describe this concept in parts of the world where icebergs are unknown (e.g., "ears of the hippopotamus," "crocodile's nose").

ICHPPC See INTERNATIONAL CLASSIFICATION OF HEALTH PROBLEMS IN PRIMARY CARE.

ICIDH International Classification of Impairments, Disabilities, and Handicaps.

ICMJHE International Committee of Medical Journal Editors. www.icmje.org.

ICRC International Commission of the Red Cross, Red Crescent.

IDENTIFICATION NUMBER, IDENTIFYING NUMBER Unique number given to every individual at birth or at some other milestone. The Nordic and Baltic nations have a system based on a sequence of digits for birth date, sex, birthplace, and additional digits for each individual. Other systems (e.g., National Insurance number in the United Kingdom, Social Security number in the United States, and Social Insurance number in Canada) are sometimes used but are neither universal nor unique, being sometimes applied to whole families or at least to more than one individual. See also HOGBEN NUMBER; SOUNDEX CODE.

IDIOSYNCRASY A distinctive characteristic or peculiarity of an individual. In PHARMACOEPIDEMIOLOGY, it means an abnormal reaction, sometimes genetically influenced, following the administration of a medication.

IEA International Epidemiological Association (www.dundee.ac.uk/iea), founded 1954. The aims of the IEA are to facilitate communication among those engaged in research and teaching in epidemiology throughout the world and to engage in the development and use of epidemiological methods in all fields of health including social, community, and preventive medicine and health services administration. These aims are achieved by holding scientific meetings and seminars, the publication of journals and reports, and by many other activities that take place every year on all continents. The official journal of the IEA is the *International Journal of Epidemiology* (http://ije.oxfordjournals.org).

IEA-EEF International Epidemiological Association European Epidemiology Federation. The European Epidemiology Federation (EEF) is an official group within the IEA. All members of the IEA in Europe are automatically members of the EEF. Most national associations of epidemiologists in the European region are also part of the EEF.

ILLNESS See DISEASE.

ILLNESS BEHAVIOR Conduct of persons in response to abnormal body signals. Such behavior influences the manner in which people monitor their bodies, define and interpret their symptoms, take remedial actions, and use the health care system. See also HEALTH BEHAVIOR.

IMMUNITY, ACQUIRED Resistance acquired by a host as a result of previous exposure to a natural PATHOGEN or foreign substance for the host, e.g., immunity to measles resulting from a prior infection with measles virus.

IMMUNITY, ACTIVE Resistance developed in response to stimulus by an antigen (infecting agent or vaccine) and usually characterized by the presence of antibody produced by the host.

IMMUNITY, NATURAL Species-determined inherent resistance to a disease agent, e.g., resistance of humans to the virus of canine distemper.

IMMUNITY, PASSIVE Immunity conferred by an antibody produced in another host and acquired naturally by an infant from its mother or artificially by administration of an antibody-containing preparation (antiserum or immune globulin).

IMMUNITY, SPECIFIC A state of altered responsiveness to a specific substance acquired through immunization or natural infection. For certain diseases (e.g., measles, chickenpox), this protection generally lasts for the life of the individual.

IMMUNIZATION (Syn: vaccination) The artificial induction of active immunity by introducing into a vulnerable host the specific antigen of a pathogenic organism. Protection of susceptible individuals from communicable disease by administration of a living modified agent (as in yellow fever), a suspension of killed organisms (as in whooping cough), or an inactivated toxin (as in tetanus). Temporary passive immunization can be produced by administration of antibody in the form of immune globulin in some conditions.

IMMUNIZATION, LATENT The process of developing immunity by a single or repeated inapparent asymptomatic infection. Not necessarily related to latent infection. See also IMMUNITY, ACQUIRED.

IMMUNOGENICITY The ability of an infectious agent to induce specific immunity.

IMPACT FACTOR See BIBLIOGRAPHIC IMPACT FACTOR (BIF).

IMPACT FRACTION A generalization of POPULATION ATTRIBUTABLE FRACTION that accommodates both hazardous and protective exposures, multiple levels of exposure, incomplete elimination of exposure, diffusion, or response to exposure. To define this measure, let IF be the impact fraction, let p' and p'' be the prevalences of an exposure level before and after an intervention program, and let RR be the risk ratio or rate ratio (properly adjusted for bias) relative to a common reference level, depending on whether impact on risks or rates is being estimated. Then the impact fraction is given by

$$\text{IF} = \frac{\Sigma(p' - p'')\text{RR}}{\Sigma p' \text{ RR}} \text{(with decreasing risk)}$$

$$\text{or IF} = \frac{\Sigma(p'' - p')\text{ RR}}{\Sigma p' \text{ RR}} \text{(with increasing risk)}$$

where the sums are over all exposure categories; in the reference category, RR = 1.

IMPACT NUMBERS Four quantities related to ATTRIBUTABLE RISK, used to communicate risk in terms relevant to four groups (total population, diseased, exposed, and exposed with disease). Expands the concept of NUMBER NEEDED TO TREAT. (1) Population impact number (PIN) is the number of subjects in the total population among whom one case is attributable to the RISK FACTOR. (2) Case impact number (CIN) is the number of people with the disease or outcome among whom one case is attributable to the risk factor. (3) Exposure impact number (EIN) is the number of people with the exposure among whom one case is attributable to the risk factor. (4) Exposed cases impact number (ECIN) is the number of exposed people with the disease or outcome among whom one case is attributable to the risk factor.[242]

IMPAIRMENT A physical or mental defect at the level of a body system or organ. See also INTERNATIONAL CLASSIFICATION OF IMPAIRMENTS, DISABILITIES, AND HANDICAPS for the official WHO definition.

IMPRINTING

1. A form of learning behavior (e.g., the expression of affection) in a critical period of development early in a young animal's life, including the life of a human; it may result from the interaction between mother and infant. The imposition of a stable behavior pattern in a young animal by exposure, during a particular period in its development, to one of a restricted set of stimuli.[243]
2. An EPIGENETIC phenomenon in which the expression of a gene varies depending on whether it is inherited from the mother or the father.

INAPPARENT INFECTION (Syn: subclinical infection) The presence of infection in a host without occurrence of recognizable clinical signs or symptoms. Of epidemiologic significance because hosts so infected, although apparently well, may serve as silent or inapparent disseminators of the infectious agent. See also DISEASE, PRECLINICAL; DISEASE, SUBCLINICAL; VECTOR-BORNE INFECTION.

INCEPTION COHORT A group of individuals identified and assembled for subsequent study at an early and uniform point in the course of the specified health condition; e.g., near the onset (inception) of symptoms, soon after diagnosis, at detection of a clinically significant pathological event. Thus, subjects who succumbed to or completely recovered from the disorder are included with those whose disease persisted.[62,63,81] Failure to select an inception cohort often severely biases studies on the NATURAL HISTORY OF DISEASE. See also STUDY BASE.

INCEPTION RATE The rate at which new spells of illness occur in a population. A term applied principally to short-term spells of illness, such as acute respiratory infections, and preferred by some epidemiologists because an annual incidence rate for such conditions may exceed the numbers in the population at risk.

INCIDENCE The number of instances of illness commencing, or of persons falling ill, during a given period in a specified population. More generally, the number of new health-related events in a defined population within a specified period of time. It may be measured as a frequency count, a rate, or a proportion.

INCIDENCE DENSITY The average person-time incidence rate. Sometimes used to describe the hazard rate. See FORCE OF MORBIDITY; INCIDENCE RATE.

INCIDENCE-DENSITY RATIO (IDR) The ratio of two incidence densities. See also RATE RATIO.

INCIDENCE PROPORTION (Syn: cumulative incidence) Incidence expressed as a proportion of the population at risk. A measure of risk. The time duration must be specified for it to be meaningful. It approximates to the INCIDENCE RATE multiplied by the time duration when that product is small. The proportion of a CLOSED POPULATION at risk for a disease that develops the disease during a specified interval.

INCIDENCE RATE The rate at which new events occur in a population. The numerator is the number of new events that occur in a defined period or other physical span. The denominator is the population at risk of experiencing the event during this period, sometimes expressed as person-time; it may instead be in other units, such as passenger-miles. The incidence rate most often used in public health practice is calculated from the formula

$$\frac{\text{Number of new events in specified period}}{\text{Average number of persons exposed to risk during this period}} \times 10^n$$

Strictly speaking, this ratio is neither a rate nor a proportion but is instead the rate multiplied by the length of the specified period. If the period is a year, the ratio is nonetheless often called the annual incidence rate. The average size of the population is often the estimated population size at the midperiod. The ratio divided by the length of the period is an estimate of the person-time incidence rate (i.e., the rate per 10^n person-years). If the ratio is small, as with many chronic diseases, it is also a good estimate of the cumulative incidence over the period (e.g., a year). If the number of new cases during a specified period is divided by the sum of the person-time units at risk for all persons during the period, the result is the person-time incidence rate.

INCIDENCE RATE RATIO The incidence rate in the exposed group divided by the incidence rate in the unexposed group. Often referred to as the rate ratio.

INCIDENCE STUDY See COHORT STUDY.

INCIDENT NUMBER See INCIDENCE.

INCLEN Acronym for International Clinical Epidemiology Network, which consists of *clinical epidemiology units* (CEUs) in about 30 countries, mostly developing nations. Each CEU includes clinical epidemiologists, statisticians, economists, and social scientists. The network began at the initiative of Kerr L. White (b. 1916), with financial support from the Rockefeller Foundation.

INCUBATION PERIOD

1. The time interval between invasion by an infectious agent and appearance of the first sign or symptom of the disease in question. See also LATENT PERIOD.
2. In a VECTOR, the period between entry of the infectious agent into the vector and the time at which the vector becomes infective; i.e., transmission of the infectious agent from the vector to a fresh final host is possible (extrinsic incubation period).

INDEPENDENCE, STATISTICAL Two events are said to be (statistically) independent if the occurrence of one is in no way predictable from the occurrence of the other.

Two variables are said to be independent if the distribution of values of one is the same for all values of the other. *Independence* is the antonym of ASSOCIATION.

INDEPENDENT VARIABLE

1. The characteristic being observed or measured that is hypothesized to influence an event or manifestation (the dependent variable) within the defined area of relationships under study; that is, the independent variable is not influenced by the event or manifestation but may cause or contribute to variation of the event or manifestation.
2. In REGRESSION ANALYSIS, an independent variable is one of (perhaps) several variables that appear as arguments in a regression equation; a regressor or covariate.[20,31] See also DEPENDENT VARIABLE; REGRESSAND; REGRESSOR.

INDEX

1. In epidemiology and related sciences, this word usually means a rating scale, e.g., a set of numbers derived from a series of observations of specified variables. Examples include the many varieties of health status index, scoring systems for severity or stage of cancer, heart murmurs, mental retardation, etc.
2. One way to present a measurement with adjustment to the results of other measurements; e.g., the Quetelet Index II, now called body-mass index (BMI), is an index of this type (weight is corrected for height).

INDEX CASE The first case in a family or other defined group to come to the attention of the investigator. See also PROPOSITUS.

INDEX GROUP (Syn: index series)

1. In an experiment, the group receiving the experimental regimen
2. In a case-control study, the cases
3. In a cohort study, the exposed group

INDICATOR VARIABLE In statistics, a variable taking only one of two possible values, one (usually 1) indicating the presence of a condition, and the other (usually zero) indicating absence of the condition. Used mainly in REGRESSION ANALYSIS.

INDIRECT ADJUSTMENT See STANDARDIZATION.

INDIRECT COSTS See COST, INDIRECT.

INDIRECT OBSTETRIC DEATH See MATERNAL MORTALITY.

INDIVIDUAL THINKING In medicine, it is the ability to make the best prediction in terms of diagnosis and prognosis for the individual patient and to adapt the management and treatment to the unique characteristics of an essentially unpredictable person. Medicine is the art of individual thinking.[10,61–63] See also ATOMISTIC FALLACY; CLINICAL STUDY; ECOLOGICAL FALLACY; POPULATION THINKING; PREVENTION PARADOX; STRATEGY, "HIGH-RISK."

INDIVIDUAL VARIATION Two types are distinguished:

1. *Intraindividual variation:* The variation of biological variables within the same individual, depending upon circumstances such as the phase of certain body rhythms and the presence or absence of emotional stress. These variables do not have a precise value but rather a range. Examples include diurnal variation in body temperature, fluctuation of blood pressure, blood sugar, etc.
2. *Interindividual variation:* As used by Darwin, the term means variation *between* individuals. This is the preferred usage; the first usage is better described as personal variation.

INDUCTION

1. Any method of rational or logical analysis that proceeds from the particular to the general. Although no infallible method of logical reasoning exists, general theories require induction. Conceptually bright ideas and breakthroughs and ordinary statistical inference belong to the realm of induction. Contrast DEDUCTION. See also HYPOTHETICO-DEDUCTIVE METHOD; INDUCTIVE LOGIC; INFERENCE.
2. Causation of the initiating events of a disease process (e.g., induction of initiating mutations at the beginning of CARCINOGENESIS).

INDUCTION PERIOD The interval between initiation of exposure to the causal agent and initiation of the health process; e.g., from onset of exposure to the disease-causing agent to initiation of the disease. See also CARCINOGEN; INCUBATION PERIOD; LATENCY PERIOD.

INDUCTIVE LOGIC Logic that seeks to reach generalizations by reasoning from an assembly of particular observations. Francis Bacon was its first proponent as applied to science. It remains an important mode of (and a collection of methods for) scientific reasoning. Its status as a "logic" has long been debated, and many authors prefer to use the term INDUCTION instead. Scholars have argued that statistical theories are attempts to put induction on a logically sound footing.[6–12] Nonetheless, epidemiology challenges these attempts insofar as epidemiologic reasoning must go beyond statistics. See also HYPOTHETICO-DEDUCTIVE METHOD; INFERENCE.

INDUSTRIAL HYGIENE The science devoted to recognition, evaluation, and control of those environmental factors or stresses arising from or in the workplace that may cause sickness, impaired health and well-being, or significant discomfort and inefficiency among workers or among persons in the community. Alternatively, the profession that anticipates and controls unhealthy conditions of work to prevent illness among employees. See also OCCUPATIONAL HEALTH.

INEQUALITIES IN HEALTH The virtually universal phenomenon of variation in health indicators (e.g., infant and maternal mortality rates, mortality and incidence rates of many diseases) in association with socioeconomic status and ethnicity. It has been observed since the vital statistics of England and Wales were examined by William Farr (1807–1883) and reported annually from 1840. The gap between best and worst health experience has widened in recent decades in many rich nations.

INFANT MORTALITY RATE (IMR) A measure of the yearly rate of deaths in children less than 1 year old. The denominator is the number of live births in the same year. Defined as

$$\text{Infant Mortality rate} = \frac{\begin{array}{c}\text{number of deaths in a year of}\\ \text{children less than 1 year of age}\end{array}}{\text{number of live births in the same year}} \times 1000$$

This is often cited as a useful indicator of the level of health in a community. The denominator is an approximation of the population at risk.

INFECTIBILITY The host characteristic or state in which the host is capable of being infected. See also INFECTIOUSNESS; INFECTIVITY.

INFECTION (Syn: colonization) The entry and development or multiplication of an infectious agent in the body of man or animals. *Infection* is not synonymous with *infectious disease*; the result may be inapparent or manifest. The presence of living infectious agents on exterior surfaces of the body is called "infestation" (e.g., pediculosis, scabies). The presence of living infectious agents upon articles of apparel or soiled articles is not infection, but represents CONTAMINATION of such articles. See also INAPPARENT INFECTION; TRANSMISSION OF INFECTION.

INFECTION, GRADIENT OF The range of manifestations of illness in the host reflecting the response to an infectious agent, which extends from death at one extreme to inapparent infection at the other. The frequency of these manifestations varies with the specific infectious disease. For example, human infection with the virus of rabies is almost invariably fatal, whereas a high proportion of persons infected in childhood with the virus of hepatitis A experience a subclinical or mild clinical infection.

INFECTION, LATENT PERIOD OF The time between initiation of infection and first shedding or excretion of the agent.

INFECTION, SUBCLINICAL See INAPPARENT INFECTION.

INFECTION RATE The incidence rate of manifest plus inapparent infections (the latter determined by seroepidemiology).

INFECTION TRANSMISSION PARAMETER (r) The proportion of total possible contacts between infectious cases and susceptibles that lead to new infections.

INFECTIOUS DISEASE See COMMUNICABLE DISEASE.

INFECTIOUSNESS A characteristic of a disease that concerns the relative ease with which it is transmitted to other hosts. A droplet spread disease, for instance, is more infectious than one spread by direct contact. The characteristics of the portals of exit and entry are thus also determinants of infectiousness, as are the agent characteristics of ability to survive away from the host and of infectivity.

INFECTIVITY

1. The characteristic of the disease agent that embodies capability to enter, survive, and multiply in the host. A measure of infectivity is the secondary attack rate.
2. The proportion of exposures, in defined circumstances, that results in infection.

INFERENCE The process of passing from observations and axioms to generalizations. In statistics, the development of generalization from sample data, usually with calculated degrees of uncertainty. CAUSAL INFERENCE from observational data is a key task of epidemiology and other sciences as sociology, education, behavioral sciences, demography, economics, or health services research; these disciplines share methodological frameworks for causal inference.

INFESTATION The development on (rather than in) the body of a pathogenic agent; e.g., body lice. Some authors use the term also to describe invasion of the gut by parasitic worms.

INFLUENCE ANALYSIS Methods to determine the ROBUSTNESS of an assessment by examining the extent to which results are affected by changes in recorded measurements and variables. The aim is to identify recorded values that made the largest contribution to the results or to find a solution that is relatively stable for the most commonly occurring values of these variables. See also OUTLIERS; SENSITIVITY ANALYSIS.

INFORMATICS The study of information and the ways to handle it, especially by means of information technology, i.e., computers and other electronic devices for rapid transfer, processing, and analysis of large amounts of data.

INFORMATION Facts that have been arranged and/or transformed to provide the basis for interpretation and conversion into knowledge.

INFORMATION BIAS (Syn: observational bias)

1. A flaw in measuring exposure, covariate, or outcome variables that results in different quality (ACCURACY) of information between comparison groups.[10,12,14,31,95] The occurrence of information biases may not be independent of the occurrence of SELECTION BIASES.
2. Bias in an estimate arising from measurement errors.

INFORMATION SYSTEM As applied in epidemology, a combination of vital and health statistical data from multiple sources, used to derive information about the health needs, health resources, costs, use of health services, and outcomes of use by the population of a specified jurisdiction. The term may also describe the automatic release from computers of stored information in response to programmed stimuli. For example, parents can be notified when their children are due to receive booster doses of an immunizing agent against infectious disease.

INFORMATION THEORY Mathematical theory dealing with the nature, effectiveness, and ACCURACY of information transfer.

INFORMED CONSENT Voluntary consent given by a subject or a responsible proxy (e.g., a parent) for participation in a study, immunization program, treatment regimen, etc., after being informed of the purpose, methods, procedures, potential benefits and potential harms, and, when relevant, the degree of uncertainty about such outcomes. The essential criteria of informed consent are that the subject has both knowledge and comprehension, that consent is freely given without duress or undue influence, and that the right of withdrawal at any time is clearly communicated to the subject. Other aspects of informed consent in the context of epidemiological and biomedical research, and criteria to be met in obtaining it, are specified in *International Ethical Guidelines for Epidemiological Studies* (Geneva: CIOMS/WHO, 2008) and *International Ethical Guidelines for Biomedical Research Involving Human Subjects* (Geneva: CIOMS/WHO, 2002).[244] See also ETHICS.

INGELFINGER RULE Rule developed by Franz Ingelfinger (1910–1980), former editor of the *New England Journal of Medicine*, as follows: "The Journal undertakes review with the understanding that neither the substance of the article nor the figures or tables have been published or will be submitted for publication during the period of review. This restriction does not apply to abstracts published in connection with scientific meetings or to news reports based on public presentations at such meetings."[245]

A revision of the rule imposed a news embargo[246] until the pertinent article is published. The Ingelfinger rule (or modifications of it) has been adopted by many high-quality peer-reviewed biomedical and science journals. The aims of the rule are to eliminate duplicate publication and reduce uncritical acceptance of original work prior to peer review and publication.[247]

INHERITANCE In the biological sciences, pattern followed by the transmission from generation to generation of a given phenotype (e.g., a disease). There are several types of complex inheritance (non-Mendelian) and of Mendelian inheritance (dominant, recessive, sex-linked).[23] See also EPIGENETIC INHERITANCE; HEREDITY.

INHERITANCE, CULTURAL The transfer from one generation to another of values, beliefs, and customs (e.g., solidarity values, patriotic feelings, leisure habits). Process through which individuals receive, learn, and adopt norms and behaviors (e.g., on smoking and alcohol use, exercise, sleeping and dietary patterns, symptom reporting, meaning-making) from the family, in school, or in other spheres of society.[248–251]

INJURY The transfer of one of the forms of physical energy (mechanical, chemical, thermal) in amounts or at rates that exceed the threshold of human tolerance. It may also result from lack of essential energy such as oxygen (e.g., drowning) or heat (e.g., hypothermia).[252]

INOCULATION See VACCINATION.

INPUT

1. The sum total of resources and energies purposefully engaged (e.g., in a health program) in order to intervene in the spontaneous operation of a system.
2. The basic resources required in terms of manpower, money, materials, and time.

INSERM Institut National de la Santé et de la Recherche Médicale (France). The French national institute for medical and health research.

INSTANTANEOUS INCIDENCE RATE See FORCE OF MORBIDITY.

INSTITUTIONAL REVIEW BOARD (IRB) The term used in the United States to describe the standing committee in a medical school, hospital, or other health care facility that is charged with ensuring the safety and well-being of human subjects involved in research. The IRB is responsible for ethical review of research proposals. Many synonyms are used in other countries, e.g., *Ethical Review Committee, Research Ethics Board.* All research, including EPIDEMIOLOGIC RESEARCH, that involves human subjects must be approved by an institutional review board or equivalent body.

INSTRUMENTAL ERROR Error due to faults arising in any or in all aspects of a measuring instrument, i.e., CALIBRATION, ACCURACY, PRECISION, etc. Also applied to error arising from impure reagents, wrong dilutions, etc.

INSTRUMENT

1. A device or questionnaire used to obtain measurements
2. An instrumental variable

INSTRUMENTAL VARIABLE See INSTRUMENTAL VARIABLE ANALYSIS.

INSTRUMENTAL VARIABLE ANALYSIS Method originally used in econometrics and some social sciences that, under certain assumptions, allows the estimation of causal effects even in the presence of unmeasured confounding for the exposure and effect of interest. An instrumental variable, or instrument, has to meet the following conditions: (1) it is associated with the exposure, (2) it affects the outcome only through the exposure, and (3) it does not share any (uncontrolled) common cause with the outcome.[253] See also CONFOUNDING BIAS; RESIDUAL CONFOUNDING.

INTEGRATION

1. The action or process of integrating. To integrate: to make a new whole; to combine parts into a new system and get them to interact so that the system expresses functions unavailable to the parts. The organizing of elements to form a coherent whole or system. Integration of knowledge from different scientific disciplines yields knowledge that no discipline alone achieves.
2. In HEALTH PROMOTION and disease PREVENTION, strategies that target several risk factors, use multiple STRATEGIES at various levels of influence, and require INTERSECTORAL ACTION. Integration entails multiplicity (more than one risk factor, level, sector, agent), and synergy resulting from multiplicity.
3. In mathematics, the process of finding an antiderivative of a given function, or its value over a specified interval.
4. In neurophysiology, the blending together of the excitatory and inhibitory nerve impulses that arrive through the thousands of synapses at a nerve cell body.

5. In medicine, the coordination within the brain of different nervous processes (e.g., sensory information from the inner ear and the eye must be integrated by the brain with other stimuli for the sense of balance and to control posture). (This definition can be a METAPHOR for INTEGRATIVE RESEARCH in many scientific fields).
6. In economics, the merging and fusion of companies or national economies.

Integration is no less crucial to science than to the functioning of postmodern societies. Examples: quality public transportation favors integration of disabled individuals and disadvantaged groups into society; integration of racial and ethnic minorities into the educational system; integration of preventive services into clinical care; political and economic processes favor integration into the European Union of Eastern European states. Synonyms, analogies and metaphors are here useful as well: *integration* involves and refers to interaction, dialogue, complicity, performance, symbiosis, sharing, pooling, porousness, amalgamation, merging, coalescing, fusing, welding, blending, weaving ...

INTEGRATIVE RESEARCH Research that integrates knowledge, data, methods, techniques, reasoning, and other scientific and cultural referents from multiple disciplines, approaches, and levels of analysis to generate knowledge that no discipline alone could achieve. For instance, research that integrates cultural, economic, and other "macro-level" or contextual factors with individual factors, as in MUTILEVEL ANALYSIS; analyses of the relationships among gene structure, expression, and function; research on the relationships among molecular pathways, pathophysiology, and clinical phenotypes, as in clinical pharmacology and clinical genetics; research that integrates interactions among environmental, genetic, and epigenetic processes.[173,254] Epidemiology is an inherently integrative discipline, and so are many of its branches, subspecialities, and approaches, like CLINICAL and MOLECULAR EPIDEMIOLOGY, SOCIAL EPIDEMIOLOGY or ENVIRONMENTAL EPIDEMIOLOGY; DEVELOPMENTAL AND LIFE COURSE EPIDEMIOLOGY, for instance, attempts to integrate biological and social risk processes.[16] See also CLINICAL STUDY; PUBLIC HEALTH IMPACT ASSESSMENT; TRANSDISCIPLINARITY; REDUCTIONISM.

INTENTION-TO-TREAT ANALYSIS A fundamental way to analyze subjects in a randomized controlled clinical trial[255,256]: all patients allocated to each arm of the treatment regimen are analyzed together "as intended" upon randomization, whether or not they actually received or completed the prescribed regimen. Failure to follow this step defeats the main purpose and advantage of RANDOM ALLOCATION and can cause serious bias. This approach is virtually always required in studies aiming to influence clinical or public health practice. It may be complemented by an explanatory analysis, in which some participants (e.g., poor compliers) are excluded from analyses.[14] Because of its pragmatic approach, intention-to-treat analysis can underestimate drug efficacy; INSTRUMENTAL VARIABLE ANALYSIS and G-ESTIMATION can be used to address this bias while making use of the random allocation. See also EFFECTIVENESS; PRAGMATIC STUDY.

INTERACTION

1. The interdependent operation of two or more causes to produce, prevent, or control an effect. *Biological interaction* means the interdependent operation of two or more biological causes to produce, prevent, or control an effect. See also ANTAGONISM; SYNERGISM.
2. Differences in the effect measure for one factor at different levels of another factor. See also EFFECT MODIFICATION; EFFECT MODIFIER.
3. The necessity for a product term in a linear model (Syn: statistical interaction).

INTERMEDIATE VARIABLE [Syn: contingent variable, intervening (causal) variable, mediator variable] A variable that occurs in a causal pathway from a causal (independent) variable to an outcome (dependent) variable. It causes variation in the outcome variable and itself is caused to vary by the original causal variable. Such a variable will be associated with both the causal and the outcome variables.

INTERNAL VALIDITY See VALIDITY, STUDY.

INTERNATIONAL CLASSIFICATION OF DISEASES (ICD) The classification of specific conditions and groups of conditions determined by an internationally representative group of experts who advise the World Health Organization, which publishes the complete list in periodic revisions. Every disease entity is assigned a number. There are 21 major divisions *(chapters)* and a hierarchical arrangement of subdivisions *(rubrics)* within each in the tenth revision. Some chapters are "etiological," e.g., Infective and Parasitic Conditions; others relate to body systems, e.g., Circulatory System; and some to classes of condition, e.g., neoplasms, injury (violence). The heterogeneity of categories reflects prevailing uncertainties about causes of disease (and classification in relation to causes). The tenth revision of the manual *(ICD-10)* was published by WHO in 1990, after ratification in 1989. See also INTERNATIONAL STATISTICAL CLASSIFICATION OF DISEASES AND RELATED HEALTH PROBLEMS (ICD-10).

INTERNATIONAL CLASSIFICATION OF HEALTH PROBLEMS IN PRIMARY CARE (ICHPPC) See INTERNATIONAL CLASSIFICATION OF PRIMARY CARE, SECOND EDITION REVISED (ICPC-2-R).

INTERNATIONAL CLASSIFICATION OF IMPAIRMENTS, DISABILITIES, AND HANDICAPS (ICIDH) First published by WHO in 1980, this is an attempt to produce a systematic TAXONOMY of the consequences of injury and disease.

An *impairment* is defined in ICIDH as any loss or abnormality of psychological, physiological, or anatomical structure or function. It is concerned with abnormalities of body structure and appearance and with organ or system function resulting from any cause; in principle, impairments represent disturbances at the organ level.

A *disability* is defined in ICIDH as any restriction or lack (resulting from an impairment) of ability to perform an activity in a manner or within the range considered normal for a human being. The term *disability* reflects the consequences of impairment in terms of functional performance and activity by the individual; disabilities thus represent disturbances at the level of the person.

A *handicap* is defined in ICIDH as a disadvantage for a given individual, resulting from an impairment or a disability, that limits or prevents the fulfillment of a role that is normal (depending on age, sex, and social and cultural practice) for that individual. The term *handicap* thus reflects interaction with and adaptation to the individual's surroundings.[22] ICIDH has been superseded by the International Classification of Functioning, Disability and Health.

INTERNATIONAL CLASSIFICATION OF PRIMARY CARE, SECOND EDITION REVISED (ICPC-2-R) The official classification of the World Organization of Family Doctors (WONCA).[257,258] WONCA is also known as the World Organization of Family Doctors. ICPC includes three elements of the doctor-patient encounter: the REASON FOR ENCOUNTER (RFE), the diagnosis, and the treatment or other action or intervention. It is a biaxial classification system based on chapters and components. It uses three-digit alphanumeric codes with mnemonic qualities to facilitate its day-to-day use. Chapters, each with an alpha code, form one axis; components with rubrics having a two-digit numeric code form the second axis. The components deal with symptoms and complaints, diagnoses and therapeutic interventions, administrative procedures and diseases. ICPC includes a detailed conversion system for linking with ICD-10 codes. See also PROBLEM-ORIENTED MEDICAL RECORD.

INTERNATIONAL COMPARISONS In epidemiology and public health, comparing regions or nations of the world in terms of disease DETERMINANTS or OUTCOMES, as in tables that show the rank order of vital statistics such as infant mortality rates, death or incidence rates for cancer, heart disease, etc. The dangers of making comparisons include the shifting tides of diagnostic fashion and the varying criteria and definitions that prevail from one nation to another. Only after ensuring that like is truly being compared with like can the comparisons be trusted, and even then only with reservations about VALIDITY. See also CROSS-CULTURAL STUDY.

INTERNATIONAL FORM OF MEDICAL CERTIFICATE OF CAUSES OF DEATH In adopting the tenth revision of *ICD* in 1990, the World Health Assembly resolved that causes of death to be entered on the medical certificate of cause of death are all those diseases, morbid conditions, or injuries that either resulted in or contributed to death and the circumstances of the accident or violence that produced such injuries. Antecedent causes and other significant conditions are also to be recorded. See DEATH CERTIFICATE.

INTERNATIONAL NOMENCLATURE OF DISEASES (IND) Since 1970, the Council for International Organizations of the Medical Sciences (CIOMS) and the WHO have collaborated in preparing an International Nomenclature of Diseases (IND). This is a complement to the ICD. The purpose of the IND is to provide a single recommended name for every disease entity. The criteria for selection are that the name should be specific, unambiguous, as self-descriptive and as simple as possible, and based on cause whenever feasible. A list of synonyms is appended to each definition.

INTERNATIONAL STATISTICAL CLASSIFICATION OF DISEASES AND RELATED HEALTH PROBLEMS The tenth revision, known in short as *ICD-10*, was approved by the International Conference for the Tenth Revision in 1989 and by the 43rd World Health Assembly in 1990. It is the latest in a series of international classifications dating back to the BERTILLON CLASSIFICATION (i.e., the International List of Causes of Death, 1893); *ICD-10* came into effect at the beginning of 1993, exactly 100 years after the original. The tenth revision has 21 chapters and uses an alphanumeric coding system in order to provide a larger coding frame than previously, leaving room for future expansion. The chapters of *ICD-10* are as follows:

I (A00–B99): Certain infectious and parasitic diseases
II (C00–C97): Neoplasms
III (D50–D89): Diseases of the blood and blood-forming organs and certain disorders involving the immune mechanism
IV (E00–E90): Endocrine, nutritional, and metabolic diseases
V (F00–F99): Mental and behavioral disorders
VI (G00–G99): Diseases of the nervous system
VII (H00–H59): Diseases of the eye and adnexa
VIII (H60–H95): Diseases of the ear and mastoid process
IX (I00–I99): Diseases of the circulatory system
X (J00–J99): Diseases of the respiratory system
XI (K00–K93): Diseases of the digestive system
XII (L00–L99): Diseases of the skin and subcutaneous tissue

XIII (M00–M99): Diseases of the musculoskeletal system and connective tissue
XIV (N00–N99): Diseases of the genitourinary system
XV (000–099): Pregnancy, childbirth, and the puerperium
XVI (P00–P96): Certain conditions originating in the perinatal period
XVII (Q00–Q99): Congenital malformations, deformations, and chromosomal abnormalities
XVIII (R00–R99): Symptoms, signs, and abnormal clinical and laboratory findings not elsewhere classified
XIX (S00–T98): Injury, poisoning, and certain other consequences of external causes
XX (V01–Y99): External causes of morbidity and mortality
XXI (Z00–Z99): Factors influencing health status and contact with health services

INTERPOLATE, INTERPOLATION To predict the value of variates within the range of observations; the resulting prediction.

INTERPRETIVE BIAS (Syn: interpretative bias, bias of interpretation)

1. Error arising from inference and speculation. Among others, two sources of the error are (a) failure of the investigators to consider all relevant and rationally defensible interpretations coherent with the facts and to assess the scientific support of each interpretation and (b) mishandling of cases that constitute exceptions to some general conclusion.
2. Errors that can occur in interpretative and evaluative processes of scientific evidence.[34]

The interpretive process is a necessary and inevitable aspect of science. Science commonly has subjective and cultural components.[259] Although unbiased interpretation of data is as important as performing rigorous experiments, evaluative processes are seldom totally objective or completely independent of scientists' convictions and theoretical apparatus. Good science inevitably embodies a tension between concrete data and deeply held convictions. Subjectivity is always alive at the cutting edge of scientific progress, where new ideas develop.[260] Lack of objective measures for the subjective components of interpretation makes no less important the interaction between data and judgment. Recognition of interpretative processes in epidemiology should not lead to a naive relativism or to deem all claims to knowledge equally valid because of subjectivity. A view that science is totally objective is mythical and ignores the human element of epidemiological inquiry.[34,127] See also AUXILIARY HYPOTHESIS BIAS; COGNITIVE DISSONANCE BIAS; CONFIRMATION BIAS; MECHANISTIC BIAS; PUBLICATION BIAS; RESCUE BIAS; "TIME WILL TELL" BIAS.

INTERSECTORAL ACTION (Syn: intersectoral collaboration) Activities and STRATEGIES involving several components of the body politic (e.g., the health sector, the education sector, the housing sector) that, working together, can enhance health conditions more effectively than when working independently of one another. See also HEALTH IN ALL POLICIES; HEALTHY PUBLIC POLICIES.

INTERVAL The set containing all numbers between two given numbers.

INTERVAL ESTIMATE An interval within which a parameter under study (such as a RELATIVE RISK) is stated to lie with a particular degree of confidence, likelihood, or probability based on an analysis of a study or multiple studies. See also CONFIDENCE INTERVAL; LIKELIHOOD INTERVAL; POSTERIOR INTERVAL.

INTERVAL INCIDENCE DENSITY See PERSON-TIME INCIDENCE RATE.

INTERVAL SCALE See MEASUREMENT SCALE.

INTERVENING CAUSE See INTERMEDIATE VARIABLE.

INTERVENING VARIABLE

1. Synonym for INTERMEDIATE VARIABLE
2. A variable whose value is altered in order to block or alter the effect(s) of another factor

See also CAUSALITY.

INTERVENTION INDEX An estimate of the impact of a therapeutic or preventive intervention.[261] It is the ratio of the number of persons whose risk level must change to prevent one premature death to the total number at risk. See also ABSOLUTE RISK REDUCTION (ARR); IMPACT NUMBERS; NUMBER NEEDED TO TREAT (NNT); RELATIVE RISK REDUCTION (RRR).

INTERVENTION STUDY An investigation involving intentional change in some aspect of the status of the subjects, e.g., introduction of a preventive or therapeutic regimen or an intervention designed to test a hypothesized relationship; usually an EXPERIMENT such as a RANDOMIZED CONTROLLED TRIAL.

INTERVIEWER BIAS Systematic error due to interviewers' subconscious or conscious gathering of selective data or influencing subject response.

INTERVIEW SCHEDULE The precisely designed set of questions used in an interview. See also SURVEY INSTRUMENT.

INTRACLASS CORRELATION

1. In sibship studies in genetics, the variance of genotypes as a proportion of the variance of phenotypes.
2. In surveys and group-randomized studies, the extent to which members of a group (cluster) resemble each other more than they resemble members of other groups (clusters). See DESIGN EFFECT.

INVERSE PROBABILITY WEIGHTING A method for the estimation of causal effects under the assumption of no unmeasured confounders. An extension of inverse weighting methods used in survey sampling and missing data analysis. Individuals in the study population are weighted by the inverse of their probability of having the level of exposure they actually have given their covariates, creating a pseudopopulation in which, theoretically, there is no confounding by the covariates used to estimate the weights.[262] See also G-ESTIMATION; MARGINAL STRUCTURAL MODELS.

INVOLUNTARY SMOKING (Syn: passive smoking) Exposure to secondhand tobacco smoke, a mixture of exhaled mainstream smoke and sidestream smoke released from a smoldering cigarette or other smoking device (e.g., cigar, pipe, bidi) and diluted with ambient air. It involves inhaling carcinogens and other toxic components present in secondhand tobacco smoke; the latter is sometimes referred to as "ENVIRONMENTAL" TOBACCO SMOKE (ETS). It includes both smoke exhaled by smokers and smoke released directly from burning tobacco into ambient air; the latter is called SIDESTREAM SMOKE and contains higher proportions of carcinogenic substances and other toxic agents than exhaled smoke. The adjective *involuntary* is preferable to *passive*, as the latter may imply acquiescence. Involuntary smoking (exposure to secondhand or "environmental" tobacco smoke) is carcinogenic to humans (group 1 of IARC).

ISLAND POPULATION A group of individuals isolated from larger groups and possessing a relatively limited gene pool; alternatively, a group that is immunologically isolated and may therefore be unduly susceptible to infection with alien pathogens.

ISEE International Society for Environmental Epidemiology (www.iseepi.org).

ISODEMOGRAPHIC MAP (Syn: density-equalizing map) A diagrammatic method of displaying administrative jurisdictions of a country in two-dimensional "maps" with areas directly proportional to the population of the jurisdictions. Thus densely populated urban regions occupy large areas of the map and sparsely inhabited rural regions occupy small areas. Additional data—such as incidence or mortality rates within each jurisdiction—can be superimposed in colors or shading to represent rates.

ISOLATE (noun)

1. In genetics, a subpopulation, generally small, in which matings take place exclusively with other members of the same subpopulation
2. In microbiology, a pure culture of an organism

ISOLATION

1. In microbiology, the separation of an organism from others, usually by making serial cultures.
2. Separation, for the period of communicability, of infected persons or animals from others under such conditions as to prevent or limit the transmission of the infectious agent from those infected to those who are susceptible or who may spread the agent to others. The *CDC Guidelines for Isolation Precautions in Hospitals* (1990) expanded on the blood and body fluid precautions described below. *Control of Communicable Disease Manual* [52] lists seven categories of isolation:
   a. *Strict isolation:* To prevent transmission of highly contagious or virulent infections that may be spread by both air and contact. The specifications include a private room and the use of masks, gowns, and gloves for all persons entering the room. Special ventilation requirements with the room at negative pressure to surrounding areas are desirable.
   b. *Contact isolation:* For less highly transmissible or serious infections and diseases or conditions that are spread primarily by close or direct contact. A private room is indicated but patients infected with the same pathogen may share a room. Masks are indicated for those who come close to the patient, gowns are indicated if soiling is likely, and gloves are indicated for touching infectious material.
   c. *Respiratory isolation:* To prevent transmission of infectious diseases over short distances through the air, a private room is indicated, but patients infected with the same organism may share a room. In addition to the basic requirements, masks are indicated for those who come in close contact with the patient; gowns and gloves are not indicated.
   d. *Tuberculosis isolation (AFB isolation):* For patients with pulmonary tuberculosis who have a positive sputum smear or chest x-rays that strongly suggest active tuberculosis. Specifications include use of a private room with special ventilation and closed door. Masks are used only if the patient is coughing and does not reliably and consistently cover the mouth. Gowns are used to prevent gross CONTAMINATION of clothing. Gloves are not indicated.
   e. *Enteric precautions:* For infections transmitted by direct or indirect contact with feces. Specifications include use of a private room if patient hygiene is poor. Masks are not indicated; gowns should be used if soiling is likely, and gloves are to be used for touching contaminated materials.
   f. *Drainage/secretion precautions:* To prevent infections transmitted by direct or indirect contact with purulent material or drainage from an infected body site.

A private room and masking are not indicated; gowns should be used if soiling is likely and gloves used for touching contaminated materials.

g. *Blood/body fluid precautions:* To prevent infections that are transmitted by direct or indirect contact with infected blood or body fluids. In addition to the basic requirements, a private room is indicated if patient hygiene is poor; masks are not indicated; gowns should be used if soiling of clothing with blood or body fluids is likely. Gloves should be used for touching blood or body fluids. Blood and body fluid precautions should be used consistently for all patients regardless of their blood-borne infection status ("universal blood and body fluid precautions"). These are intended to prevent parenteral, mucous membrane, and nonintact-skin exposure of health care workers to blood-borne pathogens. Protective barriers include gloves, gowns, masks, and protective eyewear. See also UNIVERSAL PRECAUTIONS. See also QUARANTINE.

ISOMETRIC CHART A chart or graph that portrays three dimensions on a plane surface.

IVDU Intravenous drug user, a high-risk group for transmission of blood-borne infection, especially HIV and hepatitis C.

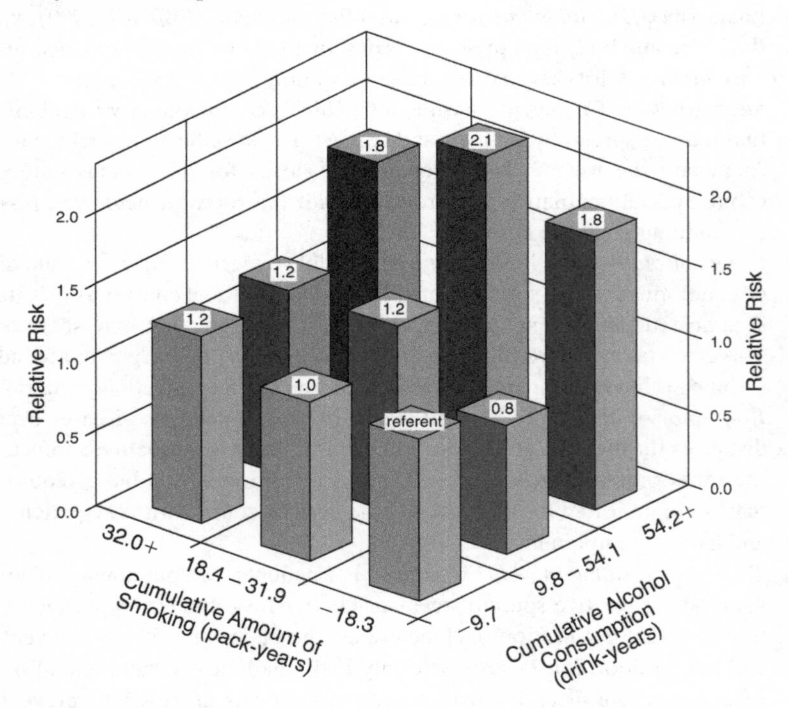

Isometric chart. Relative risks of hepatocellular carcinoma according to cumulative alcohol consumption and amount of smoking. From Tanaka K, Hirohata T. *Jpn J Epidemiol.* 1992; 2:2(Suppl):S-167. With permission.

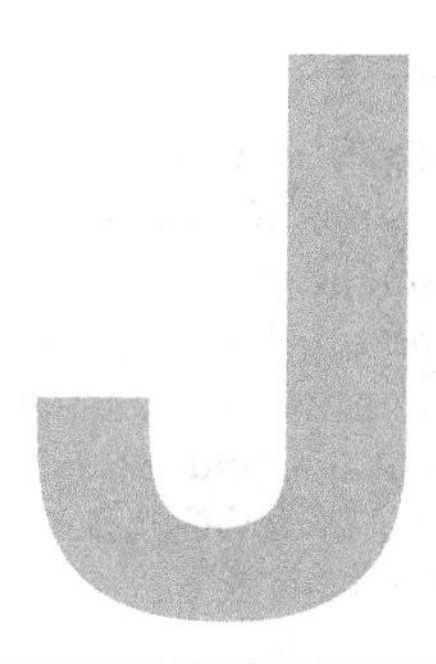

JACKKNIFE A technique for estimating the variance and the bias of an estimator. If the sample size is n, the estimator is applied to each subsample of size $n - 1$, obtained by dropping a measurement from analysis. The sum of squared differences between each of the resulting estimates and their mean, multiplied by $(n - 1)/n$, is the jackknife estimate of variance; the difference between the mean and the original estimate, multiplied by $(n - 1)$, is the jackknife estimate of bias.

JARGON Words and expressions used by a particular group, commonly members of a profession or trade (e.g., doctors, lawyers, astronauts, police). Derived from late Middle English *iargouon*, Old French, *jargoun*, meaning twittering of birds, incomprehensible sounds. Fowler's *Modern English Usage* and Sir Ernest Gowers's *Plain Words* remark adversely and at length on jargon, but perhaps the best description is Murphy's, reproduced in the preface of earlier editions of this dictionary: "obscure and/or pretentious language, circumlocutions, invented meanings, and pomposity delighted in for its own sake."[263] Murphy distinguishes between jargon and technical vocabulary, which expresses complex abstract thoughts with high resolution and precision, whereas jargon merely obfuscates. Medicine and its specialties, including epidemiology, are infested with jargon. Some can be detected in the words and phrases defined in this book. Although jargon can have legitimate uses among members of a group all of whom understand its exact meaning, it is always preferable to abide by Gowers's admonition and use plain words whenever they are sufficiently precise.

JARMAN SCORE An index of community-wide social deprivation, used mainly by general practitioners in the United Kingdom.[264] Unlike the TOWNSEND SCORE, the Jarman score has no theoretical basis; it uses weighted values for percentages of elderly persons living alone; children aged under 5 years; single-parent families; social class V (unskilled workers); the unemployed; overcrowded dwellings; changed address in the past year; ethnic minorities. The Jarman score correlates quite well with other indexes as a measure of group socioeconomic status in administratively defined jurisdictions such as urban areas. See also GINI COEFFICIENT; OVERCROWDING; TOWNSEND SCORE.

JELLINEK FORMULA A formula to estimate the prevalence of alcohol-related disease, based on the assumption that a predictable proportion of persons addicted to alcohol die of cirrhosis of the liver (confirmed by necropsy).[265] The formula fails to allow for biases (e.g., in autopsy series), for the frequency of other causes of cirrhosis, and for variations in the dose response and end-organ damage produced by alcohol abuse. It is therefore flawed.

JOB EXPOSURE MATRIX (JEM) A cross-classification of jobs and occupational exposures. Some matrices are based on tasks instead of jobs. JEMs may be based on the assessment by experts of likely occupational exposures (chemical, physical, biological, and psychosocial agents) for an open or fixed list of jobs (or tasks), usually coded according to some established national or international classification system. Some JEMs also include information for different calendar time periods.[266]

JOB STRAIN MODELS Models to explain work-related stress based on dimensions as job demands (e.g., psychological conflicts related to work pace or workload) and job control (or job decision latitude, defined as the combination of the worker's job decision-making authority and use of skills on the job). Jobs characterized by high "psychological workload demands" and low "decision latitude" increase risk for psychological job strain. Research in occupational epidemiology has shown that increased decision latitude is often preferable to reduced job demand so as to reduce mental strain. A third dimension is workplace social support (given by workmates, supervisors, employers), which may act as an effect modifier over the other two dimensions.[266]

JONES CRITERIA A set of clinical and laboratory findings for the diagnosis of rheumatic fever. The criteria include presence of group A hemolytic streptococcal infection; major manifestations (carditis, polyarthritis, etc.); minor manifestations (fever, arthralgia, etc.); ancillary tests (raised erythrocyte sedimentation rate, C-reactive protein, etc.).

JUSTICE

1. A morally defensible distribution of benefits and rewards in society. Equity or fairness—e.g., regarding the fair distribution in the population of benefits and risks of research, health care, or other goods. There is a diversity of views among epidemiologists worlwide with respect to the idea that health is a basic need and therefore an issue of social justice. See also HEALTH EQUITY.
2. In law, the successful administration of the rule of law.

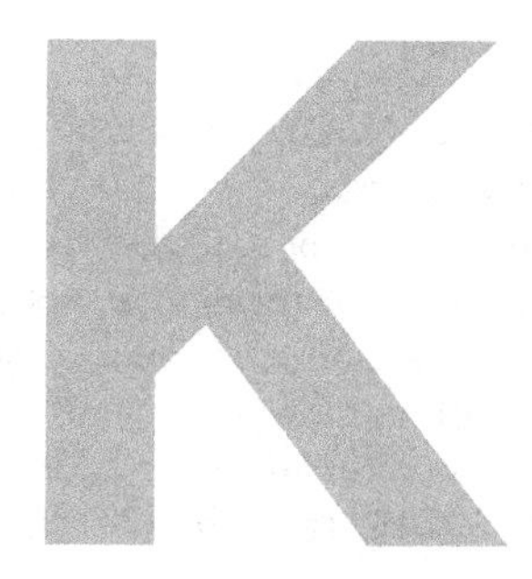

KAP (KNOWLEDGE, ATTITUDES, PRACTICE) SURVEY A formal survey, using face-to-face interviews, in which people are asked standardized pretested questions dealing with their knowledge of, attitudes toward, and use of contraceptive methods. Detailed reproductive histories and attitudes toward desired family size are also elicited. Analysis of responses provides much useful information on family planning and gives estimates of possible future trends in population structure. The term has sometimes been used to describe other varieties of surveys of knowledge, attitudes, and practice (e.g., health promotion in general or, in particular, cigarette smoking).

KAPLAN-MEIER ESTIMATE (Syn: product-limit method) A nonparametric method of estimating survival probabilities from LIFE TABLES.[267] This combines calculated probabilities of survival and estimates to allow for CENSORED observations, which are assumed to occur randomly. The intervals are defined as ending each time an event (death, withdrawal) occurs; they may therefore be unequal.

KAPPA A measure of the degree of nonrandom agreement between observers or measurements of the same categorical variable

$$\kappa = \frac{P_0 - P_e}{1 - P_e}$$

where P_0 is the proportion of times the measurements agree and P_e is the proportion of times they can be expected to agree by chance alone. If the measurements agree more often than expected by chance, kappa is positive; if concordance is complete, kappa = 1; if there is no more nor less than chance concordance, kappa = 0; if the measurements disagree more than expected by chance, kappa is negative.

KENDALL'S TAU See CORRELATION COEFFICIENT.

KNOWLEDGE CONSTRUCTION A production-oriented approach to the understanding of science. Analyses of how knowledge is created identify strategies that scientists employ in their work, discursive fact production, features of fact construction shared across contemporary sciences and EPISTEMIC COMMUNITIES, devices of representation, laboratory cultures, object reconfiguration in the laboratory, knowledge cultures and their "epistemic machineries" (i.e., their machineries of knowledge production), or social mechanisms of consensus formation. Interest in the process of knowledge production has led to an improved understanding of science as a practical accomplishment.[268] See also SOCIOLOGY OF SCIENTIFIC KNOWLEDGE.

KOCH'S POSTULATES See HENLE-KOCH POSTULATES. See also CAUSALITY; EVANS'S POSTULATES.

KRIGING A method first used in the earth sciences to smooth data from spatially scattered point measurements (e.g., drill sites). It is used in geographic epidemiology.[269] The method relies on analysis of the spatial variability of the data and allows representation of the variable under study as a continuous process throughout the country. The method is named for its developer, D. G. Krige.

KURTOSIS The extent to which a unimodal distribution is peaked.

LARGE-SAMPLE METHOD (Syn: asymptotic method) Any statistical method based on an approximation that becomes more accurate as sample size increases. Examples include chi-square tests on a set of frequencies and normal tests of estimates from frequency data.

LATE MATERNAL DEATH See MATERNAL MORTALITY.

LATENT CLASS ANALYSIS A type of statistical analysis used to group variables or observations into distinct clusters, based on the assumption that there are underlying "latent classes" within the data. Analysis can be cross-sectional or longitudinal, i.e., it can identify clusters of distinct variables at a point in time or patterns in a variable over a period of time.

LATENT HETEROGENEITY Epidemiological data that are too heterogeneous to be described by a simple MATHEMATICAL MODEL such as the binomial or Poisson distribution, suggestive of the effect of unidentified risk factors.

LATENT IMMUNIZATION See IMMUNIZATION, LATENT.

LATENT INFECTION Persistence of an infectious agent within the host without symptoms (and often without demonstrable presence in blood, tissues, or bodily secretions of the host).

LATENCY PERIOD (Syn: latent period, latency) Two mutually incompatible definitions are commonly used in the health and life sciences:

1. The interval from initiation of the disease to clinical emergence of the disease (e.g., appearance of manifestations) or to disease detection. Thus, according to this definition, the latency period begins when the INDUCTION PERIOD ends, at the initiation of the disease. In infectious disease epidemiology, the period between exposure and the onset of infectiousness (which may be shorter or longer than the INCUBATION PERIOD).
2. The interval between initiation of exposure to the causal agent and appearance or detection of the health process; e.g., from onset of exposure to the disease-causing agent to appearance of manifestations of the disease. Thus, according to this definition, the latency period begins when the INDUCTION PERIOD begins, at the initiation of exposure to the disease-causing agent.

The two definitions agree that the latency period ends when the disease becomes clinically apparent and/or detectable; in the first definition, the induction period is followed by the latency period (there is no overlap), whereas in the second definition the latency period includes the entire induction period. See also SOJOURN TIME.

LATIN SQUARE One of the basic statistical designs for experiments that aim at removing from the experimental error the variation from two sources, which may be identified with the rows and columns of the square. In such a design, the allocation of k experimental treatments in the cells of a k by k (Latin) square is such that each treatment occurs exactly once in each row and column.[98] A design for a 5 × 5 square is as follows:

A B C D E
B A E C D
C D A E B
D E B A C
E C D B A

LAW OF LARGE NUMBERS This law, enunciated by Jacob Bernoulli (1654–1705), states that the accuracy of a sample mean is increased (or the standard error of a statistic is reduced) as the numbers studied increase. The larger the sample, the more likely it is to be representative of the "universe" population. This law is valid only with unbiased samples.

LEAD TIME The time gained in treating or controlling a disease when detection is earlier than usual (e.g., in the presymptomatic stage), as when screening procedures are used for EARLY DETECTION OF DISEASE.

LEAD-TIME BIAS (Syn: zero time shift) Overestimation of survival time, owing to the backward shift in the starting point for measuring survival that arises when diseases such as cancer are detected early, as by screening procedures. A systematic error arising when follow-up of groups does not begin at comparable stages in the natural history of a condition. For example, interventions for women whose breast cancer is detected by screening cannot be validly compared with interventions for women whose disease is first detected by clinical examination at a later stage of the disease.[14,62,63] See also INCEPTION COHORT; ZERO-TIME SHIFT.

LEAST SQUARES A principle of estimation, attributed to Gauss and Legendre, in which the estimates of a set of parameters in a statistical model are those quantities that minimize the sum of squared differences between the observed values of the dependent variable and the values predicted by the model.

LEDERMANN FORMULA The observation by Ledermann[270] that the frequency distribution of alcohol consumption in the population of consumers may be log-normal; the curve is sharply skewed – approximately one-third of drinkers consume more than 60% of the total amount of alcohol. Among drinkers, the proportion of persons with alcoholism remains constant at around 7%–9%. The pattern of consumption of illicit drugs among users may also be log-normal. Questions have been raised, however, about the validity of some assumptions upon which the formula is based.

LENGTH BIAS

1. A systematic error due to selection of disproportionate numbers of long-duration cases (patients who survive longest) in one group but not in another. This can occur when prevalent rather than incident cases are included in a case-control study.
2. Given that biologically and clinically aggressive diseases often have a shorter asymptomatic pre-clinical period than less aggressive diseases, a SCREENING program is more likely to detect slower progressing diseases (e.g., slow-growing tumors), which

have better prognosis (e.g., survival).[14,62,63] The screening program may thus falsely appear to improve survival as compared to a cohort including a wider spectrum of disease. See also INCEPTION COHORT; LATENCY PERIOD; SCREENING.

LENGTH OF THE GENERATION Time required for the replacement of a female generation by their daughters of reproductive age.

LEVIN'S ATTRIBUTABLE RISK See ATTRIBUTABLE FRACTION (POPULATION).

LIFE COURSE The natural history of human life. A term for conditions that evolve over a large part or all of the life span from infancy, or even from conception, through adolescence, adult life, and senescence, sometimes peaking in early adult life, sometimes in middle age, but generally progressing throughout life as a person grows older. The term arose in recognition of the fact that the natural history of many chronic diseases and the natural life span of humans are intertwined. *Life cycle* has been used in other scientific disciplines to describe a series of distinct, bounded life stages that are socially and/or biologically determined. The concept of *life span* used in psychology assumes that development and aging form a continuous process from birth to death. The distinction between *life span* and *life course* is mainly a matter of scientific history.[16,113] See also ACCUMULATION OF RISK; DEVELOPMENTAL ORIGINS HYPOTHESIS; DEVELOPMENTAL AND LIFE COURSE EPIDEMIOLOGY; ECOLOGICAL TRANSITION; SOCIAL EPIDEMIOLOGY.

LIFE CYCLE See LIFE COURSE.

LIFE EVENTS Aspects of the pattern of living that may be associated with or produce changes in health. The relationship of "life stress" and "emotional stress" to onset of several kinds of serious chronic disease, such as coronary heart disease and hypertension, has been the subject of epidemiological studies. The Rahe-Holmes Social Readjustment Rating Scale[271] was the first to be developed to assign ranks or ratings to significant life events such as death of a spouse or other close relative, loss of regular job, relocation, marriage, divorce, etc. Many other rating scales have since been developed.

LIFE EXPECTANCY See EXPECTATION OF LIFE.

LIFE EXPECTANCY FREE FROM DISABILITY (LEFD) An estimate of life expectancy adjusted for activity-limitation (data for which are derived from hospital discharge statistics, etc.). See also DISABILITY-ADJUSTED LIFE YEARS (DALYs); DISABILITY-FREE LIFE EXPECTANCY; QUALITY-ADJUSTED LIFE YEARS (QALYs).

LIFE EXPECTANCY WITH DISABILITY The average number of years an individual is expected to live with disability if current patterns of mortality and disability continue to apply. See DISABILITY-FREE LIFE EXPECTANCY.

LIFE SPAN See LIFE COURSE.

LIFESTYLE The set of habits and customs that is influenced, modified, encouraged, or constrained by the lifelong process of socialization. These habits and customs include use of substances such as alcohol, tobacco, tea, coffee; dietary habits; exercise; etc., which have important implications for health and are often the subject of epidemiological investigations.

LIFE TABLE (Syn: actuarial table) A summarizing technique used to describe the pattern of mortality and survival in populations. The survival data are time-specific and cumulative probabilities of survival of a group of individuals subject, throughout life, to the age-specific death rates in question. The life-table method can be applied to the study not only of death but also of any defined endpoint, such as the onset of disease or the occurrence of specific complication(s) of disease. The survivors to age x are denoted by the symbol l_x, the expectation of life at age x is denoted by the symbol $\mathring{e}_x$, and the proportion alive at age x who die between age x and $x + 1$ years is denoted by the symbol nq_x. The life table method is used in public health and in assessments of treatment regimens in clinical practice.

The first rudimentary life tables were published in 1693 by the astronomer Edmund Halley. These made use of records of the funerals in the city of Breslau. In 1815 in England, the first actuarially correct life table was published, based on both population and death data classified by age.

Two types of life tables may be distinguished according to the reference year of the table: the current, or period, life table and the generation, or cohort, life table.

The current life table is a summary of mortality experience over a brief period (1 to 3 years), and the population data relate to the middle of that period (usually close to the date of a census). A current life table therefore represents the combined mortality experience by age of the population in a particular short period of time.

The cohort, or generation, life table describes the actual survival experience of a group, or cohort, of individuals born at about the same time. Theoretically, the mortality experience of the persons in the cohort would be observed from their moment of birth through each consecutive age in successive calendar years until all of them die.

The clinical life table describes the outcome experience of a group, or cohort, of individuals classified according to their exposure or treatment history.

Life tables are also classified according to the length of age interval in which the data are presented. A complete life table contains data for every single year of age, from birth to the last applicable age. An abridged life table contains data by intervals of 5 or 10 years of age. See also EXPECTATION OF LIFE; SURVIVORSHIP STUDY.

LIFE TABLE, EXPECTATION OF LIFE FUNCTION, $\mathring{e}_x$ (Syn: average future lifetime) The expectation of life function is a statement of the average number of years of life remaining to persons who survive to age x.

LIFE TABLE, SURVIVORSHIP FUNCTION, l_x The survivorship function is a statement of the number of persons out of an initial population of defined size (e.g., 100,000 live births) who would survive or remain free of a defined endpoint condition to age x under the age-specific rates for the specified year. The value of l_{40}, for example, is determined by the cumulative operation of the specific death rates for all ages below 40.

LIFETIME RISK The risk to an individual that a given health effect will occur at any time after exposure without regard for the time at which that effect occurs.

LIKELIHOOD FUNCTION A function constructed from a statistical model and a set of observed data that gives the probability of the observed data for various values of the unknown model parameters. Values for the parameters that maximize this function are called MAXIMUM LIKELIHOOD ESTIMATES of the parameters.

LIKELIHOOD INTERVAL An interval containing all parameter values that have a value of the LIKELIHOOD FUNCTION greater than a certain proportion of the maximum; e.g., one seventh of the maximum, which roughly corresponds to a 95% confidence interval in most cases.

LIKELIHOOD RATIO

1. The ratio of the values of the LIKELIHOOD FUNCTION at two different parameter values or under two different data models. Usually, one of the two values is taken to be the maximum of the function (the value of the function at the maximum-likelihood estimates). See LIKELIHOOD-RATIO TEST.

2. The probability that a given test result would occur in a person with the target disorder divided by the probability that the same result would occur in a person without that disorder. It can be calculated for any level of a test result (for continuous diagnostic tests with many possible cutoff values) as the ratio of the probability of that test result among individuals with the target disorder to the probability of that same test result among individuals who are free of the target disorder. For a positive result, the likelihood ratio equals the ratio sensitivity/(1 – specificity). For a negative test result the likelihood ratio equals (1 – sensitivity)/specificity.

Likelihood ratios are used to appraise screening and diagnostic tests. See also SENSITIVITY AND SPECIFICITY.

LIKELIHOOD-RATIO TEST A statistical test based on the ratio of the maximum value of the likelihood function under one statistical model to the maximum value under another statistical model; the models differ in that one includes and the other excludes one or more parameters.

LIKERT SCALE An ordinal scale of responses to a question or statement ordered in a hierarchical sequence, such as from "strongly agree" through "no opinion" to "strongly disagree." Rensis Likert, a social psychologist, developed an empirical method for assigning numerical scores to such a scale.

LINEAR MODEL A statistical model in which the average value of a dependent variable y at a given value of a factor, x, is assumed to be equal to $\alpha + \beta x$, where α and β are unknown constants.

LINEAR REGRESSION REGRESSION ANALYSIS using linear models.

LINKAGE See GENETIC LINKAGE; RECORD LINKAGE.

LINKAGE DISEQUILIBRIUM A condition in which alleles at two loci or genes are found together in a population at a greater frequency than predicted simply by the product of their individual allele frequencies. Alleles at markers near disease-causing genes tend to be in linkage disequilibrium in the affected individuals.[23]

LIVE BIRTH WHO definition adopted by the Third World Health Assembly, 1950: "Live birth is the complete expulsion or extraction from its mother of a product of conception, irrespective of the duration of the pregnancy, which, after such separation, breathes or shows any other evidence of life, such as beating of the heart, pulsation of the umbilical cord, or definite movement of voluntary muscles, whether or not the umbilical cord has been cut or the placenta is attached; each product of such a birth is considered live born."

In the *Report of WHO Expert Committee on Prevention of Perinatal Mortality and Morbidity* (Technical Report Series 457, 1970), it is noted that the above definition requires the inclusion as live births of very early and patently nonviable fetuses and that accordingly it is not strictly applied. The committee suggested, therefore, that the WHO should introduce a viability criterion into the definition so that very immature fetuses surviving for very short periods were excluded, even though they showed one or more of the transitory signs of life. The Conference for the Tenth Revision of the International Classification of Diseases (*ICD-10*) recommended that the above definitions, adopted for *ICD-9*, should remain unchanged.

LOCUS

1. The position of a point, as defined by the coordinates on a graph
2. The position that a gene occupies on a chromosome

LOD SCORE In genetics, the log odds ratio of observed to expected distribution of genetic markers.

LOGIC The branch of philosophy and science that deals with canons of thought and criteria of validity in reasoning. Logic relies on precise definition of tangible objects, terms, and concepts; rational classification; application of fundamental principles of the underlying field of scholarship (mathematics, physics, ethics, etc.); and minimal use of axioms and assumptions. Properly done, epidemiology applies logic to arrive at conclusions about cause-and-effect relationships.[180,263] See also HYPOTHETICO-DEDUCTIVE METHOD.

LOGICAL FRAMEWORK (LOGFRAME) ANALYSIS A method of project or program planning that uses a matrix of the goal, purpose, expected results, and activities on the vertical axis and the performance indicators, means of verification, and assumptions on the horizontal axis. The approach is often conducted in a group setting with facilitation, so as to promote teamwork and ownership of the plan. The matrix can be used also for project monitoring and evaluation and may be updated in response to changes in the timetable, performance, or feasibility of component activities. Logframe planning is favored by some international development agencies.

LOGISTIC MODEL A statistical model for an individual's risk (probability of disease y) as a function of a risk factor x:

$$P(y|x) = \frac{1}{1+e^{-\alpha-\beta x}} = \text{expit}(\alpha+\beta x)$$

where e is the (natural) exponential function and expit is the logistic function. This model has a desirable range, 0 to 1 and other attractive statistical features. In the multiple logistic model, the term βx is replaced by a linear term involving several factors, e.g., $\beta 1 x_1 + \beta 2 x_2$ if there are two factors x_1 and x_2.

LOGIT (Syn: log-odds) The natural logarithm of the ratio of the ODDS.

LOGIT MODEL A linear model for the logit (natural log of the odds) of disease as a function of one or more fctors X:

$$\text{Logit (disease given } X = x) = \alpha+\beta x$$

This model is mathematically equivalent to the LOGISTIC MODEL.

LOG-LINEAR MODEL A statistical model that uses a LINEAR MODEL for the logarithms of frequency counts in contingency tables.

LOG-NORMAL DISTRIBUTION If a variable Y is such that the natural log of Y is normally distributed, it is said to have log-normal distribution. This is a SKEW DISTRIBUTION. See also NORMAL DISTRIBUTION.

LONGITUDINAL STUDY See COHORT STUDY.

LOST TO FOLLOW-UP Study subjects in a COHORT STUDY whose outcomes are unknown (e.g., because they could not or did not wish to attend follow-up visits). See also ATTRITION; CENSORING; COHORT.

LOW BIRTH WEIGHT See BIRTH WEIGHT.

"LUMPING AND SPLITTING" Derisive term describing the propensity of some researchers to group related phenomena or to separate phenomena that hitherto had been grouped.

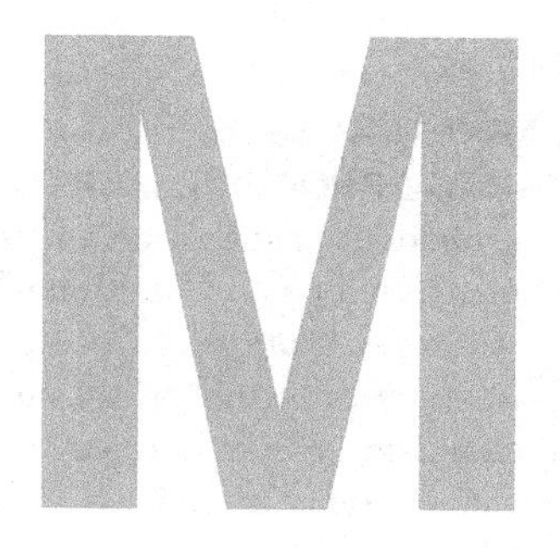

MACHINE LEARNING The ability of a program to learn from experience—i.e., to modify its execution on the basis of newly acquired information. In epidemiology and bioinformatics, examples include artificial neural networks, support vector machines, Bayesian networks, and other methods that update their procedures as new data are provided.[176]

MANN-WHITNEY TEST A test that compares two groups of ordinal scores, showing the probability that they form parts of the same distribution. It is a nonparametric equivalent of the *t*-test.

MANTEL-HAENSZEL ESTIMATE, MANTEL-HAENSZEL ODDS RATIO Mantel and Haenszel provided an adjusted ("summary") ODDS RATIO estimate that may be derived from grouped and matched sets of data.[272] It is now known as the Mantel-Haenszel estimate, one of the few eponymous terms of modern epidemiology.

The statistic may be regarded as a type of weighted average of the individual odds ratios, derived from dividing a sample into a series of strata. Ideally, the strata would be internally homogeneous with respect to confounding factors. The Mantel-Haenszel method can also be extended to the summarization of rate ratios and rate differences from follow-up studies.

MANTEL-HAENSZEL TEST (SYN: COCHRAN-MANTEL-HAENSZEL TEST) A summary CHI-SQUARE TEST developed by Mantel and Haenszel for stratified data and used when controlling for CONFOUNDING. It is a slight modification of an earlier test by William Gemmel Cochran.

MANTEL'S TREND TEST A regression test of the ODDS RATIO against a numerical variable representing ordered categories of exposure. It generalizes the MANTEL-HAENSZEL TEST can be used to analyze results of any study, including a CASE-CONTROL STUDY.

MARGINAL STRUCTURAL MODELS Statistical models that use INVERSE PROBABILITY WEIGHTING for the estimation of causal effects in longitudinal studies in which there are time-varying confounders affected by prior exposure.[273] Marginal structural models aim, for instance, to control for the effects of time-dependent confounders affected by prior treatment. These models cannot be used to estimate the effects of dynamic treatment regimes. They can, however, be used to estimate the effect of a nondynamic treatment regime when the data are derived from a cohort study in which the treatment regime is dynamic. They can be an alternative to G-ESTIMATION of structural nested models.

MARGINALS The row and column totals of a contingency table.

MARGIN OF SAFETY An estimate of the ratio of the no-observed-effect level (NOEL) to the level accepted in regulations. See also NO-OBSERVED-ADVERSE-EFFECT LEVEL.

MARKETING See SOCIAL MARKETING.

MARKOV PROCESS, MARKOV CHAIN A stochastic process such that the conditional probability distribution for the state at any future instant, given the present state, is unaffected by any additional knowledge of the past history of the system. Invented by Andrei A. Markov (1856–1922). A family of regression models for correlated data used to study event histories that include transitions between several states; e.g., Markov chains are a common way of modeling the progression of a chronic disease through various severity states; for these models, a transition matrix with the probabilities of moving from one state to another for a specific time interval is usually estimated from cohort data. Several types of Markov models (e.g., "hidden Markov models") are applied in health services research, health economics, clinical epidemiology, infectious disease epiemiology, genetic epidemiology, and systems biology. See also MONTE-CARLO STUDY.

MASKED STUDY See BLIND(ED) STUDY.

MASKING (Syn: blinding) Procedures intended to keep participants in a study from knowing some facts or observations that might bias or influence their actions or decisions regarding the study.

MASS ACTION PRINCIPLE A fundamental principle of epidemic theory:[274,275] the incidence of an infectious disease one SERIAL INTERVAL in the future is dependent on the product of the current prevalence and the number of susceptibles in the population:

$$C_{t+1} = C_t \times S_t \times r$$

where

C_{t+1} = the number of new cases one serial interval in the future
C_t = the number of current cases
S_t = the number of susceptibles
r = the INFECTION TRANSMISSION PARAMETER

MATCHED CONTROLS See CONTROLS, MATCHED.

MATCHING The process of making a study group and a comparison group similar or identical with respect to their distribution of extraneous factors.[12,31,97] Several kinds of matching can be distinguished:

1. *Caliper matching* is the process of matching comparison group subjects to study group subjects within a specified distance for a continuous variable (e.g., matching age to within 2 years).
2. *Frequency matching* requires that the frequency distributions of the matched variable(s) be similar in study and comparison groups.
3. *Category matching* is the process of matching study and control group subjects in prespecified categories, such as occupational groups or age groups.
4. *Individual matching* relies on identifying individual subjects for comparison, each resembling a study subject on the matched variable(s).
5. *Pair matching* is individual matching in which study and comparison subjects are paired.

MATERNAL MORTALITY Several definitions related to maternal mortality have been agreed upon by internationally representative groups under the auspices of the WHO.

A *maternal death* is death of a woman while pregnant or within 42 days of termination of pregnancy, irrespective of the duration and the site of pregnancy, from any cause related to or aggravated by the pregnancy or its management but not from accidental or incidental causes.

A *late maternal death* is the death of a woman from direct or indirect obstetric causes more than 42 days but less than 1 year after termination of pregnancy.

A *pregnancy-related death* is death of a woman while pregnant or within 42 days of termination of pregnancy, irrespective of the cause of death.

Direct obstetric deaths are those resulting from obstetric complications of the pregnant state (pregnancy, labor, and the puerperium) from interventions, omissions, incorrect treatment, or a chain of events resulting from any of the above.

Indirect obstetric deaths are those resulting from previous existing disease that developed during pregnancy and not due to direct obstetric causes but aggravated by the physiological effects of pregnancy.

In order to improve the quality of maternal mortality data and provide alternative methods of collecting data on deaths during pregnancy or related to it, as well as to encourage the recording of deaths from obstetric causes occurring more than 42 days following termination of pregnancy, the 43rd World Health Assembly in 1990 adopted the recommendation that countries consider the inclusion on death certificates of questions regarding current pregnancy and pregnancy within 1 year preceding death.

MATERNAL MORTALITY (RATE) The risk of dying from causes associated with childbirth. The numerator is the deaths arising during pregnancy or from puerperal causes (i.e., deaths occurring during and/or due to deliveries, complications of pregnancy, childbirth, and the puerperium). Women exposed to the risk of dying from puerperal causes are those who have been pregnant during the period. Their number being unknown, the number of live births is used as the conventional denominator for computing comparable maternal mortality rates. The formula is:

$$\text{Annual maternal mortality rate} = \frac{\begin{array}{c}\text{number of deaths from puerperal}\\ \text{causes in a given geographic area}\\ \text{during a given year}\end{array}}{\begin{array}{c}\text{number of live births that}\\ \text{occurred among the population of}\\ \text{the given geographic area during}\\ \text{the same year}\end{array}} \times 1000 \text{ (or 100,000)}$$

There is variation in the duration of the postpartum period in which death may occur and be certified as due to "puerperal causes," i.e., MATERNAL MORTALITY. Although the WHO defines maternal mortality as death during pregnancy or within 42 days of delivery, in some areas a period as long as a year is used. Maternal deaths may be subdivided into two groups: direct obstetric deaths and indirect obstetric deaths.

MATHEMATICAL MODEL A representation of a system, process, or relationship in mathematical form in which equations are used to simulate the behavior of the system or process under study. The model usually consists of two parts: the mathematical structure itself (e.g., Newton's inverse square law or Gauss's "normal" law), and the particular constants or parameters associated with them (such as Newton's gravitational constant or the Gaussian standard deviation). A mathematical model is fully DETERMINISTIC if the dependent variables involved take on values not allowing for any play of CHANCE.

A model is said to be stochastic, or RANDOM, if random variation is allowed to enter the picture. See also MODEL.

MATRIX

1. In epidemiology and biostatistics, a display of data in columns and rows.
2. In human biology, a formative tissue.

MAXIMUM ALLOWABLE CONCENTRATION (MAC) See SAFETY STANDARDS.

MAXIMUM LIKELIHOOD ESTIMATE The value for an unknown parameter in a model that maximizes the probability of obtaining exactly the data that were observed. Most often used to find estimates of coefficients in LOGISTIC MODELS.

M-BIAS Bias in collider (C)-specific or C-adjusted exposure (E) - disease (D) associations arising from an "M pattern" within the underlying causal structure (in which all or part of the C–E association arises from shared causes A of C and E, and all or part of the C–D association arises from shared causes B of C and D).[82] It is called "M" because of the M shape of the corresponding CAUSAL DIAGRAM, the "M diagram", in which events are temporally ordered from top (earliest) to bottom (latest), C is a COLLIDER on the "back-door" path from E to D passing through A, C and B (a back-door path from E to D is a path that begins with an arrow pointing to E; such paths are sources of confounding). Like other collider-stratification bias, M-bias arises from adjustment for a variable C that numerically behaves like a classical confounder (in that the effect estimate changes upon adjustment for C). Unlike other collider-stratification bias, M-bias attributable to C-adjustment may not be apparent from the time order of the events, for C may be determined before E or D; hence, one may be led to adjust for C (and thus introduce bias) if one uses traditional confounder-selection criteria, even if one takes care to not adjust for variables affected by E or D.[82] See also CONFOUNDING BIAS.

MCNEMAR'S TEST A form of the CHI-SQUARE TEST for matched-pairs data. It is a special case of the MANTEL-HAENSZEL TEST.

MDR (MULTIDRUG RESISTANT) See DRUG RESISTANCE, MULTIPLE.

MEAN, ARITHMETIC The sum of all the individual values in a set of measurements divided by the number of values in the set. A MEASURE OF CENTRAL TENDENCY. See also AVERAGE.

MEAN-DIFFERENCE PLOT (Syn: Tukey mean-difference plot) A scatter plot that shows changes in the percentiles of the distribution of a measure from samples obtained at two time points. The differences of each percentile from the earlier to the later time points are plotted on the vertical axis, and the means of the two values of each percentile are on the horizontal axis. Data are typically shown for the 2.5, 5, 10, 20, 30, 40, 50, 60, 70, 80, 90, 95, and 97.5 percentile points. Departure of the plotted points from a horizontal line indicates change of shape of the distribution.

MEAN, GEOMETRIC A MEASURE OF CENTRAL TENDENCY. This is calculated by adding the logarithms of the individual values, calculating their arithmetic mean, and converting back by taking the antilogarithm. Can be calculated only for positive quantities.

MEAN, HARMONIC A MEASURE OF CENTRAL TENDENCY computed by summing the reciprocals of all the individual values and dividing the resulting sum into the number of values.

MEASUREMENT The procedure of applying a standard scale to a variable or to a set of values.

MEASUREMENT BIAS

1. Systematic error (BIAS) in a measurement.

2. Systematic error arising from inaccurate measurements (or classification) of subjects on study variable(s). See INFORMATION BIAS.

MEASUREMENT, TERMINOLOGY OF There is sometimes ambiguity about the terms used to describe the properties of measurement: *accuracy, precision, validity, reliability, repeatability*, and *reproducibility. Accuracy* and *precision* are often used synonymously, *validity* is defined variously, and *reliability, repeatability*, and *reproducibility* are often used interchangeably. Etymologies are helpful in making a case for preferred usages, but they are not always decisive. *Accuracy* is from the Latin *cura* (care), and while this may be of interest to those in the health field, it does not illuminate the origins of the standard definition, that is, "conforming to a standard or a true value" *(OED). Accuracy* is distinguished from *precision* in this way: A measurement or statement can reflect or represent a true value without detail; e.g., a temperature reading of 37.5°C may be accurate, but it may not be precise if a thermometer that registers 37.527°C is taken as the reference. See also ACCURACY.

Precision (from Latin *praecidere*, cut short) is the quality of being sharply defined through exact detail. A faulty measurement may be expressed precisely but may not be accurate. Measurements should be both accurate and precise, but the two terms are not synonymous. See also PRECISION.

Consistency or *reliability* describes the property of measurements or results that conform to themselves.

Reliability (Latin *religare*, to bind) is defined by the *OED* as a quality that is sound and dependable. Its epidemiological usage is similar; a result or measurement is said to be reliable when it is stable (i.e., when repetition of an experiment or measurement gives the same results). The terms *repeatability* and *reproducibility* are synonymous (the *OED* defines each in terms of the other), but they do not refer to a quality of measurement—rather, only to the action of performing something more than once. Thus, a way of discovering whether or not a measurement is reliable is to repeat or reproduce it. The terms *repeatability* and *reproducibility*, formed from their respective verbs, are used inaccurately when they are substituted for *reliability*, a noun that refers to the measuring procedure rather than the attribute being measured. However, in common usage, both *repeatability* and *reproducibility* refer to the capacity of a measuring procedure to produce the same result on each occasion in a series of procedures conducted under identical conditions.

Validity is used correctly when it agrees with the standard definition given by the *OED:* "sound and sufficient." If, in the epidemiological sense, a test measures what it purports to measure (it is sufficient) then the test is said to be valid. See also ACCURACY; PRECISION; RELIABILITY; REPEATABILITY; VALIDITY; VALIDITY, STUDY.

MEASUREMENT SCALE The range of possible values for a measurement (e.g., the set of possible responses to a question, the physically possible range for a set of body weights).

Measurement scales can be classified according to the quantitative character of the scale:

1. DICHOTOMOUS SCALE (Syn: binary scale): One that arranges items into either of two mutually exclusive categories; e.g., yes/no, alive/dead.
2. NOMINAL SCALE (Syn., polytomous scale, polytomy): Classification into unordered qualitative categories; e.g., race, religion, and country of birth. Measurements of individual attributes are purely nominal scales, as there is no inherent order to their categories.

3. ORDINAL SCALE: Classification into ordered qualitative categories, e.g., social class (I, II, III, etc.), where the values have a distinct order but their categories are qualitative in that there is no natural (numerical) distance between their possible values. See also RANKING SCALE.
4. INTERVAL SCALE: An (equal) interval involves assignment of values with a natural distance between them, so that a particular distance (interval) between two values in one region of the scale meaningfully represents the same distance between two values in another region of the scale. Examples include Celsius and Fahrenheit temperature, date of birth.
5. RATIO SCALE: A ratio is an interval scale with a true zero point, so that ratios between values are meaningfully defined. Examples are absolute (Kelvin) temperature, weight, height, blood count, and income, as in each case it is meaningful to speak of one value as being so many times greater or less than another value.

Dichotomous, nominal, and ordinal scales are sometimes called qualitative or "categorical," but the latter term has other meanings, such as *discrete* (as opposed to continuous). An example of a categorical scale that is also a ratio scale is household size (1, 2, 3, ...). Interval and ratio scales are sometimes called quantitative scales.

MEASURE OF ASSOCIATION A quantity that expresses the strength or degree of association between variables. Commonly used measures of association are ratios and differences between means, proportions, risks, or rates, and correlation and regression coefficients.

MEASURE OF EFFECT See EFFECT MEASURE.

MEASURES OF CENTRAL TENDENCY A general term for several values of the distribution of a set of values or measurements located at or near the middle of the set. The principal measures of central tendency are the MEAN (AVERAGE), MEDIAN, and MODE.

MECHANICAL TRANSMISSION Transmission of pathogens by a vector (e.g., a housefly) without biological development in or dependence on the vector. Many fecal-oral infections are spread by this means. See also VECTOR-BORNE INFECTION.

MECHANISM In epidemiology and other health, life, and social sciences, the way in which a particular health-related event or outcome occurs, often described in terms of the agents and steps involved. Whereas the focus is often on biological mechanisms, environmental, social, and cultural mechanisms are also relevant to epidemiology, public health, medicine, and related disciplines.

MECHANISTIC BIAS A form of INTERPRETIVE BIAS that occurs if interpretation of scientific evidence is less rigorous when basic science furnishes credibility for the putative mechanisms underlying the findings than when it does not.[34] See also BIOLOGICAL PLAUSIBILITY; COHERENCE.

MECHANISTIC EPIDEMIOLOGY Epidemiological research that focuses on MECHANISMS underlying and explaining associations between DETERMINANTS and health-related events or states. It is not a formal branch or specialty of epidemiology, nor is it an epidemiological method or philosophy. Loosely, the opposite of "BLACK-BOX EPIDEMIOLOGY." See also APPLIED EPIDEMIOLOGY.

MEDIAN A MEASURE OF CENTRAL TENDENCY. The simplest division of a set of measurements is into two parts – the lower and the upper half. The point on the scale that divides the group in this way is called the "median."

MEDIATOR (MEDIATING) VARIABLE See INTERMEDIATE VARIABLE.

MEDICAL AUDIT A health service evaluation procedure in which selected data from patients' charts are summarized in tables displaying such data as average length of stay or duration of an episode of care, the frequency of diagnostic and therapeutic procedures, and outcomes of care arranged by diagnostic category. These are often compared with predetermined norms.

MEDICAL CARE See HEALTH CARE.

MEDICAL GEOGRAPHY (Syn: geographical pathology). A branch of science concerned with the spatial variations in environmental conditions related to health and disease. It combines biology, ecology, medicine, epidemiology, and geography and applies techniques such as mapping to medical and health problems.[276,277] Satellite imaging and remote sensing have facilitated mapping the distribution of epidemiologically important biota, such as phytoplankton and zooplankton, and have strengthened the integration of epidemiology, ecology, and geography in studies of medical geography and geographical medicine. Cartographic methods such as CHOROPLETHIC and ISODEMOGRAPHIC maps provide a useful visual display of the geographical variations in the distribution of disease, medical and other health care facilities, etc. See also GEOGRAPHIC INFORMATION SYSTEM; GEOMATICS.

MEDICAL RECORD A file of information relating to a transaction(s) in personal health care. In addition to facts about a patient's illness, medical records nearly always contain other information. The information in medical records includes the following:

1. Clinical, i.e., diagnosis, treatment, progress, etc.
2. Demographic, i.e., age, sex, birthplace, residence, etc.
3. Sociocultural, i.e., language, ethnic origin, religion, etc.
4. Sociological, i.e., family (next of kin), occupation, etc.
5. Economic, i.e., method of payment (fee-for-service, indigent, etc.).
6. Administrative, i.e., site of care, provider, etc.
7. "Behavioral," e.g., records of broken appointment may indicate dissatisfaction with service provided.

MEDICAL STATISTICS The branch of BIOSTATISTICS concerned with medical problems and research.

MEDICALIZATION The process by which problems traditionally considered nonmedical come to be defined and treated as medical issues. The process of identification of a personal or social condition as a medical issue subject to medical intervention. The expansion of medical profession's influence and authority into the domains of everyday existence.[108,143,144,207,217] See also GENETIZATION; INTEGRATION; REDUCTIONISM.

MENDELIAN RANDOMIZATION

1. An approach or "strategy" of observational epidemiology that uses findings from association studies of well-characterized functional genetic variants to assess CAUSAL INFERENCES about modifiable environmental exposures. One of the INSTRUMENTAL VARIABLE approaches for making causal inferences from observational data in the face of uncontrolled confounders.[212,278] It is based on the fact that inheritance of one genetic trait is independent of (i.e., *randomized* with respect to) other unlinked traits. Functional variants will not be associated with other genetic variants apart from those with which they are in LINKAGE DISEQUILIBRIUM; this assumption follows from the law of independent assortment (sometimes referred to as Mendel's second law), hence the term Mendelian randomization. At a population level, traits influenced by genetic variants are generally not associated with the social, behavioral, and

environmental factors that confound relationships in conventional epidemiological studies. Thus genetic variants can serve as an indicator of the action of environmentally modifiable exposures. Example: studies have pointed out that the autosomal dominant condition of lactase persistence is positively associated with drinking milk; thus protective associations of lactase persistence with osteoporosis, bone mineral density, or fracture risk provide evidence that milk drinking protects against these conditions. Mendelian randomization may help to avoid confounding, bias due to reverse causation or reporting tendency, and underestimation of associations due to variability in behaviors and phenotypes. Factors limiting the inferential power of Mendelian randomization include confounding of associations between genotype, intermediate phenotype, and disease through linkage disequilibrium or population stratification; pleiotropy and the multifunctionality of genes; canalization and developmental stability; and lack of suitable polymorphisms for studying modifiable exposures of interest.[212,278]

2. Originally, random assortment of genetic variants at conception, used to provide an unconfounded study design for estimating treatment effects for childhood malignancies.

MENDEL'S LAWS Derived from the pioneering genetic studies of Gregor Mendel (1822–1884). Mendel's first law states that genes are particulate units that segregate; i.e., members of the same pair of genes are never present in the same gamete, but always separate and pass to different gametes. Mendel's second law states that genes assort independently; i.e., members of different pairs of genes move to gametes independently of one another.

META-ANALYSIS A statistical analysis of results from separate studies, examining sources of differences in results among studies, and leading to a quantitative summary of the results if the results are judged sufficiently similar to support such synthesis. In the biomedical sciences, the systematic, organized, and structured evaluation of a problem of interest, using information (commonly in the form of statistical tables or other data) from a number of independent studies of the problem. A frequent application is the pooling of results from a set of randomized controlled trials, which in aggregate have more statistical power to detect differences at conventional levels of statistical significance. Meta-analysis has a qualitative component (i.e., classification of studies according to predetermined characteristics capable of influencing results, such as study design, completeness and quality of data, absence of biases), and a quantitative component (i.e., extraction and analysis of the numerical information). The aim is to integrate the findings, if possible, and to identify overall trends or patterns in the results.[279] Studies must be subject to critical appraisal, and various biases in the selection of subjects, detection of events, or presentation of results (e.g., PUBLICATION BIAS) must be assessed.[14,106,280]
See also SYSTEMATIC REVIEW.

METAPHOR A word, image, expression, concept, or symbol used as a cognitive device to convey or comprehend an idea – sometimes an abstract or complex concept. In epidemiology, a classic example is the "WEB OF CAUSATION." Metaphors are important in many scientific and professional endeavors, including many epidemiology-related activities (e.g., HEALTH PROMOTION, RISK ASSESSMENT, risk communication); and, of course, in teaching epidemiology.[143,144,169,216,217] They may inspire or otherwise form the basis of subsequent formal developments (e.g., CAUSAL DIAGRAMS partly stem from and formalize the web-of-causation metaphor).

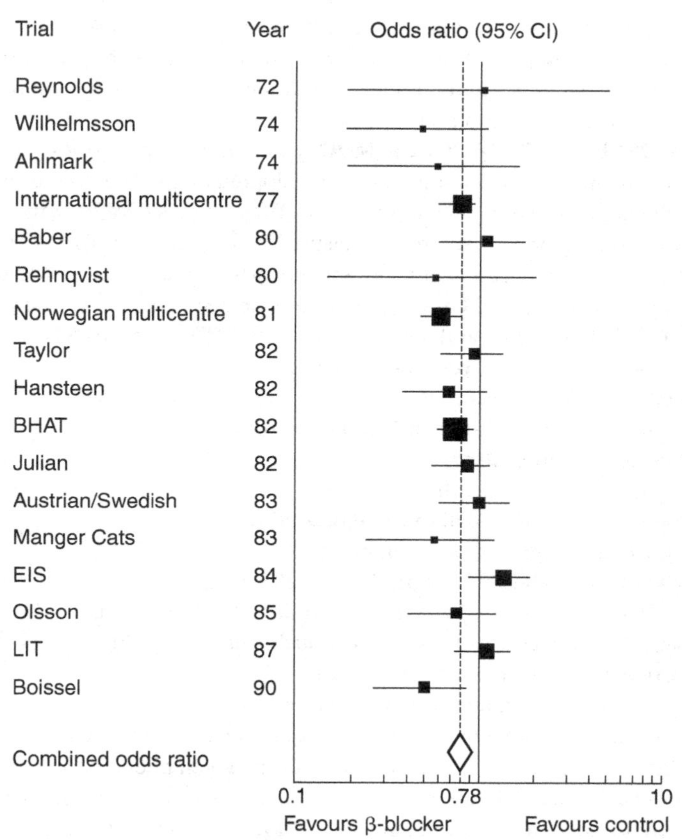

Meta-analysis of mortality results from 17 studies of β-blockade in secondary prevention after acute myocardial infarction. The size of the "box" in each box-and-whiskers plot is proportional to the numbers in the study, and the combined odds ratio is represented by the diamond shape in the bottom row of the diagram. Figures like this have been called meta-analysis plots, Cochrane plots, or Chalmers plots. They most often appear without an eponymous name. From Davey Smith, G, Eggar M, Phillips AN. Metaanalysis and data synthesis in medical research. In Detels R, Holland WW, McEwen J, Omenn G, eds. *Oxford Textbook of Public Health*, 3rd ed. Vol 2. New York: Oxford University Press, 1997, p. 636.

METHODOLOGY The scientific study of methods. Methodology should not be confused with methods. The word *methodology* is all too often used when the writer means *method*.

MIASMA THEORY An explanation for the origin of epidemics, the "miasma theory" was implied by many ancient writers and made explicit by Lancisi in *De noxiis paludum effluviis* (1717). It was based on the notion that when the air was of a "bad quality" (a state that was not precisely defined but that was supposedly due to decaying organic matter), the persons breathing that air would become ill. Malaria ("bad air") is the classic example of a disease that was long attributed to miasmata. "Miasma" was believed to pass from cases to susceptibles in those diseases considered contagious.

MIGRANT STUDIES Studies taking advantage of migration to one country by those from other countries with different physical and biological environments, cultural background, and/or genetic makeup, and different morbidity or mortality experience.

Comparisons are made between the mortality or morbidity experience of the migrant groups with that of their current country of residence and/or their country of origin. Sometimes the experiences of a number of different groups who have migrated to the same country have been compared.

MILLENNIUM DEVELOPMENT GOALS (MDGs) drawn from the actions and targets contained in the Millenium Declaration, which was adopted by 189 nations during the United Nations Millennium Summit in September 2000. To be achieved by 2015, the eight MDGs break down into 18 quantifiable targets measured by 48 indicators. The MDGs recognize the interdependence between health, growth, poverty reduction, and sustainable development; they acknowledge that development rests on democratic governance, the rule of law, respect for human rights, and peace and security.[281] The eight MDGs are:

Goal 1: Eradicate extreme poverty and hunger.

Goal 2: Achieve universal primary education.

Goal 3: Promote gender equality and empower women.

Goal 4: Reduce child mortality.

Goal 5: Improve maternal health.

Goal 6: Combat HIV/AIDS, malaria, and other diseases.

Goal 7: Ensure environmental sustainability.

Goal 8: Develop a Global Partnership for Development.

MILL'S CANONS In *A System of Logic* (first edition 1843), John Stuart Mill (1806–1873) devised logical strategies ("canons") from which causal relationships may be inferred. Four in particular are pertinent to epidemiology:[10]

Method of agreement (first canon): "If two or more instances of the phenomenon under investigation have only one circumstance in common, the circumstance in which alone all the instances agree, is the cause (or effect) of the given phenomenon."

Method of difference (second canon): "If an instance in which the phenomenon under investigation occurs, and an instance in which it does not occur, have every circumstance in common save one, that one occurring only in the former, the circumstance in which alone the two instances differ is the effect, or cause or a necessary part of the cause, of the phenomenon."

Method of residues (fourth canon): "Subduct from any phenomenon such part as is known by previous inductions to be the effect of certain antecedents, and the residue of the phenomenon is the effect of the remaining antecedents."

Method of concomitant variation (fifth canon): "Whatever phenomenon varies in any manner whether another phenomenon varies in some particular manner, is either a cause or an effect of that phenomenon, or is connected with it through some fact of causation."

See also CAUSAL CRITERIA.

MINIMAL CLINICALLY IMPORTANT DIFFERENCE The smallest effect of a treatment that patients perceive as beneficial and that, in the absence of unacceptable side effects, inconvenience, and costs, mandates that the treatment be given. A term used in clinical trials.

MINIMUM DATA SET (Syn: uniform basic data set) A widely agreed upon and generally accepted set of terms and definitions constituting a core of data acquired for medical records and employed for developing statistics suitable for diverse types of analyses and users. Such sets have been developed for birth and death certificates, ambulatory care, hospital care, and long-term care. See also BIRTH CERTIFICATE; DEATH CERTIFICATE; HOSPITAL DISCHARGE ABSTRACT SYSTEM.

MISCLASSIFICATION The erroneous classification of an individual, a value, or an attribute into a category other than that to which it should be assigned.[12,31,97] The probability of misclassification given the true value may be the same in all study groups (nondifferential misclassification) or may vary between groups (differential misclassification, e.g., accuracy of diagnoses of cases depends on their alcohol consumption).[254] It is wrong to assume that nondifferential misclassification can produce only bias toward the null in measures of association or effect; other conditions must also be satisfied in order to ensure that bias is toward the null, most prominently that the misclassification must be independent of (unrelated to) the occurrence of other errors.[12] Such independence is rare in clinical and epidemiological research.

MISSION The purpose for which an organization exists. See also GOAL, OBJECTIVE, TARGET.

MMWR *Morbidity and Mortality Weekly Report*. A publication of the U.S. Centers for Disease Control and Prevention (www.cdc.gov/mmwr).

MOBILITY, GEOGRAPHIC Movement of persons from one permanent place of residence (country or region) to another.

MOBILITY, SOCIAL Movement from one defined socioeconomic group to another, either upward or downward. Downward social mobility, which can be related to impaired health (e.g., alcoholism, schizophrenia, mental retardation), is sometimes referred to as "social drift."

MODE The most frequently occurring value in a set of observations. One of the MEASURES OF CENTRAL TENDENCY. See also AVERAGE.

MODEL

1. An abstract representation of the relationship between logical, analytical, or empirical components of a system. See also MATHEMATICAL MODEL.
2. A formalized expression of a theory or the causal situation regarded as having generated observed data.
3. (Animal) model: an experimental system that uses animals because humans cannot be used for ethical or other reasons.
4. A small-scale simulation, e.g., by using an "average region" with characteristics resembling those of the whole country.

In epidemiology, the use of models began with an effort to predict the onset and course of epidemics. In the second report of the Registrar-General of England and Wales (1840), William Farr developed the beginnings of a predictive model for communicable disease epidemics. He had recognized regularities in the smallpox epidemics of the 1830s. By calculating frequency curves for these past outbreaks, he estimated the deaths to be expected. See also DEMONSTRATION MODEL; MATHEMATICAL MODEL; THEORETICAL EPIDEMIOLOGY.

MODEL LIFE TABLE Simulated life table constructed for a country, used mainly when vital statistics are deficient. The model may be based on averaging of empirical data or on more sophisticated methods. The Coale-Demeny method is a range of models for life expectancies ranging from 20 to 80+ years with four variations of mortality patterns.

MODIFYING FACTOR See EFFECT MODIFIER.

MOLECULAR EPIDEMIOLOGY An approach to study the molecular mechanisms, pathophysiology, and etiology of disease; less frequently, early detection, treatment and prognosis. A way of practicing INTEGRATIVE RESEARCH; sometimes, a level of measurement—but not really a discipline with substantive research content.[23,282–285] From an instrumental viewpoint, the use in EPIDEMIOLOGICAL RESEARCH of the techniques of molecular and cellular biology, genetics, systems biology, proteomics and other "omics" approaches to analyze BIOMARKERS.[192,193] Molecular techniques are used in CANCER EPIDEMIOLOGY to identify, characterize, and measure molecular changes involved in CARCINOGENESIS (xenobiotic DNA adducts, somatic genetic mutations); metabolic polymorphisms; and many other genetic and EPIGENETIC processes. Molecular epidemiology is making valuable contributions to biomedical, clinical, and population sciences; e.g., research on the role of gene-environment interactions in the etiology of many diseases is generating knowledge about biological mechanisms as well as about primary prevention.[80] See also HuGENet.

MONITORING

1. The intermittent performance and analysis of measurements aimed at detecting changes in the health status of populations or in the physical or social environment. In principle, it is different from SURVEILLANCE, which is often a continuous process, although surveillance techniques are used in monitoring. It may also imply intervention in the light of observed measurements and analysis of the effect of the intervention (e.g., on the health status of a population or on an environmental compartment). The process of collecting and analyzing information about the implementation and effects of a public health program.
2. In management, the episodic oversight of the implementation of an activity, seeking to ensure that input deliveries, work schedules, targeted outputs, and other required actions are proceeding according to plan.

MONOGENIC DISEASES Diseases in which a genetic variant of high PENETRANCE confers a high risk of developing the disease and may thus be thought to be the sole cause of the disease, although the penetrance and expressivity of the gene are sometimes regulated by other genes or even by lifestyle and environmental exposures (e.g., diet, access to effective medical treatment). An antonym of POLYGENIC DISEASES.

MONOTONIC SEQUENCE A sequence is said to be monotonically increasing if each value is greater than or equal to the previous one and monotonically decreasing if each value is less than or equal to the previous one. If equality of values is excluded, we speak of a strictly (increasing or decreasing) monotonic sequence. A sequence that is monotonic in either direction is said to be monotone, or to display monotonicity.

MONTE-CARLO STUDY, TRIAL Complex relationships that are difficult to solve by mathematical analysis are sometimes studied by computer experiments that simulate and analyze a sequence of events using random numbers. Such experiments are called Monte Carlo trials or studies, in recognition of Monte Carlo as one of the gambling capitals of the world. See also MARKOV PROCESS; SIMULATION.

MOOSE Meta-analysis Of Observational Studies in Epidemiology. A consensus checklist to improve the quality of reports of META-ANALYSES of observational studies. It contains specifications on background, search strategy, methods, results, discussion, and conclusion.[95,106,286] See also CONSORT; QUADAS; QUOROM; STARD; STROBE; TREND.

MORBIDITY

1. Any departure, subjective or objective, from a state of physiological or psychological well-being. In this sense *sickness, illness*, and *morbid condition* are similarly defined and synonymous (but see DISEASE).
2. The WHO Expert Committee on Health Statistics noted in its sixth report (1959) that morbidity could be measured in terms of three units:

a. Persons who were ill
b. The illnesses (periods or spells of illness) that these persons experienced
c. The duration (days, weeks, etc.) of these illnesses

See also HEALTH INDEX; INCIDENCE RATE; NOTIFIABLE DISEASE; PREVALENCE.

MORBIDITY RATE A term, preferably avoided, used to refer to the incidence rate and sometimes (incorrectly) to the prevalence of disease.

MORBIDITY SURVEY A method for estimating the prevalence and/or incidence of disease in a population. A morbidity survey is usually designed simply to ascertain the facts as to disease distribution and not to test a hypothesis. See also CROSS-SECTIONAL STUDY; HEALTH SURVEY.

MORTALITY:INCIDENCE RATIO See CANCER MORTALITY:INCIDENCE RATIO.

MORTALITY RATE See DEATH RATE.

MORTALITY STATISTICS Statistical tables compiled from the information contained in DEATH CERTIFICATES. Most administrative jurisdictions in all nations produce tables of mortality statistics. These may be published at regular intervals; they usually show numbers of deaths and/or rates by age, sex, cause, and sometimes other variables.

MOVING AVERAGES (Syn: rolling averages) A set of methods for smoothing irregularities in trend data, such as long-term secular trends in incidence or mortality rates. Graphical display of (say, 3- or 5-year) moving averages makes it easier to discern long-term trends in rates that otherwise might be obscured by short-term fluctuations. The span over which the average is taken is sometimes called the *window width*. Within that window, the averages may be weighted by proximity to the point at which the rate is being estimated. This weighting function is sometimes called a "kernel function," and the process is then called *kernel smoothing*.

MRC Medical Research Council (UK, Canada, other countries) Oversight government-appointed groups that define and set policies for research in all aspects of medical science and usually implement policies by allocating funds for research training, research programs, and research projects.

MSM Men who have sex with men. In this group, high-risk practices for HIV infection may occur.

MULTICOLLINEARITY In multiple regression analysis, a situation in which at least some of the regressors (independent variables) are highly correlated with each other. Such a situation can result in inaccurate or undefined estimates of the parameters in the regression model.[12,20]

MULTIDRUG-RESISTANT (MDR) See DRUG RESISTANCE, MULTIPLE.

MULTIFACTORIAL ETIOLOGY See MULTIPLE CAUSATION.

MULTILEVEL ANALYSIS (Syn: contextual analysis, hierarchical analysis) Integration of contextual, group, or macrolevel factors with individual-level factors in epidemiological analyses of health states and outcomes. The rationale is that the distribution of health and disease in populations is not explained only by characteristics of individuals.[287] Methodologies that analyze outcomes in relation to determinants simultaneously measured at different levels (e.g., individual, workplace, neighborhood, region). One aim of multilevel analyses is to explain how group- and individual-level variables interact in shaping health. Such analyses require one to select the appropriate contextual units and contextual variables, to correctly specify the model, and to account for residual correlation between individuals within contexts.[120,137]

MULTILEVEL MODEL (Syn: hierarchical model) A REGRESSION MODEL in which the coefficients of the regressors are themselves modeled as functions of properties of the regressors. For example, in a regression of colon cancer incidence in relation to food intakes, the food coefficients may be modeled as functions of their nutrient contents. In a regression of lung-cancer incidence in relation to occupation, an occupational coefficient may be modeled as a function of the chemical exposures in the occupation. The properties used to model the coefficients are called second-level or second-stage co-variates. Multilevel models are equivalent to *random-coefficient models* or *mixed models* in which the second-level covariates have random coefficients.

MULTINOMIAL DISTRIBUTION The probability distribution associated with the classification of each of a sample of individuals into one of several mutually exclusive and exhaustive categories, assuming that the individual classifications are independent of one another. When the number of categories is two, the distribution is called BINOMIAL DISTRIBUTION.

MULTIPHASE SAMPLING Method of sampling that gathers some information from a large sample and more detailed information from subsamples within this sample, either at the same time or later. Contrast to MULTISTAGE SAMPLING.

MULTIPHASIC SCREENING See SCREENING.

MULTIPLE CAUSATION (Syn: multifactorial etiology) The concept that a given health state or health-related process may have more than one cause. A combination of causes or alternative combinations of causes is often required to produce the health outcome. See also CAUSAL DIAGRAM; DISEASES OF COMPLEX ETIOLOGY; PROBABILITY OF CAUSATION; RISK FACTOR; WEB OF CAUSATION.

MULTIPLE CAUSE THEORY A theory coherent with MULTIPLE CAUSATION, i.e., with the fact that multiple coexisting causes may influence the occurrence of disease and other health outcomes. By contrast, HENLE-KOCH POSTULATES do not admit multiple causes of a single disorder, nor do they contemplate causal relations not susceptible to experimentation. Early in the twentieth century, German scientists raised questions about the limitation of such postulates and paved the way for new ideas on multifactorial causality.[288] Consensus about MULTIPLE CAUSATION coalesced a half-century later, when chronic noninfectious disease had become a leading public health concern. Thereafter, the theory permeated epidemiology up to the present time.[6–11,66,67,120,169,253,262,273]

MULTIPLE COMPARISON PROBLEMS Problems that arise from the fact that the greater the number of conventional statistical tests of significance conducted on a data set, the greater the probability that at least one or more tests will falsely reject the NULL HYPOTHESIS solely because of the play of chance. Adjustment of the ALPHA LEVEL in this situation is a debatable option; it has been strongly criticized because it will dramatically raise the false-negative rate (rate of TYPE-II ERROR, failure to reject a false null).[12] See also *P* VALUE; SIGNIFICANCE, STATISTICAL.

MULTIPLE COMPARISON TECHNIQUES Statistical procedures to adjust for differences in probability levels in setting up simultaneous confidence limits involving several distributions or sets of data or in comparing the means of several groups. *Tukey's method* is the most conservative; this uses the difference between the largest and smallest means as a measure of their dispersion; the q statistic, based on the α level (acceptable rate of TYPE-I ERROR), and the number of groups are used as multipliers of the standard deviation. The *Bonferroni correction* adjusts the α error level to compensate for multiple comparisons between three or more groups or two or more response variables.

Such conventional multiple comparisons techniques are problematic because they raise the false-negative rate (rate of TYPE-II ERROR, failure to reject a false null), often to the point that it may become impossible to detect any true effects. Modern techniques that attempt to address both type-I and type-II error have been developed, especially under the topic of EMPIRICAL-BAYES METHODS and SHRINKAGE ESTIMATION.

MULTIPLE LOGISTIC MODEL See LOGISTIC MODEL.

MULTIPLE OF THE MEDIAN A simple method of adjusting for variables such as age and sex in direct proportion to the magnitude of the original measurements; the method is not much affected by variation in measurement errors. However, the method is criticized because the multiple of the median is affected by the distribution of results used to determine the median, and there is no correction for the spread of the data. For these reasons the Z SCORE is preferable.

MULTIPLE REGRESSION TECHNIQUES Techniques for REGRESSION ANALYSIS that allow the inclusion of multiple regressors (independent variables).[20]

MULTIPLE RISK Where more than one RISK FACTOR for the development of a disease or other outcome is present and their combined presence results in an increased risk, we speak of "multiple risk." The increased risk may be due to the additive effects of the risks associated with the separate risk factors, or to SYNERGISM. See also MULTIPLE CAUSATION.

MULTIPLICATIVE MODEL A model in which the joint effect of two or more causes is the product of their individual effects. For instance, if factor X multiplies risk by the amount x in the absence of factor Y, and factor Y multiplies risk by the amount y in the absence of factor X, then the multiplicative risk model states that the two factors X and Y together will multiply the risk by $x \times y$. See also ADDITIVE MODEL.

MULTISTAGE MODEL A mathematical model, mainly for carcinogenesis, based on the theory that a specific carcinogen may affect any one of several stages in the development of cancer.

MULTISTAGE SAMPLING Selection, random or otherwise, of entities (such as geographical regions, schools, workplaces) followed by random sampling of persons within each sampled group. The method has advantages such as convenience and FEASIBILITY, but it complicates analysis. Contrast to MULTIPHASE SAMPLING.

MULTIVARIATE ANALYSIS A set of techniques used when the variation in several variables has to be studied simultaneously. In statistics, any analytical method that allows the simultaneous study of two or more DEPENDENT VARIABLES (regressands).[12,20,31,97]

MUTAGEN A physical or chemical agent that raises the frequency of mutation above the spontaneous rate. Any substance that can cause genetic mutations. Mutagens cause mutations in several different ways.

MUTAGENIC That which causes mutations. Contrast CLASTOGENIC and ANEUGENIC.

MUTATION Any change in a DNA sequence. In a clinical sense, any such change that disrupts the information contained in DNA and leads to disease. Many types of mutations and mechanisms leading to mutations exist.[23] Change in the genetic material not caused by genetic segregation or recombination that is transmitted to daughter cells and to succeeding generations provided that it is not a dominant lethal factor.

MUTATION RATE The frequency with which mutations occur per gene or per generation.

NATIONAL DEATH INDEX A computerized central registry of deaths in the United States, started in 1979 and operated by the U.S. National Center for Health Statistics, which facilitates mortality follow-up. See also CANADIAN MORTALITY DATABASE.

NATURAL EXPERIMENT Naturally occurring circumstances in which subsets of the population have different levels of exposure to a supposed causal factor in a situation resembling an actual experiment, where human subjects would be randomly allocated to groups. The presence of persons in a particular group is typically nonrandom; yet for a natural experiment, it suffices that their presence is independent of (unrelated to) potential confounders. See also EXPERIMENT; EXPERIMENTAL EPIDEMIOLOGY; OBSERVATIONAL STUDY.

Investigation by John Snow (1813–1858) of the distribution of cholera cases in London in relation to the sources of water supply is an excellent example of a natural experiment. It would have been unethical for Snow to allocate subjects to groups exposed to a lethal infection; but tracing the source of their drinking water, using what is now sometimes called SHOE-LEATHER EPIDEMIOLOGY, gave him the opportunity to make crucially important observations. "To turn this grand experiment to account, all that was required was to learn the supply of water to each individual house where a fatal attack of cholera might occur .... I resolved to spare no exertion which might be necessary to ascertain the exact effect of the water supply on the progress of the epidemic, in the places where all the circumstances were so happily adapted for the inquiry.... I had no reason to doubt the correctness of the conclusions I had drawn from the great number of facts already in my possession, but I felt that the circumstances of the cholera-poisoning passing down the sewers into a great river, and being distributed through miles of pipes, and yet producing its specific effects was a fact of so startling a nature, and of so vast importance to the community, that it could not be too rigidly examined or established on too firm a basis."[289]

NATURAL FOCUS OF INFECTION (Syn: natural nidality of disease). A focus existing outside a human population (e.g., in domestic or wild animals) often transmitted by a vector; humans can be infected if they enter such a biotype. The concept was developed and studied by the Soviet-era Russian epidemiologist A. D. Pavlovsky.

NATURAL HISTORY OF DISEASE The course of a disease from pathological onset or inception to resolution. Many diseases have certain relatively well-defined stages that, taken all together, are referred to as the "natural history of the disease" in question. These stages are as follows:

1. Stages of pathological onset. They are constantly being changed in many diseases; "onset," in particular, tends to be redefined in increasingly smaller microbiological (e.g., molecular and genetic) terms.
2. Presymptomatic stage: from initiation of disease to the first appearance of symptoms and/or signs.
3. Clinically manifest disease, which may progress inexorably to a fatal termination, be subject to remissions and relapses, or regress spontaneously, leading to recovery.

The nature and borders of these broad stages varies vastly across diseases. Some diseases have precursors. For example, elevated serum cholesterol is among the precursors of coronary heart disease. Precursor lesions may long precede the stage of pathological onset, but many alterations will be reversible or of unknown prognostic significance. An intense search is presently taking place for genetic, biochemical, or peptidomic "precursors" or "markers" of many diseases; a common aim is to market tests for EARLY DETECTION, which should be able to alter the natural history of the disease if they are promptly followed by effective interventions (e.g., surgical treatment). Studies on precursor and prognostic factors must integrate evidence on the putative biochemical or molecular markers with clinical, anatomopathological, and pathophysiological reasoning.

Often it is more a model or framework than a reality: the presentation and course of human disease tends to vary a lot in different individuals and contexts. The term *natural* should not be taken as a synonym of *biological*, since the course of disease in humans is not influenced only by biological and health care processes but also by social and cultural interactions (e.g., by cultural beliefs and norms on health care seeking, attributions of meaning to symptoms, economic barriers to treatment).[124] The term has also been used to mean "descriptive epidemiology of disease." See also SICKNESS "CAREER"; EARLY CLINICAL DETECTION; CLINICAL STUDY; INCUBATION PERIOD; INDUCTION PERIOD; LATENCY PERIOD; SCREENING.

NATURAL HISTORY STUDY A study, generally longitudinal, designed to yield information about the natural course of a disease or condition. See also INCEPTION COHORT.

NATURAL RATE OF INCREASE (DECREASE) See GROWTH RATE OF POPULATION.

NCHS National Center for Health Statistics (United States) (www.nchs.gov).

NEAREST NEIGHBOR METHOD A means of analyzing the spatial patterns of a free-living population. A term from veterinary epidemiology. Random sampling points are located throughout an area and the distance from each point to the nearest individual is measured; alternatively, individuals are selected at random and, from each of these, the distance to the nearest neighbor is measured.

NECESSARY CAUSE A causal factor whose presence is required for the occurrence of the effect. See also ASSOCIATION; CAUSALITY; CAUSATION OF DISEASE, FACTORS IN; COMPONENT CAUSES; DISEASES OF COMPLEX ETIOLOGY; EVANS'S POSTULATES; HILL'S CRITERIA OF CAUSATION; INTEGRATION; SUFFICIENT CAUSE.

NEEDLE STICK Puncture of the skin by a needle that may have been contaminated by contact with an infected patient or fluid. See also SHARPS.

NEED(S) In health economics, the minimum amount of resources required to exhaust an individual's or a specified population's capacity to benefit from an intervention.[1] In other contexts, need is variously and often vaguely defined. Sociologists allude to *perceived need*, meaning the beliefs or perceptions of health care providers or users about their requirements. Physicians speak of *professionally defined needs*, meaning undiagnosed and/or untreated conditions ranging from dangers to the public health, such as the risk of TB posed by persons who are excreting tubercle bacilli in sputum, to mild myopia or astigmatism in persons who would benefit from wearing corrective lenses.

NEEDS ASSESSMENT A systematic procedure for determining the nature and extent of problems experienced by a specified population that affect their health either directly or indirectly. Needs assessment makes use of epidemiological, sociodemographic, and qualitative methods to describe health problems and their environmental, social, economic, and behavioral determinants. The aim is to identify unmet health care needs and make recommendations about ways to address these needs, whether they are explicit health problems such as untreated diseases or "problems waiting to happen," such as inadequate housing, ignorance due to low literacy levels, domestic violence, lack of access to long-term care, etc. Needs assessment is either a routine or an ad hoc activity in many local public health departments.[290]

NEGATIVE PREDICTIVE VALUE See PREDICTIVE VALUE, NEGATIVE.

NEGATIVE STUDY Often taken to mean a study that fails to find evidence for an effect. It is a somewhat confusing term because it also suggests a "negative effect," which in turn may mean a preventive or a deleterious effect. See also CONFOUNDING, NEGATIVE; FALSE NEGATIVE; NULL STUDY.

NEONATAL MORTALITY RATE

1. In VITAL STATISTICS, the number of deaths in infants under 28 days of age in a given period, usually a year, per 1000 live births in that period.
2. In obstetrical and perinatal research, the term *neonatal mortality rate* is often used to denote the cumulative mortality rate of live-born infants within 28 days of age. See DEATH RATE.

NESTED CASE-CONTROL STUDY An important type of case-control study in which cases and controls are drawn from the population in a fully enumerated COHORT. Typically, some data on some variables are already available about both cases and controls; thus concerns about differential (biased) MISCLASSIFICATION of these variables can be reduced (e.g., environmental or nutritional exposures may be analyzed in blood from cases and controls collected and stored years before disease onset). A set of controls is selected from subjects (i.e., noncases) at risk of developing the outcome of interest at the time of occurrence of each case that arises in the cohort.[12,31,97,291]

NESTED DESIGN A study design that is applied to a population already identified in an existing population or study; an example is a nested case-control study, in which cases and controls are drawn from a fully enumerated cohort, which may already be under investigation in a cohort study.

NET MIGRATION The numerical difference between immigration and emigration.

NET MIGRATION RATE The net effect of immigration and emigration on an area's population, expressed as an increase or decrease per 1000 population of the area in a given year.

NET REPRODUCTION RATE (NRR) The average number of female children born per woman in a cohort subject to a given set of age-specific fertility rates, a given set of age-specific mortality rates, and a given sex ratio at birth. This rate measures replacement fertility under given conditions of fertility and mortality: it is the ratio of daughters to mothers assuming continuation of the specified conditions of fertility and mortality. It is a measure of population growth from one generation to another under constant conditions. This rate is similar to the gross reproduction rate but takes into account that some women will die before completing their childbearing years. An NRR of 1.00 means that each generation of mothers is having exactly enough daughters to replace itself in the population. See also GROSS REPRODUCTION RATE; REPLACEMENT-LEVEL FERTILITY.

NET REPRODUCTIVE RATE (R) (Syn: case reproduction rate) In infectious disease epidemiology, the average number of secondary cases that will occur in a mixed host population of susceptibles and nonsusceptibles when one infected individual is introduced. Its relationship to the BASIC REPRODUCTIVE RATE (R_0) is given by

$$R = R_0 x$$

where x is the proportion of the host population that is susceptible.

NEUROEPIDEMIOLOGY A branch or subspecialty of epidemiology that studies factors influencing the occurrence of disorders and diseases affecting the nervous system, like Parkinson's disease and multiple sclerosis. Primary outcomes include incidence, prevalence, survival, and mortality from neurological diseases. As mentioned above, this dictionary includes definitions for just a few branches of EPIDEMIOLOGY.

NGO Nongovernmental organization.

NHANES National Health and Nutrition Examination Survey (of the National Center for Health Statistics).

NHMRC National Health and Medical Research Council (Australia) (www.nhmrc.gov.au).

NIDUS A focus of infection. The term can be used to describe any heterogeneity in the distribution of a disease, but it is usually applied to a small area in which conditions favor occurrence and spread of a communicable disease. Also, the site of origin of a pathological process.

NIH National Institutes of Health (United States) (www.nih.gov).

NIOSH National Institute for Ocupational Safety and Health (United States) (www.niosh.gov).

NNT See NUMBER NEEDED TO TREAT.

NNH See NUMBER NEEDED TO HARM.

NNS See NUMBER NEEDED TO SCREEN.

NOCEBO An unpleasant or adverse effect attributable to administration of a PLACEBO.

N-OF-ONE STUDY (Syn: single-patient trial) A variation of a randomized controlled CROSSOVER CLINICAL TRIAL, in which a sequence of alternative treatments is randomly allocated to only one patient. Changes in signs and symptoms (or other reversible outcomes) experienced by the patient are compared, with the aim of deciding on the optimal regimen for the patient.[292–294]

NOISE (IN DATA) This term is used when extraneous uncontrolled variables and/or errors influence the distribution of measurements made in a study, thus rendering difficult or impossible the determination of relationships between variables under scrutiny.

NOMENCLATURE A list of all approved terms for describing and recording observations.

NOMINAL SCALE See MEASUREMENT SCALE.

NOMOGRAM A form of line chart showing scales for the variables involved in a particular formula in such a way that corresponding values for each variable lie on a straight line intersecting all the scales.

NONCONCURRENT STUDY See HISTORICAL COHORT STUDY.

NONDIFFERENTIAL MISCLASSIFICATION See MISCLASSIFICATION.

NONEXPERIMENTAL STUDY See OBSERVATIONAL STUDY.

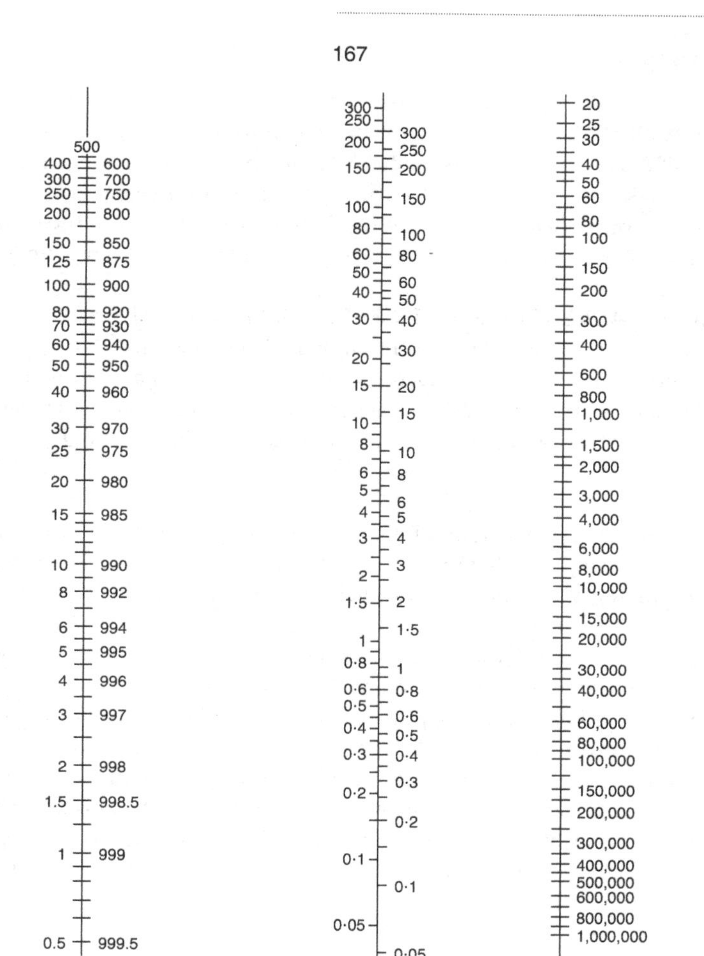

Nomogram of confidence limits to a rate. From Rosenbaum R. Nomograms for rates per 1000. *Br Med J* 1963; 1:169–170.

NONGENOTOXIC CARCINOGENS Carcinogens that do not cause direct damage to the DNA. Nongenotoxic processes and mechanisms include induction of inflammation, immunosuppression, formation of reactive oxygen species (ROS), activation of receptors such as the arylhydrocarbon receptor (AhR) or estrogen receptor (ER), and EPIGENETIC silencing. Together, GENOTOXIC and nongenotoxic mechanisms can alter signal-transduction pathways, finally resulting in hypermutability, genomic instability, loss of proliferation control, and resistance to apoptosis—features characteristic of cancer cells. At early stages of tumorigenesis the nongenotoxic effects are reversible and may require continuous presence of the compound. Long-term exposure to low doses of GENOTOXIC carcinogens also contributes to nongenotoxic alterations. Some nongenotoxic environmental carcinogens weaken cell-cycle checkpoint functions, thus leading to genetic instability or to heritable alterations of the genome.[219,295]

NONMALEFICENCE The ethical principle of causing no harm. See also PRECAUTIONARY PRINCIPLE.

NONPARAMETRIC METHODS See DISTRIBUTION-FREE METHOD.

NONPARAMETRIC TEST See DISTRIBUTION-FREE METHOD.

NONPARTICIPANTS (Syn: nonresponders) Members of a study sample or population who do not take part in the study for whatever reason, or members of a target population who do not participate in an activity. Differences between participants and nonparticipants have been demonstrated repeatedly in studies of many kinds, and this is often a source of BIAS.

NO-OBSERVED-ADVERSE-EFFECT LEVEL (NOAEL) The highest dose at which no adverse health effects are detected in an animal population. A NOAEL-SF is a no-observed-effects level with an added safety factor for human exposures; it is used in setting human safety standards. In practice, the safety factor added is commonly two or more orders of magnitude (i.e., a hundredfold or a thousandfold greater than the NOAEL).

NORM

1. What is usual; e.g., the range into which blood pressure values usually fall in a population group, the dietary or infant feeding practices that are usual in a given culture, or the way that a given illness is usually treated in a given health care system.
2. What is desirable; e.g., the range of blood pressures that a given authority regards as being indicative of present good health or as predisposing to future good health, the dietary or infant feeding practices that are valued in a given culture, or the health care procedures or facilities for health care that a given authority regards as desirable. In the latter sense, norms may be used as criteria in evaluating health care in order to determine the degree of conformity with what is desirable (e.g., the average length of stay of patients in hospital). Behavior that is considered culturally desirable and appropriate and therefore expected from members that belong to the community.

NORMAL

1. Within the usual range of variation in a given population or group. Frequently occurring in a given population or group. In this sense, "normal" is frequently defined as "within a range extending from two standard deviations below the mean to two standard deviations above the mean," or "between specified percentiles of the distribution" (e.g., the 10th and 90th percentiles).
2. Indicative or predictive of good health or conducive to good health. For a diagnostic or screening test, a "normal" result is one in a range within which the probability of a specific disease is low. See also NORMAL LIMITS
3. (Of a distribution) Gaussian distribution or NORMAL DISTRIBUTION.

NORMAL DISTRIBUTION (Syn: Gaussian distribution) The continuous frequency distribution of infinite range whose PROBABILITY DENSITY is given by the equation

$$f(x) = \frac{1}{(2\pi\sigma^2)^{1/2}} e^{-(x-\mu)^2/2\sigma^2}$$

where x is the abscissa, $f(x)$ is the ordinate, μ is the mean, $e \approx 2.718$ is the base of the natural logarithm, and σ the standard deviation. All possible values of the variable are displayed on the horizontal axis. The relative frequency (relative probability) of each value is displayed on the vertical axis, producing the graph of the normal distribution.

The properties of a normal distribution include the following:

1. It is a continuous, symmetrical distribution; both tails extend to infinity.
2. The arithmetic mean, mode, and median are identical.
3. Its shape is completely determined by the mean and standard deviation.
4. In common situations found in epidemiology, it is the approximate distribution for sums and means of variables provided that there are enough variables being summed or averaged, no one variable dominates the sum or average, and the variables are not too highly correlated among themselves. Then this is so even if the component variables are not themselves normal. An example is the mean of independent binary variables; the individual variables are far from normal, but the distribution of their mean gets close to normal even if there are as few as five of them. This property is sometimes called the *central limit* property.

NORMAL LIMITS The limits of the "normal" range of a test or measurement, in the sense of being indicative of or conducive to good health. One way to determine normal limits is to compare the values obtained when the measurements are made in two groups, one that is healthy and has been found to remain healthy and another that is ill or subsequently found to become ill. The result may be two overlapping distributions. Outside the area where the distributions overlap, a given value clearly identifies the presence or absence of disease or some other manifestation of poor health. If a value falls into the area of overlap, the individual may belong either to the normal or the abnormal group. The choice of the normal limits depends upon the relative importance attached to the identification of individuals as healthy or unhealthy. See also FALSE NEGATIVE; FALSE POSITIVE; SENSITIVITY AND SPECIFICITY.

NORMATIVE Pertaining to the normal, usual, accepted standards or values. See also NORM.

NOSOCOMIAL Relating to a hospital. Arising while a patient is in a hospital or as a result of being in a hospital. Denoting a new disorder (unrelated to the patient's primary condition) associated with being in a hospital.

NOSOCOMIAL INFECTION (Syn: hospital-acquired infection) An infection originating in a medical facility; e.g., occurring in a patient in a hospital or other health care facility in whom the infection was not present or incubating at the time of admission.[52,57] Includes infections acquired in the hospital but appearing after discharge; it also includes such infections among staff. See also HOSPITAL EPIDEMIOLOGY.

NOSOGRAPHY, NOSOLOGY Classification of ill persons into groups, whatever the criteria for their CLASSIFICATION, and agreement as to the boundaries of the groups. The assignment of names to each disease entity in the group results in a nomenclature of disease entities, or nosography.[296]

NOTIFIABLE DISEASE A disease that, by statutory requirements, must be reported to the public health authority in the pertinent jurisdiction when the diagnosis is made. A disease deemed of sufficient importance to the public health to require that its occurrence be reported to health authorities.

The reporting to public health authorities of communicable diseases is, unfortunately, very incomplete. The reasons for this include diagnostic inexactitude; the desire of patients and physicians to conceal the occurrence of conditions carrying a social stigma (e.g., sexually transmitted diseases); and the indifference of physicians to the usefulness of information about such diseases as hepatitis, influenza, and measles. Yet notifications are extremely important. They provide the starting point for investigations into the failure of preventive measures, such as immunizations, for tracing sources of infection, finding common vehicles of infection, describing the geographic CLUSTERING of infection, and various other purposes, depending upon the particular disease.

N.S., n.s. Abbreviation, usually written lower case, for *not statistically significant*. See also SIGNIFICANCE.

NUCLEOPHILIC Having an affinity for positive charge; molecules that behave as electron donors. Nucleophilic or chemically inert compounds such as aromatic and heterocyclic amines, aminoazo dyes, polycyclic aromatic hydrocarbons (PAHs), N-nitrosamines, and others represent the great majority of human CARCINOGENS; because these chemicals do not react directly with cellular constituents—they require enzymatic conversion into their ultimate carcinogenic forms—they are termed PROCARCINOGENS. See also ELECTROPHILIC.

NULL HYPOTHESIS The statistical hypothesis that one variable has no association with another variable or set of variables, or that two or more population distributions do not differ from one another. In statistical terms, the null hypothesis states that the differences observed in a study or test occurred as a result of the operation of chance alone. See also TEST HYPOTHESIS.

NULL STUDY A study that fails to find evidence for an association or effect (e.g., coffee drinking does not increase or decrease the risk of colon cancer). The term is more precise than the often used synonym NEGATIVE STUDY.

NUMBER NEEDED TO HARM (NNH) (Syn: Number Needed to be treated to Harm one person)

1. The number of persons needed to be treated, on average, to produce one more adverse event (e.g., occurrence of a disease, complication, adverse reaction, relapse). The number of persons who need to receive the treatment for one of them to experience an adverse effect. It is a clinically oriented way of expressing the risk of one intervention over another and takes the absolute risk of the event into account. It is used to summarize results of studies and to assist in clinical decision making.
2. The reciprocal of the ABSOLUTE RISK INCREASE. Let ARC be the absolute risk of events in the control group and ART the absolute risk of events in the treatment group; then the absolute risk increase (ARI) = ART – ARC and NNH = 1 / ARI. It may also be calculated as 100 divided by the ARI to express it as a percentage.[14,15] Example: the occurrence of adverse outcomes in a clinical trial was 10% (0.10) in the treated group and 4% (0.04) in the placebo group; hence, the ARI was 0.06 and 1 / 0.06 = 16.7; i.e., on average, about 17 patients have to be treated in order to increase the number having an adverse outcome by 1.

Definitions 1 and 2 look equivalent but are not the same unless the treatment acts independently of other background factors leading to the harm. See also ABSOLUTE RISK REDUCTION (ARR); NUMBER NEEDED TO TREAT (NNT); RELATIVE RISK REDUCTION (RRR).

NUMBER NEEDED TO SCREEN (NNS) The average number of persons who must undergo a SCREENING test and the ensuing diagnostic and therapeutic procedures in order to prevent one case of the disease of interest:

$$NNS = NNT / PrC$$

where NNT is the NUMBER NEEDED TO TREAT and PrC is the prevalence of carriers of the variant of interest in the population screened. When the NNT is to be used to compute the NNS, computation of the NNT is based, as usual, on the reciprocal of the ABSOLUTE RISK REDUCTION (ARR) (i.e., NNT = 1 / ARR); yet in GENETIC SCREENING, the ARR is the lifetime risk of the disease among carriers of the genetic variant of interest minus the risk of the disease achieved once the carriers are identified, diagnosed, and treated with the available means. A reasonable (low) NNS is attained only by screening for highly penetrant genetic variants in high-risk families, not for such mutations in the general population or for low-penetrant polymorphisms.[213] See also GENETIC PENETRANCE; MONOGENIC DISEASES; POLYGENIC DISEASES; SCREENING.

NUMBER NEEDED TO TREAT (NNT) (Syn: Number Needed to be Treated)

1. The number of persons needed to be treated, on average, to prevent one more event (e.g., occurrence of a disease to be prevented, complication, adverse reaction, relapse). It is a clinically meaningful way of expressing the benefit of an intervention over another; it takes the absolute risk of the event into account. It is used to summarize results of studies and to assist in clinical decision making.[297,298]
2. The reciprocal of the ABSOLUTE RISK REDUCTION. Let ARC be the absolute risk of events in the control group and ART the absolute risk of events in the treatment group; then the absolute risk reduction (ARR) = ARC – ART and the NNT = 1 / ARR. It may also be calculated as 100 divided by the ARR expressed as a percentage. Example: the occurrence of adverse outcomes in a clinical trial was 10% (0.10) in the placebo group and 4% (0.04) in the treated group; hence the ARR was 0.06 and 1 / 0.06 = 16.7 (i.e., on average, about 17 patients have to be treated in order to prevent one of them from having an adverse outcome or to reduce the number having an adverse outcome by 1). The ARR is higher and the NNT lower in groups with higher absolute risks.[14,15]

Definitions 1 and 2 seem equivalent but are not so unless the treatment acts independently of other background factors leading to the harm. See also MEASURE OF ASSOCIATION; NUMBER NEEDED TO HARM; RELATIVE RISK REDUCTION (RRR).

NUMERATOR The upper portion of a fraction, used to calculate a rate or a ratio. See also DENOMINATOR.

NUMERICAL TAXONOMY The construction of homogeneous groupings or taxa using numerical methods.

OBJECTIVE

1. (n.) The precisely stated end to which efforts are directed, specifying the population outcome, variable(s) to be measured, etc. See also GOAL; TARGET.
2. (adj.) A perspective or method that is free of prejudice, bias, favoritism, special interest. Some authors believe that such perspectives do not exist in reality and that at best an objective view is simply an ideal to strive for.

OBSERVATIONAL EPIDEMIOLOGY The application of epidemiological reasoning, knowledge and methods to studies, and activities that are nonexperimental. Epidemiological studies and programs (e.g., SURVEILLANCE) in which main conditions (e.g., exposures) are not under the direct control of the epidemiologist.

OBSERVATIONAL STUDY (Syn: nonexperimental study) A study that does not involve any intervention (experimental or otherwise) on the part of the investigator.[8–12,31,81,97] A study with RANDOM ALLOCATION is inherently experimental or nonobservational. Observations are not just a haphazard collection of facts; in their own way, observational studies must apply the same rigor as experiments.[61,95] Many important epidemiological, clinical, and microbiological studies are completely observational or have large observational components. See also CASE REPORTS; CLINICAL STUDY.

OBSERVATIONAL EPIDEMIOLOGICAL STUDY Epidemiological study that does not involve any intervention (experimental or otherwise) on the part of the investigator; e.g., a population study in which changes in health status are studied in relation to changes in other characteristics. Most analytical epidemiological designs (e.g, CASE-CONTROL and COHORT STUDIES) are properly called observational because investigators observe without intervention other than to record, classify, count, and statistically analyze results.

OBSERVER BIAS Systematic difference between a true value and the value actually observed due to OBSERVER VARIATION.

OBSERVER VARIATION (ERROR) Variation (or error) due to failure of the observer to measure or to identify a phenomenon accurately. Observer variation erodes scientific credibility whenever it appears. Sir Thomas Browne, in *Pseudodoxia Epidemica* (1646), subtitled "Enquiries into very many commonly received tenents and presumed truths," recognized several sources of error: "the common infirmity of human nature, the erroneous disposition of the people, misapprehension, fallacy or false deduction, credulity, obstinate adherence to authority, the belief in popular conceits, the endeavours of Satan."

All observations are subject to variation. Discrepancies between repeated observations by the same observer and between different observers are to be expected; these can be diminished but probably never absolutely eliminated.

Variation may arise from several sources. The observer may miss an abnormality or think that one has been found where none is present; a measurement or a test may give incorrect results due to faulty technique or incorrect reading and recording of the results; or the observer may misinterpret the information. Two varieties of observer variation are interobserver variation (the amount observers vary from one another when reporting on the same material) and intraobserver variation (the amount one observer varies between observations in reporting more than once on the same material).

OCCAM'S RAZOR The philosophical principle of scientific parsimony (parsimony is used here in the sense of unwillingness to use unnecessary resources, frugality, austerity). An ancient principle often attributed the philosopher and Franciscan friar William of Occam (c.1285–1349), who said: *Entia non sunt multiplicanda praeter necessitatem* (i.e., assumptions to explain a phenomenon must not be multiplied beyond necessity). In *The Grammar of Science* (1892), Karl Pearson called this the most important canon in the whole field of logical thought. This maxim does not contradict the conclusion that multiple causes may operate in a system. The number of possible causes implicated depends upon the frame of reference of the investigator and the scope of the inquiry. The principle is also important in MULTIVARIATE ANALYSIS (i.e., models should not be complicated beyond necessity).[20,93,97] Its primacy in statistics has been challenged by modern computing developments, in which highly complex models, augmented by computer-intensive fitting and validation methods (such as CROSS-VALIDATION, SHRINKAGE, and the BOOTSTRAP), can greatly outperform parsimonious methods developed in the precomputer era when many variables are available for the analysis. See also OVERFITTING.

OCCUPATIONAL EPIDEMIOLOGY The study of the effects of workplace exposures on the frequency and distribution of diseases and injuries in the population. The application of epidemiological knowledge to populations of workers. Occupational epidemiological research studies workers under a variety of working conditions, including exposure to psychosocial, chemical, biological, or physical (e.g., noise, heat, radiation) agents to determine if the exposures cause adverse health outcomes.[266,299]

OCCUPATIONAL HEALTH The specialized practice of medicine, public health, and other health professions in an occupational setting or with a focus on the work determinants of health. Its aims are to promote health as well as to prevent occupationally related diseases and injuries and the impairments arising therefrom—and, when work-related injury or illness occurs, to treat these conditions. This field combines preventive and therapeutic health services and, as the numbers of persons in many occupations are known fairly precisely, provides good opportunities for epidemiological studies.[300] Bernadino Ramazzini (1633–1714) is regarded as the "father of occupation medicine," having published *De Morbis Artificum* (*On the Diseases of Workers*) in 1700.

OCCURRENCE In epidemiology, a general term describing the frequency of a disease or other attribute or event in a population; it does not distinguish between INCIDENCE and PREVALENCE. The term is also used to allude to processes that lead to disease or that influence the incidence of disease.

ODA See Official Development Assistance.

ODDS The ratio of the probability of occurrence of an event to that of nonoccurrence, or the ratio of the probability that something is one way to the probability that it is another way. If 60% of smokers develop a chronic cough and 40% do not, the odds among smokers in favor of developing a cough are 60 to 40, or 1.5; this may be contrasted with the probability or risk that smokers will develop a cough, which is 60 over 100 or 0.6. See also LOGIT.

ODDS RATIO (Syn: cross-product ratio, relative odds) The ratio of two odds. The term *odds* is defined differently according to the situation under discussion. Consider the following notation for the distribution of a binary exposure and a disease in a population or a sample:

	Exposed	Unexposed
Disease	*a*	*b*
No disease	*c*	*d*

The odds ratio (cross-product ratio) is *ad/bc*.

The *exposure-odds ratio* for a set of case-control or cross-sectional data is the ratio of the odds in favor of exposure among the cases *(a/b)* to the odds in favor of exposure among noncases *(c/d)*. This reduces to *ad/bc*. In a case-control study with incident cases, unbiased subject selection, and a "rare" (uncommon) disease, *ad/bc* is an approximate estimate of the RISK RATIO; the accuracy of this approximation is proportional to the cumulative incidence of the disease. With incident cases, unbiased subject selection, and DENSITY SAMPLING of controls, *ad/bc* is an estimate of the ratio of the person-time incidence rates (FORCE OF MORBIDITY) in the exposed and unexposed (no rarity assumption is required for this).

The *disease-odds ratio* for a cohort or cross-sectional study is the ratio of the odds in favor of disease among the exposed *(a/c)* to the odds in favor of disease among the unexposed (*b/d*). This reduces to *ad/bc* and hence is equal to the exposure-odds ratio for the cohort or cross section.

The *prevalence-odds ratio* refers to an odds ratio derived cross-sectionally, as, for example, an odds ratio derived from studies of prevalent (rather than incident) cases.

The *risk-odds ratio* is the ratio of the odds in favor of getting disease if exposed to the odds in favor of getting disease if not exposed. The odds ratio derived from a cohort study is an estimate of this ratio. See also CASE-CONTROL STUDY; RARE-DISEASE ASSUMPTION.

OECD Organization for Economic Co-operation and Development (www.oecd.org).

OFFICE OF POPULATION CENSUSES AND SURVEYS (OPCS) (United Kingdom) Now the Office for National Statistics (www.gro.gov.uk).

OFFICIAL DEVELOPMENT ASSISTANCE (ODA) The term used by international development agencies for material and financial support provided by governments in high-income countries to those in low-income countries.

ONCOGENE A gene that can cause neoplastic transformation of a cell; oncogenes are slightly transformed equivalents of normal genes.

ONE-TAILED TEST A statistical test based on the assumption that only one direction of departure from the TEST HYPOTHESIS is of interest.

ONTOLOGY The study of what is the form and nature of reality and what can be known about it. The set of things whose existence is acknowledged by a particular theory or system of thought; it is in this sense that some experts speak of the ontology of a theory. The natural sciences embody implicit ontological schemes that cannot be wholly justified on purely empirical grounds and can engender theoretical perplexities.[301] See also EPISTEMOLOGY.

OPCS See Office of Population Censuses and Surveys.

OPEN-ENDED QUESTION A question that allows respondents to answer in their own words rather than according to a predetermined set of possible responses, i.e., a closed-ended question. Open-ended questions can be difficult to code and classify for statistical analysis.

OPERATIONAL DEFINITION A definition embodying criteria used to identify and classify individual members of a set or concept to facilitate classification and counting.

OPERATIONAL RESEARCH The systematic study, by observation and experiment, of the working of a system (e.g., health services), with a view to improvement.

OPERATIONS RESEARCH

1. The fitting of models to data or the designing of models
2. Synonym for OPERATIONAL RESEARCH

OPPORTUNISTIC INFECTION Infection with organism(s) that are normally innocuous (e.g., commensals in the human) but become pathogenic when the body's immunological defenses are compromised, as in the acquired immunodeficiency syndrome (AIDS).

OPPORTUNITY COST The benefit foregone, or value of opportunities lost, by engaging resources in a service; usually quantified by considering the benefit that would accrue by investing the same resources in the best alternative manner. The concept of opportunity cost derives from the notion of scarcity of resources.

ORDINAL SCALE See MEASUREMENT SCALE.

ORDINATE The distance of a point, P, from the horizontal or x axis of a graph, measured along the vertical or y axis. See also ABSCISSA; GRAPH; AXIS.

OUTBREAK An epidemic limited to localized increase in the incidence of a disease, e.g., in a village, town, or closed institution; *upsurge* is sometimes used as a euphemism for outbreak.

OUTCOME RESEARCH Research on outcomes of interventions. This is a large part of the work of clinical epidemiologists and epidemiologists involved in health services research.

OUTCOMES All the possible results that may stem from exposure to a causal factor or from preventive or therapeutic interventions. All identified changes in health status arising as a consequence of the handling of a health problem. See also CAUSALITY; CAUSATION OF DISEASE, FACTORS IN; DEPENDENT VARIABLE.

OUTLIERS Observations differing so widely from the rest of the data as to lead one to suspect that a gross error may have been committed, or suggesting that these values come from a population different from that giving rise to the bulk of the observations.

OUTPUT The immediate result of professional or institutional health care activities, usually expressed as units of service (e.g., patient hospital days, outpatient visits, laboratory tests performed).

OVERADJUSTMENT Statistical adjustment by an excessive number of variables or parameters, uninformed by substantive knowledge (e.g., lacking coherence with biological, clinical, epidemiological, or social knowledge). It can obscure a true effect or create an apparent effect when none exists. See also CAUSAL DIAGRAM; CONFOUNDING BIAS; CONFOUNDING, NEGATIVE; OVERMATCHING.

OVERCROWDING This sociodemographic term is variously defined. The UK Office of Population Censuses and Surveys (OPCS) uses an *index of overcrowding*, defined as the number of persons in private households living at a density greater than one person per room as a proportion of all persons in private households.

OVERFITTING Fitting a statistical model with a large number of parameters relative to the amount of data available and the fitting method used. It contradicts the principle of scientific parsimony, or OCCAM'S RAZOR. Chance error produced when large numbers of potential predictors are used to discriminate among a small number of outcome events and discrimination cannot be reproduced in a different sample. Genomic-based diagnostic research has been seen to be particularly prone to this type of error.[192] Statistical methods such as CROSS-VALIDATION, EMPIRICAL-BAYES METHODS, and SHRINKAGE can be used to address this problem without oversimplifying the model. See also CROSS VALIDATION; DATA DREDGING.

OVERMATCHING An undesirable result from matching comparison groups too closely or on too many variables. Several varieties can be distinguished:

1. The MATCHING procedure partially or completely obscures evidence of a true causal association between the independent and dependent variables. Overmatching may occur if the matching variable is involved in—or is closely connected with—the mechanism whereby the independent variable affects the dependent variable. The matching variable may be an intermediate cause in the causal chain under study, or it may be strongly affected by such an intermediate cause or a consequence of it.
2. The matching procedure uses one or more unnecessary matching variables (e.g., variables that have no causal effect or influence on the dependent variable) and hence cannot confound the relationship between the independent and dependent variables but reduces PRECISION.
3. The matching process is unduly elaborate, involving the use of numerous matching variables and/or insisting on very close similarity with respect to specific matching variables. This leads to difficulty in finding suitable controls. See also MATCHING.

OVERVIEW See META–ANALYSIS; SYSTEMATIC REVIEW.

OVERWINTERING See VECTOR-BORNE INFECTION.

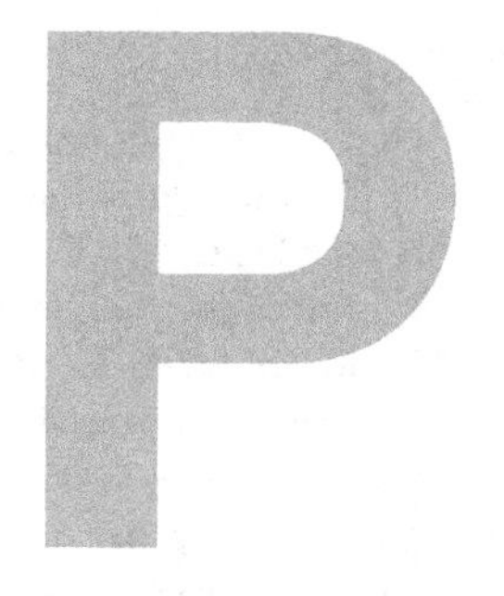

P See *P* VALUE.

PAHO See Pan American Health Organization.

PAIRED SAMPLES In a CLINICAL TRIAL, pairs of subject patients may be studied. One member of each pair receives the experimental regimen and the other receives a suitably designated control regimen. Pairing should be based on a prognostic variable, such as age.

Pairing may similarly be used in a CASE-CONTROL STUDY or in a COHORT STUDY. See also MATCHING.

PAN AMERICAN HEALTH ORGANIZATION (PAHO) The autonomous division of the WORLD HEALTH ORGANIZATION (WHO) that deals with the health affairs of North, Central, and South America (www.paho.org).

PANDEMIC An epidemic occurring worldwide or over a very wide area, crossing international boundaries, and usually affecting a large number of people.

PANEL STUDY A combination of cross-sectional and cohort methods in which the investigator conducts a series of cross-sectional studies of the same individuals or study sample. This method of study permits changes in one variable to be related to changes in other variables.

PARADIGM A broad intellectual framework or set of assumptions used to analyze a scientific issue or a field of scientific inquiry. Loosely, a pattern of thought or conceptualization—an overall way of regarding phenomena within which scientists normally work. In the particular sense used by Thomas Kuhn, paradigms are governing concepts of cause in a given science during a given period. Paradigms reflect causal concepts operative in current or so-called "normal" science. In Kuhn's influential view (one not accepted by all philosophers of science), such paradigms can be displaced only by scientific revolutions.[302] The causal theories of disease governing the thought of successive eras reflect different paradigms (e.g., miasma, germs, MULTIPLE CAUSATION). The inductive methods of Aristotle in the fourth century B.C. and of Bacon in the seventeenth century were rejected by David Hume in the eighteenth century and again by Karl Popper in the twentieth. However, they have been given modern forms in the machine-learning, artificial intelligence, and Bayesian literature. A paradigm may dictate what form of explanation will be found acceptable or well supported, but a science may change paradigms.[7,196] See also DEDUCTIVE LOGIC; HYPOTHETICO-DEDUCTIVE METHOD; INDUCTIVE LOGIC.

PARAMETER In mathematics, a quantity in a formula or model that is assumed not to vary within the system under study. In statistics and epidemiology, a measureable characteristic of a population that is often estimated by a statistic, e.g., mean, standard deviation, regression coefficients.

PARAMETRIC TEST A statistical test that depends upon assumption(s) about the distribution of the data (e.g., that these are normally distributed).

PARAMUTATION In EPIGENETICS, an interaction between two alleles of a single locus, resulting in a heritable change of one allele that is induced by the other allele. Paramutation violates Mendel's first law, which states that in the process of the formation of the gametes (egg or sperm) the allelic pairs separate, one going to each gamete, and that each gene remains completely uninfluenced by the other. In paramutation, an allele in one generation heritably affects the other allele in future generations, even if the allele causing the change is itself not transmitted. What may be transmitted in such a case are different types of RNAs, which may be packaged in egg or sperm and cause paramutation upon transmission to the next generation. This may mean that RNA is a molecule of inheritance, just like DNA. Paramutation can result in a single allele of a gene controlling a spectrum of phenotypes. See also EPIGENETIC INHERITANCE.

PARASITE An animal or vegetable organism that lives on or in another and derives its nourishment therefrom. An obligate parasite is one that cannot lead an independent nonparasitic existence. A facultative parasite is one that is capable of either parasitic or independent existence.

PARASITE COUNT See WORM COUNT.

PARASITE DENSITY The collective degree of parasite load (or of parasitemia) in a population. Calculated by the geometric mean or the weighted average of the individual parasite counts (e.g., by using a frequency distribution based on a geometric progression).

PARASITEMIA Presence of parasites in the blood. The term can also be used to express the quantity of parasites in the blood (e.g., "a parasitemia of 2%").

PARATENIC HOST (Syn: transport host) A second, third, or subsequent intermediate host of a parasite, in which the parasite does not undergo any development or replication but remains, usually encysted, until the paratenic host is ingested by the definitive host of the parasite.

PARITY The status of a woman with regard to having borne viable children. The number of full-term children previously borne by a woman, excluding miscarriages and abortions in early pregnancy but including stillbirths.

PARTICIPANT Person upon whom research is conducted. The term *research participant* is suggested in preference to *research subject* on the grounds that *subject* may be demeaning, but this can be ambiguous, because members of research teams are also called participants. *Volunteer* may be an alternative, but this too can be misleading, because not all persons upon whom research is conducted are volunteers. The term *research subject* is less ambiguous. The most suitable term differs according to the setting and should be selected for both clarity and for acceptability in that setting.

PARTICIPANT OBSERVATION A method used in the social sciences in which the research worker (observer) is (or pretends to be) a member of the group being studied. Epidemiologists distrust the method on the grounds that objectivity of the observations may be compromised.

PARTICULARIZATION A method of analysis opposite to generalization or abstraction. It focuses on the specificity of a number of facts and illustrates an issue through the use of example.

PASSAGE The transfer of microorganisms from human to animal host(s) either directly or via laboratory culture; in the laboratory, this procedure is used to check for conformity with the HENLE–KOCH POSTULATES.

PASSENGER VARIABLE A variable that varies systematically with the dependent (outcome) variable under study without having a direct causal relation to it.[22] A third (explanatory) variable, the common cause of both the dependent and the passenger variable, "explains," or accounts for, their association.

PASSIVE SMOKING See INVOLUNTARY SMOKING; ENVIRONMENTAL TOBACCO SMOKE.

PASTEURIZATION The process of heat-treating milk or other perishable foodstuffs to kill pathogens. Developed by and named for the great French bacteriologist Louis Pasteur (1822–1895).

PATH ANALYSIS A mode of analysis involving assumptions about the direction of causal relationships between linked sequences and configurations of variables. This permits the analyst to construct and test the appropriateness of alternative models (in the form of a path diagram) of the causal relations that may exist within the array of variables included in the finite system studied. Identification of the less probable sequences of causal pathways may permit them to be eliminated from further consideration.

PATH DIAGRAM See CAUSAL DIAGRAM.

PATHOGEN An organism capable of causing disease (literally, causing a pathological process).

PATHOGENESIS The mechanisms by which a cause or etiological agent produces disease. The etiology of a disease, disability or other health state begins with causes that initiate pathogenesis or favor pathogenetic mechanisms; control of such causes favours PRIMARY PREVENTION of the disease.

PATHOGENICITY The property of an organism that determines the extent to which overt disease is produced in an infected population, or the power of an organism to produce disease. Also used to describe comparable properties of toxic chemicals, etc. Pathogenicity of infectious agents is measured by the ratio of the number of persons developing clinical illness to the number exposed to infection. See also VIRULENCE, with which pathogenicity is sometimes confused.

PEARSON'S CHI-SQUARE See CHI-SQUARE TEST.

PEARSON'S PRODUCT MOMENT CORRELATION See CORRELATION COEFFICIENT.

PEDIGREE A diagram showing the ancestral relationships and transmission of genetic traits over several generations of a family.

PEER REVIEW Process of review of research proposals, manuscripts submitted for publication, and abstracts submitted for presentation at scientific meetings, whereby these are judged for scientific and technical merit by other scientists in the same field. The term also refers to review of clinical performance when it is a form of medical AUDIT.

PENALIZED ESTIMATION See SHRINKAGE ESTIMATION.

PENETRANCE See GENETIC PENETRANCE.

PERCEIVED NEED A felt need. The term usually refers to the need for health care felt by the person or community concerned and which may not be perceived by health professionals or political authorities.

PERCENTILE The set of divisions that produce exactly 100 equal parts in a series of continuous values, such as children's heights or weights. Thus, a child above the 90th percentile has a greater value for height or weight than over 90% of all in the series.

PERFORMANCE BIAS

1. Systematic differences in the care provided to members of the different study groups other than the intervention under investigation. For instance, patients who know they are in the control group may be more likely to use other forms of care, patients who know they are in the intervention group may be more likely to experience PLACEBO EFFECTS, and health care providers may treat patients differently according to what group they are in. To prevent unintended differences in care and placebo effects, those providing and receiving care can sometimes be "blinded" so that they do not know the group to which the recipients of care have been allocated. See also BLIND(ED) STUDY.
2. It may exist when the intervention actually received by study subjects differed substantially from the intervention that was intended or planned.

PERINATAL MORTALITY Literally, mortality around the time of birth. Conventionally, this time is limited to the period between 28 weeks gestation and 1 week postnatally. However, as the following discussion indicates, other factors, especially the weight of the fetus, should be considered. The *Ninth (1975) Revision of the International Classification of Diseases* includes the following:

Perinatal mortality statistics

It is recommended that national perinatal statistics should include all fetuses and infants delivered weighing at least 500 g [or, when BIRTH WEIGHT is unavailable, the corresponding gestational age (22 weeks) or body length (25 cm crown–heel)], whether alive or dead. It is recognized that legal requirements in many countries may set different criteria for registration purposes, but it is hoped that countries will arrange the registration or reporting procedures in such a way that the events required for inclusion in the statistics can be identified easily. It is further recommended that less mature fetuses and infants should be excluded from perinatal statistics unless there are legal or other valid reasons to the contrary.

It is recommended above that national statistics would include fetuses and infants weighing between 500 g and 1000 g both for their inherent value and because their inclusion improves the completeness of reporting at 1000 g and over.

Inclusion of this group of very immature births, however, disrupts international comparisons because of differences in national practices concerning their registration. Another factor affecting international comparisons is that all live-born infants, irrespective of birth weight, are included in the calculation of rates, whereas some lower limit of maturity is applied to infants born dead.

In order to eliminate these factors, it is recommended that countries should present, solely for international comparisons, "standard perinatal statistics" in which both the numerator and denominator of all rates are restricted to fetuses and infants weighing 1000 g or more [or, where BIRTH WEIGHT is unavailable, the corresponding gestational age (28 weeks) or body length (25 cm crown–heel)].

The Conference for the tenth revision (ICD-10) made no changes to these definitions.

PERINATAL MORTALITY RATE

1. In most industrially developed nations, this is defined as

$$\text{Perinatal mortality rate} = \frac{\text{fetal deaths (28 weeks + of gestation) + postnatal deaths (first week)}}{\text{fetal deaths (28 weeks + of gestation) + live births}} \times 1000$$

2. The WHO's definition, more appropriate in nations with less well established vital records, is

$$\text{Perinatal mortality rate} = \frac{\text{late fetal deaths (28 weeks + of gestation) + postnatal deaths (first week)}}{\text{live births in a year}} \times 1000$$

Note the difference in denominator of the perinatal mortality rate as defined by the WHO and in industrially developed nations. This makes international comparison difficult. The WHO Expert Committee on the Prevention of Perinatal Mortality and Morbidity (1970) recommended a more precise formulation: "Late fetal and early neonatal deaths weighing over 1000 g at birth expressed as a ratio per 1000 live births weighing over 1000 g at birth."

PERIODICITY A repeating pattern of a phenomenon or an event, especially the repetition of comparable values, e.g., seasonal fluctuation in numbers of cases of respiratory infections.

PERIODIC (MEDICAL) EXAMINATIONS Assessment of health status conducted at predetermined intervals (e.g., annually or at specified milestones in life, such as infancy, school entry, preemployment, or preretirement). This form of medical examination generally follows a formal protocol, employing a set of structured questions and/or a predetermined set of laboratory tests.

PERIOD OF COMMUNICABILITY See COMMUNICABLE PERIOD.

PERMISSIBLE EXPOSURE LIMIT (PEL) An occupational health standard to safeguard workers against dangerous substances in the workplace. See SAFETY STANDARDS.

PERSONAL HEALTH CARE Those services to individuals that are performed on a one-to-one basis by a health care worker for the purpose of maintaining or restoring health.

PERSONAL MONITORING DEVICE An instrument attached to a person to measure the exposure of that person to hazardous substance(s).

PERSON-TIME A measurement combining persons and time as the denominator in incidence and mortality rates when, for varying periods, individual subjects are at risk of developing disease or dying. It is the sum of the periods of time at risk for each of the subjects. The most widely used measure is person-years. With this approach, each subject contributes only as many years of observation to the population at risk as the period over which that subject has been observed to be at risk of the disease; a subject observed over 1 year contributes 1 person-year, a subject observed over a 10-year period contributes 10 person-years. This method can be used to measure incidence rate over extended and variable time periods. See also CONTEXT.

PERSON-TIME INCIDENCE RATE (Syn: interval incidence density) A measure of the incidence rate of an event (e.g., a disease or death) in a population at risk, given by

$$\frac{\text{Number of events occurring during the interval}}{\text{Number of person-time units at risk observed during the interval}}$$

PERSON-TO-PERSON SPREAD OF DISEASE See TRANSMISSION OF INFECTION.

PERSON-YEARS See PERSON-TIME.

PERSPECTIVE PLOT Diagrammatic representation of the relationship among three variables, one each on the horizontal and vertical axes and the third represented by a series of lines drawn so as to convey an illusion of three dimensions. See also CONTOUR PLOT.

PHARMACOEPIDEMIOLOGY (Syn: drug epidemiology) The study of the distribution and determinants of drug-related events in populations and the application of this study to efficacious treatment. The application of epidemiological knowledge, methods, and reasoning to describe, explain, control, and predict the uses and effects (beneficial and adverse) of drugs, vaccines, and related biological products in human populations. The public health foundation of pharmacoepidemiology is that drugs and vaccines are among the factors that influence the distribution of health states in human populations. Its core lies at the intersection of two subspecialties: clinical pharmacology and CLINICAL EPIDEMIOLOGY. Pharmacoepidemiology also aids pharmacology, public health, and other health sciences by increasing knowledge about the occurrence and causes of diseases, the distribution of health states, and the functioning of the health care system[92,303,304] See also CANCER EPIDEMIOLOGY; CARDIOVASCULAR EPIDEMIOLOGY; ENVIRONMENTAL EPIDEMIOLOGY; MOLECULAR EPIDEMIOLOGY; NEUROEPIDEMIOLOGY.

PHASE I, PHASE II, PHASE III TRIAL See CLINICAL TRIAL.

PHENOTYPE The observable properties, characteristics, or form of an organism or person produced by the GENOTYPE in synergy or interaction with the environment. All aspects of a living organism other than its genetic constitution. See also GENETIC PENETRANCE.

PHYSICIAN (Syn: medical practitioner, doctor) Professional person qualified by education and authorized by law to practice medicine.

PICKLES CHARTS Day-by-day plots of new cases of infectious disease seen in the practice of a family doctor; the method was developed and used by the British general

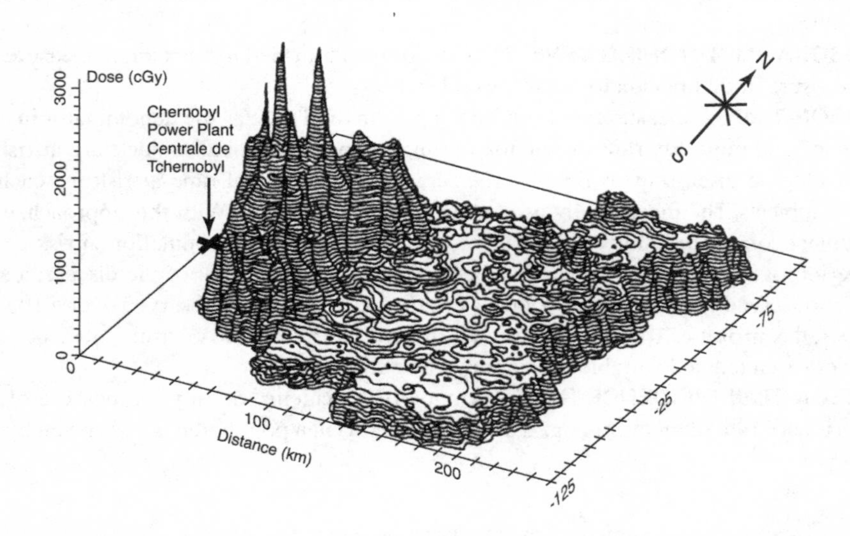

Perspective plot. Average distribution of thyroid doses of radioactive iodine, Ukraine, 1986. From *World Health Stat Q* 1996; 49:1. With permission.

practitioner and epidemiologist William Pickles (1885–1969) to demonstrate CLUSTERING in time and the progress of epidemic diseases in a small, relatively isolated, closed community. It has been used frequently by doctors and nurses in other isolated communities.[305]

PIE CHART A circular diagram divided into segments, each representing a category or subset of data. The amount for each category is proportional to the angle subtended at the center of the circle and hence to the area of the sector.

When several pie charts are used to describe several populations, the area of each circle is proportional to the size of the population it represents.

PILOT INVESTIGATION, STUDY A small-scale test of the methods and procedures to be used on a larger scale if the pilot study demonstrates that these methods and procedures can work.

PLAs Persons living with AIDS.

PLACEBO A medication or procedure that is inert (i.e., one having no pharmacological effect) but intended to give patients the perception that they are receiving treatment or assistance for their complaint. From Latin *placebo*, "I shall please."

PLACEBO EFFECT The beneficial effect resulting solely from the administration of a treatment, no matter whether strictly a placebo, an active drug, or another therapeutic procedure. Hence, placebo effects accompany also the prescription of efficacious drugs. They may be due to a variety of factors and occur through different mechanisms, including an empathic relationship between the prescribing physician and the patient or the patient's expectation of an effect (e.g., the power of suggestion). The very accomplishments of medicine, attained through scientific research, have augmented its placebo effects and metaphoric power.[127] See also HALO EFFECT; NOCEBO.

PLASTICITY The potential for change in intrinsic characteristics in response to environmental stimuli.[16] Phenotypic plasticity is a cell's ability to change its behavior in response to internal or external environmental cues.[116] The ability of a genotype to produce more than one alternative form of structure, physiological state, or behavior in response to environmental conditions. It is a quality of organisms as they develop.

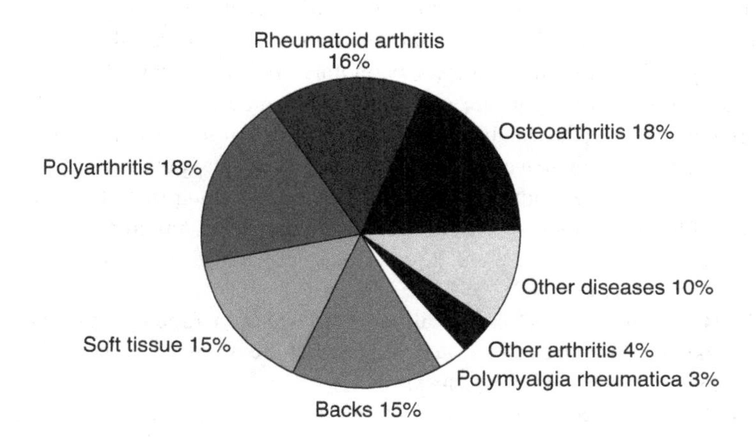

Pie chart. Percentage distribution of new outpatients in a rheumatic diseases clinic. From Silman AJ, Croft PR. Musculoskeletal diseases. In Detels R, Holland W W, McEwen J, Omenn G, eds. *Oxford Textbook of Public Health*, 3rd ed. Vol 3. New York: Oxford University Press, 1997, p. 1175. Copyright held by editors.

Within the limits imposed by genetic and mechanical constraints, each person has a range of options for his or her LIFE COURSE and final body form and function.[45] See also DEVELOPMENTAL ORIGINS HYPOTHESIS; EPIGENETICS; PROGRAMMING; SENSITIVE PERIOD.

PLAUSIBILITY See BIOLOGICAL PLAUSIBILITY; COHERENCE; HILL'S CRITERIA OF CAUSATION.

PLOT, BOX AND WHISKER See BOX-AND-WHISKERS PLOT.

PLOT, CAT AND WHISKER See CAT-AND-WHISKERS PLOT.

PLOT, FOREST See FOREST PLOT.

PLOT, FUNNEL See FUNNEL PLOT.

POINT SOURCE EPIDEMIC See EPIDEMIC, COMMON SOURCE.

POISSON DISTRIBUTION A distribution function used to describe the occurrence of rare events or the sampling distribution of isolated counts in a continuum of time or space (e.g., cases of an uncommon disease). The number of events X has a Poisson distribution with parameter λ (lambda) if the probability of observing k events ($k = 0, 1, \ldots$) is equal to

$$Pr(X = k) = \frac{e^{-\lambda}\lambda^{k}}{k!}$$

where e is the base of natural logarithm, 2.7183 .... The mean and variance of the distribution are both equal to λ. This distribution is used in modeling person-time incidence rates and caseloads.

POLICY A guide to action to change what would otherwise occur; a decision about amounts and allocations of resources; a statement of commitment to certain areas of concern; the distribution of the amount shows the priorities of decision makers. *Public policy* is policy at any level of government.[104,229] See also HEALTHY PUBLIC POLICIES.

POLITICAL EPIDEMIOLOGY The scientific study of political factors, processes, and conditions affecting the health of human populations.[306] The effects on health of the institutions derived from political power.[307] At least since Rudolf Virchow (1821–1902) proposed medicine as a political science, many epidemiologists have studied the effects on individual and community health of politically modifiable processes as democracy, political rights, and civil liberties. *Political economy* is the discipline that examines the relationships of individuals to society, economic production, and the activities of the state. *Political economy of health* is a theoretical framework used to study health inequalities; it proposes that health disparities and inequalities are caused by social structures and institutions, which create, enforce, and perpetuate poverty and privilege.[137,308] *Political ecology* is the study of the political and economic principles controlling the relations of human beings to one another and to the environment.[18]

POLLUTANT Any undesirable solid, liquid, or gaseous matter in a solid, liquid, or gaseous environmental medium.

POLLUTION Any undesirable modification of air, water, or food by substances that are toxic or may have adverse effects on health or that are offensive even if not necessarily harmful to health. See also CONTAMINATION.

POLYGENIC DISEASES Diseases in which multiple gene variants or genetic alterations jointly influence the risk of developing the disease, often through complex processes in which environmental and EPIGENETIC factors also intervene. A term sometimes used to refer to DISEASES OF COMPLEX ETIOLOGY. An antonym of MONOGENIC DISEASES.

POLYGENIC INHERITANCE The transmission of a phenotypic trait whose expression depends on the effect of multiple genes.

POLYMORPHISM, GENETIC The occurrence in a population of two or more genotypes. The existence of two or more genetic variants. A genome segment or locus in which alternate forms (alleles) are present. In population genetics, variation is polymorphic if all alleles are found at frequencies >1%. Genetic polymorphims can have opposite relations with different diseases; e.g., people with the NAT2-slow genotype are thought to have an increased risk of bladder cancer if exposed to aromatic amines (which are deactivated by acetylation) but a decreased risk of colon cancer if exposed to heterocyclic amines (activated by acetylation).[23,214–219,309]

POLYTOMOUS Divided or involving division into multiple parts. A categorical variable with three or more categories. See also MEASUREMENT SCALES.

PONDERAL INDEX The anthropometric index of body mass. Defined as height divided by the cube root of the body weight. The BODY MASS INDEX is generally regarded as a better index of body mass because it appears better correlated with tissue composition (percent body fat).

POPULATION

1. All the inhabitants of a given country or area considered together; the number of inhabitants of a given country or area.
2. In sampling, the whole collection of units (the "UNIVERSE") from which a sample may be drawn; not necessarily a population of persons – the units may be institutions, records, or events. The sample is intended to give results that are representative of the whole population; it may deviate from that goal owing to random and systematic errors. See also GENERAL POPULATION.

POPULATION ATTRIBUTABLE RISK (PAR) This term is sometimes used[62,310,311] as a synonym for ATTRIBUTABLE FRACTION (POPULATION). It is also used for the difference of the population rate or risk of disease and the rate or risk in the unexposed.

POPULATION ATTRIBUTABLE RISK PERCENT This is the attributable fraction in the population expressed as a percentage. See also ATTRIBUTABLE FRACTION (POPULATION).

POPULATIONBASED Pertaining to a general population defined by geopolitical boundaries; this population is the denominator and/or the sampling frame.

POPULATION DYNAMICS Changes in the structure of a population; loosely used as a synonym for DEMOGRAPHY.

POPULATION EXCESS RATE A measure of the number of disease cases associated with exposure to a putative cause of the disease in the population. It is the difference between the rates of disease in the entire population and among the nonexposed.

POPULATION GENETICS Study of the genetic composition of populations. The main aim is to estimate gene frequencies and detect selective factors in the environment that influence these frequencies.

POPULATION HEALTH

1. The health of the population measured by health status indicators; it is influenced by physical, biological, social, and economic factors in the environment, by personal health behavior, and by access to and effectiveness of health care services.
2. The prevailing or aspired level of health in the population of a specified country or region or in a defined subset of that population. The distinction between *population health* and PUBLIC HEALTH is that *population health* describes the condition whereas *public health* includes the policies, programs, practices, procedures, institutions,

and disciplines required to achieve the desired state of population health. The term also sometimes means the disciplines involved in studying the determinants and dynamics of a population's health status.[312]

POPULATION IMPACT NUMBER See IMPACT NUMBERS.

POPULATION MEDICINE See COMMUNITY MEDICINE.

POPULATION MOMENTUM In a growing population, the phenomenon of continuing population growth beyond the time when replacement-level fertility has been achieved because of the increasing size of childbearing and younger age cohorts resulting from higher fertility and/or falling mortality in preceding years.

POPULATION PREVENTIVE STRATEGY See STRATEGY, "POPULATION."

POPULATION PYRAMID A graphic presentation of the age and sex composition of the population. The population pyramid is constructed by computing the percentage distribution of a population simultaneously cross-classified by sex and age. The percentage that each female age group is of the total is plotted on the right and the corresponding percentages for males are plotted on the left. Sometimes the pyramid is constructed using absolute numbers, rather than proportions, in each age and sex group. A population pyramid is intended to provide a quick overall comprehension of age and sex structure in the population. A population whose pyramid has a broad base and narrow apex may be identified as a high-fertility population. Changing shape over time reflects the changing composition of the population associated with changes in fertility and mortality at each age. Since the figure is two-dimensional, the word *pyramid* is incorrectly used, but the more accurate word *profile* has never caught on.

POPULATION, SOURCE (Syn: base population) The group from which a study group is selected.

POPULATION, STUDY (Syn: study group, study sample) The group selected for investigation.

POPULATION, TARGET See TARGET POPULATION.

POPULATION THINKING By contrast to INDIVIDUAL THINKING, a mode of reasoning that consists in first observing and then predicting the experiences of a whole group of people defined in a specific way (e.g., geographically, socially, biologically).[10] Population thinking is deemed indispensable for GROUP COMPARISONS. See also CLINICAL STUDY; PREVENTION PARADOX; STRATEGY, "POPULATION."

POSITION EFFECT The effect on the expression of a gene when its location in a chromosome is changed, often by translocation. See also EPIGENETIC INHERITANCE.

POSITIVE PREDICTIVE VALUE See PREDICTIVE VALUE, POSITIVE.

POSTERIOR ODDS The odds calculated after reference to results of a study. See BAYES' THEOREM.

POSTERIOR PROBABILITY The probability calculated after reference to results of a study. See BAYES' THEOREM.

POSTMARKETING SURVEILLANCE Studies conducted after a drug or vaccine has been licensed for marketing and public use. Designed to provide information on the actual uses and effects of the product under common conditions of living, especially on the occurrence of side effects and adverse drug reactions unlikely to be detected with the lower numbers of subjects that take part in premarketing studies. It uses epidemiological and nonepidemiological designs. The latter include voluntary reporting systems of adverse events by health professionals. Postmarketing epidemiological studies may be observational and experimental.[92,303] See also CLINICAL TRIAL, PHASE IV.

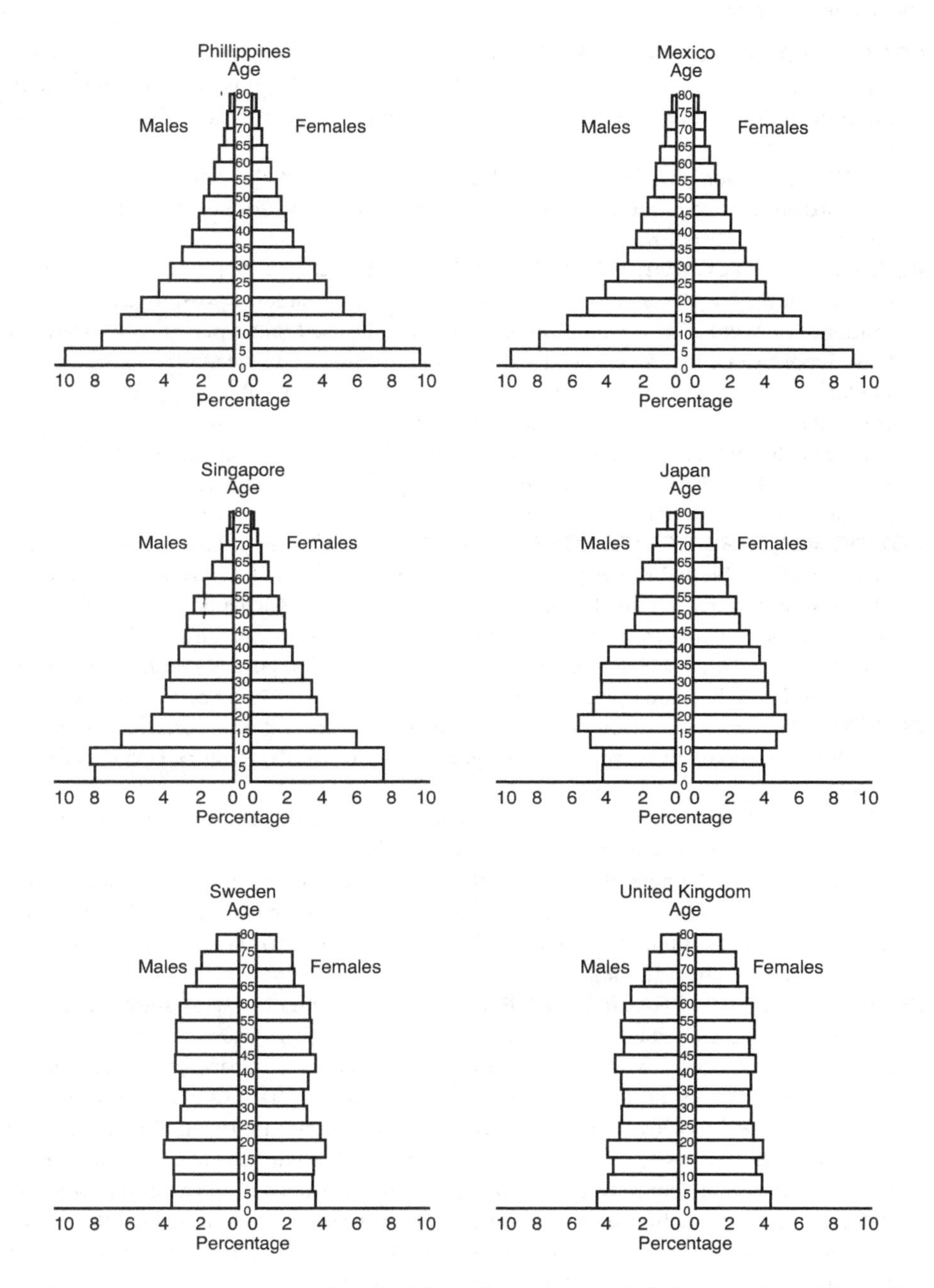

Population pyramids. Age pyramids for populations of six countries, 1965. Source: United Nations, 1973. From Basch PF, *Textbook of International Health*, 2nd ed. New York: Oxford University Press, 1999.

POSTNEONATAL MORTALITY RATE The number of infant deaths between 28 days and 1 year of age in a given year per 1000 live births in that year. It is an important rate to monitor in developing countries, where older infants frequently die of infections and malnutrition.

POTENCY The strength of a particular drug, toxin, or hazard; the ratio of the dose of a standard amount required to elicit a specific response to the dose of the test agent that elicits the same response.

POTENTIAL OUTCOMES, POTENTIAL OUTCOME MODEL A potential outcome is the outcome of a person, group, or other unit of study under a possibly hypothetical sequence of events.[91] For example, it may be hypothesized that a person will survive at least 5 more years by accepting a treatment but not survive by declining the treatment. Under this model for the person's potential outcomes, survival is a hypothesized outcome under treatment. If the person declines treatment and then dies, we will not know if indeed the model is correct because we will not observe what his or her outcome would have been had the treatment been accepted. Any further reasoning about the person's outcome under treatment will thus involve COUNTERFACTUAL LOGIC.

POTENTIAL YEARS OF LIFE LOST (PYLL) A measure of the relative impact of various diseases and lethal forces on society. PYLL highlights the loss to society as a result of youthful or early deaths. The figure for PYLL due to a particular cause is the sum, over all persons dying from that cause, of the years that these persons would have lived had they reached a specified age. The concept derives from Petty's *Political Arithmetic* (1687) and is elaborated upon in Dublin and Lotka's *Money Value of a Man* (1930).

POVERTY The individual's or group's lack of material or cultural resources. Inability to afford an adequate standard of living. See also ABSOLUTE POVERTY LEVEL; RELATIVE POVERTY LEVEL.

POWER Roughly, the ability of a study to demonstrate an association if one exists. The power of a study is determined by several factors, including the frequency of the condition under study, the magnitude of the effect, the study design, and sample size. Mathematically, power is defined as the probability that the null hypothesis will be rejected if it is false, and is equal to $1 - \beta$, where β is the probability of TYPE II ERROR (failing to reject a false null hypothesis).

PRAGMATIC STUDY, PRAGMATIC TRIAL (Syn: management trial) A study (including randomized clinical trials) whose aim is to improve health status or health care of a specified population, provide a basis for decisions about health care, or evaluate previous actions.[14,255,256] See also EXPLANATORY STUDY; COMMUNITY DIAGNOSIS; PROGRAM REVIEW.

PRECAUTIONARY PRINCIPLE The "better safe than sorry" approach to assessing and managing health risks, especially those associated with environmental hazards. Where there is sufficient evidence to believe that a risk exists, prudence and ethical norms and values require that action should be taken to reduce or eliminate that risk, even if the evidence is not conclusive. Similar in some ways the medical maxim *Primum non nocere* ("First do no harm") and the ethical principle of NONMALEFICENCE.

PRECIPITATING FACTORS See CAUSATION OF DISEASE, FACTORS IN.

PRECISION

1. Relative lack of random error. Contrast with INTERNAL VALIDITY, the relative lack of BIAS, or nonrandom error. As a principle, in etiological research, internal validity must take precedence over precision. However, sometimes a slightly biased, highly precise estimate may be preferable to an unbiased but highly imprecise estimate.

2. In statistics, one measure of precision is the inverse of the variance of a measurement or estimate. A measure of imprecision is the standard error of measurement—the standard deviation of a series of replicate determinations of the same quantity.
3. The quality of being sharply defined or stated. One measure of precision is the number of distinguishable alternatives from which a measurement was selected, sometimes indicated by the number of significant digits in the measurement. Precision does not imply ACCURACY. See also MEASUREMENT, TERMINOLOGY OF.

PRECURSOR A condition or state preceding pathological onset of a disease; sometimes detectable by SCREENING. See also RISK MARKER.

PREDICTIVE VALUE (of a screening test or of a diagnostic test) The probability of the disease given the results of the test. Predictive values of a test are determined by the SENSITIVITY and SPECIFICITY of the test and by the PREVALENCE of the condition for which the test is used. See also SCREENING.

PREDICTIVE VALUE, NEGATIVE (Syn: predictive value of a negative test) The probability that a person with a negative test result is a true negative (e.g., does not have the disease).

PREDICTIVE VALUE, POSITIVE (Syn: predictive value of a positive test) The probability that a person with a positive test result is a true positive (e.g., does have the disease).

PREDISPOSING FACTORS See CAUSATION OF DISEASE, FACTORS IN.

PREGNANCY-RELATED DEATH See MATERNAL MORTALITY.

PREMUNITION A state of resistance in a host harboring a parasite to superinfection by a parasite of the same species. The state is dependent on the continued survival of parasites in the body and disappears after their elimination; it may be complete or partial. A term used mainly in the epidemiology of parasitic diseases, especially malaria.

PREPATENT PERIOD In parasitology, the period equivalent to the incubation period of microbial infections; the corresponding phase may be biologically different from microbial multiplication when the invading organism is a multicellular parasite that undergoes developmental stages in the host.

PRESCRIPTIVE SCREENING See SCREENING.

PRESUMPTIVE TREATMENT Treatment of clinically suspected cases without, or prior to, results from confirmatory laboratory tests.

PREVALENCE A measure of disease occurence: the total number of individuals who have an attribute or disease at a particular time (it may be a particular period) divided by the population at risk of having the attribute or disease at that time or midway through the period. When used without qualification, the term usually refers to the situation at a specified point in time (point prevalence). A measure of occurrence or disease frequency, often used to refer to the proportion of individuals in a population who have a disease or condition.[12,31,97,313] It is a proportion, not a rate. Types of prevalence include the following:

Annual prevalence The proportion of individuals with the disease or attribute at any time during a year. It includes cases of the disease arising before but extending into or through the year as well as those having their inception during the year. Only occasionally used.

Lifetime prevalence The proportion of individuals who have had the disease or condition for at least part of their lives at any time during their LIFECOURSE.

One-year prevalence The proportion of individuals with the disease or condition at any time during a calendar year. It includes cases arising before and during the year.

Period prevalence The proportion of individuals with a disease or an attribute at a specified period of time. To calculate a period prevalence, the most appropriate denominator for the period must be found.

Point prevalence The proportion of individuals with a disease or an attribute at a specified point in time.

PREVALENCE POOL The diseased subset of a population.[12]

PREVALENCE STUDY See CROSS-SECTIONAL STUDY.

PREVENTABLE FRACTION (POPULATION) In a situation in which exposure to a given factor is believed to protect against a disease (or other outcome), the preventable fraction in the population is the proportion of the disease (in the population) that would be prevented if the whole population were exposed to the factor. This measure must be interpreted with caution, as part or all of the apparent protective effect may be due to other factors associated with the apparent protective factor.

In a study of a total population, the preventable fraction (population) of the incidence rate is computed as

$$(I_p - I_e) / I_p$$

where I_p is the incidence rate of the disease (or other outcome) in the population and I_e is what the incidence rate would be if everyone were exposed.

The same approach may be applied to other measures of disease frequency; e.g., the preventable caseload is

$$(A_p - A_e) / A_p$$

where A_p is the caseload in the population and A_e is what the caseload would be if everyone were exposed.

PREVENTED FRACTION (POPULATION) In a situation in which exposure to a given factor is believed to protect against a disease (or other outcome), the prevented fraction is the proportion of the hypothetical total load of disease (in the population) that has been prevented by exposure to the factor. This measure must be interpreted with caution, as part or all of the apparent protective effect may be due to other factors associated with the apparent protective factor.

In a study of a total population, the prevented fraction of the incidence rate is computed as

$$(I_u - I_p) / I_{u,} \text{or } P_e(1 - RR)$$

where I_p is the rate of the disease in the population, I_u is what the rate would be if everyone were not exposed, and P_e is the prevalence of exposure.

PREVENTION Actions that prevent disease occurrence. Actions aimed at eradicating, eliminating, or minimizing the impact of disease and disability, or if none of these is feasible, retarding the progress of disease and disability. The concept of *prevention* is best defined in the context of *levels* of prevention, traditionally called primary, secondary, and tertiary prevention. Other levels (primordial prevention, quaternary prevention) are also used. There is significant conceptual and practical overlapping among levels – largely, depending on the type of disease (e.g., on the NATURAL HISTORY OF THE DISEASE). Effective prevention STRATEGIES often interact and operate across levels.

1. PRIMORDIAL PREVENTION consists of conditions, actions, and measures that minimize hazards to health and that hence inhibit the emergence and establishment of processes and factors (environmental, economic, social, behavioral, cultural) known to increase the risk of DISEASE.[313] Primordial prevention is accomplished through many public and private HEALTHY PUBLIC POLICIES and INTERSECTORAL ACTION. It may be seen as a form of primary prevention.
2. PRIMARY PREVENTION aims to reduce the incidence of disease by personal and communal efforts, such as decreasing environmental risks, enhancing nutritional status, immunizing against communicable diseases, or improving water supplies. It is a core task of PUBLIC HEALTH, including HEALTH PROMOTION.
3. SECONDARY PREVENTION aims to reduce the prevalence of disease by shortening its duration. If the disease has no cure, it may increase survival and quality of life; it will also increase the prevalence of the disease. It seldom prevents disease occurrence; it does so only when EARLY DETECTION of a precursor lesion leads to complete removal of all such lesions. It is a set of measures available to individuals and communities for the early detection and prompt intervention to control disease and minimize disability; e.g., by the use of SCREENING programs. It is a core task of PREVENTIVE MEDICINE. Both EARLY CLINICAL DETECTION and population-based SCREENING usually aim at achieving secondary prevention. In certain diseases, these activities may also contribute to tertiary prevention.
4. TERTIARY PREVENTION consists of measures aimed at softening the impact of long-term disease and disability by eliminating or reducing impairment, disability, and handicap; minimizing suffering; and maximizing potential years or useful life. It is mainly a task of rehabilitation.
5. QUATERNARY PREVENTION consists of actions that identify patients at risk of overdiagnosis or overmedication and that protect them from excessive medical intervention.[314] Actions that prevent IATROGENESIS.

PREVENTIONIST A physician who specializes in PREVENTIVE MEDICINE and possesses specialist qualifications in this field. Loosely, a professional who practices PREVENTIVE MEDICINE.[315]

PREVENTION, CLARK'S LEVELS OF See PREVENTION.

PREVENTION LEVEL See PREVENTION.

PREVENTION PARADOX As formulated by Geoffrey Rose (1926–1993), a preventive measure that brings large benefits to the community but may offer little to each participating person.[72] For example, to prevent one death due to a motor vehicle accident, many hundreds of people must wear seat belts. Conversely, an intervention that brings much benefit to an individual may have a small impact in the population. See also STRATEGY.

PREVENTIVE MEDICINE The application of preventive measures by clinical practitioners. A specialized field of medical practice composed of distinct disciplines that utilize skills focusing on the health of defined populations in order to promote and maintain health and well-being and prevent disease, disability, and premature death.

In addition to the knowledge of basic and clinical sciences and the skills common to all physicians, the distinctive aspects of preventive medicine include knowledge of and competence in biostatistics; epidemiology; administration, including planning, organization, management, financing, and evaluation of health programs; environmental health; application of social and behavioral factors in health and disease; and the application of primary, secondary, and tertiary prevention measures within clinical medicine. See also HEALTH EDUCATION; HEALTH PROMOTION; STRATEGY.

PRIMARY CASE The individual who introduces the disease into the family or group under study. Not necessarily the first diagnosed case in a family or group. See also INDEX CASE.

PRIMARY CARE EPIDEMIOLOGY The application of epidemiological principles and methods to the study of problems arising in primary care, aimed at improving their management. This subdiscipline includes studies at and on the interface between primary care and the community (or the general population) as well as on the interfaces between primary and secondary (and tertiary) care. Much work involves studying the determinants and outcomes of consultations in primary care. Here, DETERMINANTS include also the nature of symptoms, signs, or illnesses occurring in the community and factors influencing decisions to consult or not to consult. OUTCOMES include—in addition to all other conventional outcomes—the duration, severity, and impact of illnesses and symptom complexes. They also include all aspects of primary care management (e.g., access, diagnostic investigations, referrals, treatments).[316] As mentioned above, EPIDEMIOLOGY is applied in many types of populations and health care settings; hence this dictionary includes just some examples of definitions for a few setting-based branches of epidemiology.

PRIMARY HEALTH CARE

1. Health care that begins at the time of first encounter between a patient and a provider of health care. It often is primary *medical* care.[317]
2. Primary health care is essential health care made accessible at a cost the country and the community can afford, with methods that are practical, scientifically sound, and socially acceptable.[318] Everyone in the community should have access to it. Related sectors should also be involved in it in addition to the health sector. At the very least it should include education of the community on the health problems prevalent and on methods of preventing health problems from arising or of controlling them; the promotion of adequate supplies of food and of proper nutrition; safe water and basic sanitation; maternal and child health care, including family planning; the prevention and control of locally endemic diseases; immunization against the main infectious diseases; appropriate treatment of common diseases and injuries; and the provision of essential drugs. See also COMMUNITY-ORIENTED PRIMARY HEALTH CARE.

PRIMORDIAL PREVENTION See PREVENTION.

PRINCIPAL COMPONENT ANALYSIS A statistical method to simplify the description of a set of interrelated variables. Its general objectives are data reduction and interpretation; there is no separation into dependent and independent variables; the original set of correlated variables is transformed into a smaller set of uncorrelated variables called the principal components. Often used as the first step in a factor analysis.

PRION A virus-like particle, an infectious protein, to which several so-called SLOW VIRUS diseases are attributed, including Creutzfeldt-Jakob disease and kuru in humans, bovine spongiform encephalopathy in cattle, and scrapie in sheep. Unlike viruses and bacteria, prions do not contain DNA or RNA. The word was coined in 1982 by the American neurologist Stanley B. Prusiner, from *pro*teinaceous *in*fectious particles, reversing the order of the vowels. Prusiner received the Nobel Prize in 1997 for the discovery of prions.

PRIOR ODDS The odds of disease before knowing the symptom. See BAYES' THEOREM.

PRIOR PROBABILITY Probability calculated or estimated from past data, theory, and judgment, before a study is analyzed. See BAYES' THEOREM.

PRIVACY The state of being undisturbed or free from public attention. The rules, regulations, and laws governing privacy and access to health-related information vary and change frequently. Privacy and CONFIDENTIALITY are protected by public interest groups and in some nations by privacy commissioners; the safeguards can affect EPIDEMIOLOGICAL RESEARCH requiring access to personal, private information. The concepts are increasingly important in situations where epidemiologists require access to data in medical and other records.[186,319] See also INFORMED CONSENT.

PROBABILITY

1. Frequency probability: the limit of the relative frequency of an event in a sequence of N random trials as N approaches infinity, i.e., the limit of

$$\frac{\text{Number of occurrences of the event}}{N}$$

2. Subjective probability: a measure, ranging from 0 to 1, of the degree of belief in a hypothesis or statement. Other definitions of probability exist (e.g., logical probability) but are rarely found in epidemiology, statistics, and clinical research. All probabilities obey the laws given by the axioms that:
   a. All probabilities are 0 or greater: for any event or statement A, $\Pr(A) \geq 0$.
   b. The probability of anything certain to happen is 1; i.e., if A is certain, $\Pr(A) = 1$.
   c. If two events or statements A and B, cannot both be true at once (they are mutually exclusive), then the probability of their conjunction (A or B) is the sum of their separate probabilities: $\Pr(A \text{ or } B) = \Pr(A) + \Pr(B)$.

PROBABILITY DENSITY For a continuous variable, the function that gives the rate at which its PROBABILITY DISTRIBUTION is increasing. Not to be confused with FREQUENCY DISTRIBUTION.

PROBABILITY DISTRIBUTION For a discrete random variable, the function that gives the probabilities that the variable equals each of a sequence of possible values. Examples include the binomial and Poisson distributions. For a continuous random variable, the function that gives the probability that the variable is less than or equal to any given value; but the term is often used synonymously with the probability density function.

PROBABILITY OF CAUSATION For a given case, the probability that exposure played a role in disease occurrence.[12] Although it is sometimes equated with the ATTRIBUTABLE FRACTION, the probability of causation can be much greater than that fraction. To illustrate, suppose 100 patients given an incorrect treatment each lived 8 years but would have lived 10 years each had they not received the incorrect treatment. Then the probability of causation of death by the incorrect treatment is 100%. After 10 years of follow-up, the total person-time at risk of death was 100(8) = 800; but if the incorrect treatment had not been given, it would have been 100(10) = 1000. Therefore the death rate over the 10 years was 100/800 = 0.125/year, but it would have been only 100/1000 had the incorrect treatment not been given. Thus the attributable fraction for the death rate was (0.125 – 0.100)/0.125 = 0.20 or 20%, which is far less than the probability of causation. In realistic examples the difference is less dramatic, but it still may be huge.

PROBABILITY SAMPLE (Syn: random sample) See SAMPLE.

PROBABILITY THEORY The branch of mathematics dealing with the purely logical properties of probability. Its theorems underlie most statistical methods.

PROBAND See PROPOSITUS.

PROBLEM-ORIENTED MEDICAL RECORD (POMR) A medical record in which the patient's history, physical findings, laboratory results, etc., are organized to give a cumulative record of problems (e.g., hemoptysis, rather than disease, such as pneumonia). The record includes subjective, objective, and significant negative information; discussions and conclusions; and diagnostic and treatment plans with respect to each problem. This type of record, which was developed by Lawrence Weed,[320] contrasts with the traditional medical record, which is less formally organized, usually recording all information from each source (history, physical, and laboratory findings) together without regard to the problems the information describes.

Since the problems may not be described in terms of conventional disease labels, their classification and counting for epidemiological purposes are sometimes difficult. The INTERNATIONAL CLASSIFICATION OF HEALTH PROBLEMS IN PRIMARY CARE (ICHPPC) is an attempt to overcome this difficulty.

PROCARCINOGEN The precursor of an active carcinogen. The procarcinogen itself is not usually carcinogenic but is converted to the active carcinogen after it has been metabolized by "xenobiotic metabolizing enzymes" such as cytochrome P450, dependent monooxygenases, glutathione S-transferases, sulfotransferases, and others. To elicit detrimental effects, the great majority of human chemical carcinogens require metabolic activation.[219,309] See also CARCINOGEN.

PROCATARCTIC CAUSE A term used by epidemiologists of the late nineteenth and early twentieth centuries to describe predisposing causes associated with habits of life.

PRODUCT LIMIT METHOD See KAPLAN-MEIER ESTIMATE.

PROFESSIONAL ACTIVITY STUDY (PAS) The HOSPITAL DISCHARGE ABSTRACT SYSTEM, which covers many acute short-stay hospitals in the United States. It provides regularly published statistical tables arranged according to hospital service, diagnostic category, etc., giving details on diagnostic and therapeutic procedures, length of stay, and outcome.

PROFILE PLOT (Syn: barycentric coordinates) A graphical method of data presentation used when several categories add to 100%; it permits the categories to be plotted on a plane surface using coordinates running inward at right angles from each side of an equilateral polyhedron.

PROFILE, TRIAL See CONSORT.

PROGRAM

1. A (formal) set of procedures to conduct an activity, e.g., control of malaria.
2. An ordered list of instructions directing a computer to carry out a desired sequence of operations. The objective is normally the solution of a problem.

PROGRAM EVALUATION AND REVIEW TECHNIQUES (PERT) A work-scheduling method that uses ALGORITHMS and also enunciates general principles of procedure for allocating resources. It calls for the listing of specific tasks to be completed and the resources—personnel, equipment, supplies, and other items—that will be needed, along with their costs; a time chart indicating when each component task is to begin and end; an enumeration of interim accomplishment levels during that period; and a specification of times for interim review of the progress of the plan.

PROGRAMMING The process whereby a stimulus or insult at a SENSITIVE PERIOD of development has lasting effects on the structure or function of the body. It has other meanings in other areas of science. It is no longer recommended to describe the developmental origins of adult disease.[45] See DEVELOPMENTAL ORIGINS HYPOTHESIS.

PROGRAM REVIEW An evaluative study of a specific health program operating in a specific setting that is performed to provide a basis for decisions concerning the operation of the program.

PROGRAM TRIAL An experimental or quasi-experimental evaluative study of a (health) program.

PROLECTIVE Pertaining to data collected by planning in advance. A research study may use data collected for the study purposes or RETROLECTIVE data. Two of many imaginative terms coined by Alvan R. Feinstein (1925–2001),[321,322] aiming to be more precise than the common terms *prospective* and *retrospective*. Rarely used. See also DIRECTIONALITY.

PROPENSITY SCORE Conditional probability of being treated given a certain set of measured covariates. It can be used to control confounding through matching, stratification, regression adjustment, or a combination of these methods, and it can be used along with other covariate adjustments.[323]

PROPERTIES OF A CAUSE As described by David Hume in 1739, they are ASSOCIATION (cause and effect occur together), TIME ORDER (causes precede effects), and CONNECTION or DIRECTION.[10,71] See also CAUSAL CRITERIA; CAUSALITY.

PROPHYLAXIS The preventive management of disease in individuals and populations. See also CHEMOPROPHYLAXIS.

PROPORTION A type of ratio in which the numerator is included in the denominator. The ratio of a part to the whole, expressed as a "decimal fraction" (e.g., 0.2), as a "common fraction" (1/5), or as a percentage (20%). By definition, a proportion (p) must be in the range (decimal) $0.0 \leq p \leq 1.0$. Since numerator and denominator have the same dimension, any dimensional contents cancel out, and a proportion is a dimensionless quantity. Where numerator and denominator are based on counts rather than measurements, the originals are also dimensionless, although it should be understood that proportions can be used for measured quantities (e.g., the skin area of the lower limb is x percent of the total skin area) as well as for counts (e.g., 15% of the population died). A PREVALENCE is a count-based proportion. The nondimensionality of a proportion, and its range limitations, do not necessarily apply to other kinds of ratios, of which "proportion" is a subset. See also RATE; RATIO.

PROPORTIONAL HAZARDS MODEL (Syn: Cox model) A statistical MODEL in SURVIVAL ANALYSIS proposed by Paul Sheehe in 1962 and more fully developed by D. R. Cox in 1972. It asserts that the effect of the study factors on the HAZARD RATE in the study population is multiplicative and does not change over time. For example, the model for the two factors x_1 and x_2 asserts that the rate at time t $\lambda(t)$, is given by

$$e^{\beta_1 x_1 + \beta_2 x_2} \lambda_0(t)$$

where $\lambda_0(t)$ is the rate when $x_1 = x_2 = 0$, and e is the base of the natural logarithm.

PROPORTIONAL MORTALITY-ODDS RATIO The odds of deaths from a specified condition in a defined population divided by the odds of deaths expected from this condition in a standard population, usually expressed either on an age-sex-specific basis or sex-specific after age adjustment. Often preferred to the proportional mortality ratio on the grounds that it tends to better approximate the ratio of mortality rates in the two populations.

PROPORTIONAL MORTALITY RATIO The proportion of observed deaths from a specified condition in a defined population divided by the proportion of deaths expected from this condition in a standard population, usually expressed either on an age-sex-specific basis or sex-specific after age adjustment. Unlike the STANDARDIZED MORTALITY RATIO, it does not require data on the age composition of the population but only on the deaths. The acronym PMR is preferably avoided because the same initial letters can stand for perinatal mortality rate.

PROPOSITUS (Syn: proband) The family member who first draws attention to a (genetic) pedigree of a given trait. The INDEX CASE in a genetic study.

PROSPECTIVE STUDY See COHORT STUDY.

PROTOCOL The plan, or set of steps, to be followed in a study or investigation or in an intervention program. See also ALGORITHM, CLINICAL.

PROTOPATHIC BIAS A type of BIAS that can occur if the first symptoms of the outcome of interest are the reasons for using the treatment under study.[321] See also CONFOUNDING BY INDICATION.

PROXIMAL DETERMINANT See DETERMINANT, PROXIMAL (PROXIMATE).

PSEUDO-LONGITUDINAL STUDY If a population is randomly sampled, for example annually, it is possible to identify a sequence of subsamples with age ranges increasing in step with the dates of the samples. The sequence of subsamples resembles a regularly measured cohort except that it consists of a different sample at each sampling occasion, which may overlap little if at all.

PSYCHOSOCIAL EPIDEMIOLOGY See SOCIAL EPIDEMIOLOGY.

PUBLICATION BIAS

1. The result of the tendency of authors to submit, organizations to encourage, reviewers to approve, and editors to publish articles containing "positive" findings (e.g., a gene-disease association), especially "new" results, in contrast to findings or reports that do not report statistically significant or "positive" results.
2. Tendency of authors to preferentially include in their study reports findings that conform to their preconceived notions or outcomes preferred by their institution or sponsor.

Publication bias distorts available scientific evidence on a wide range of issues. It can be a particularly important source of bias in META-ANALYSIS.[106,280] See also EPISTEMIC COMMUNITIES; KNOWLEDGE CONSTRUCTION; INTERPRETIVE BIAS; REPRESSION BIAS; SUPPRESSION BIAS; SCIENTIFIC MISCONDUCT.

PUBLIC HEALTH

1. One of the efforts organized by society to protect, promote, and restore the people's health.
2. The Acheson Report[324] offered this definition: "The science and art of preventing disease, prolonging life, and promoting health through organized efforts of society."
3. The combination of sciences, skills, and beliefs that is directed to the maintenance and improvement of the health of all the people through collective or social actions.

The programs, services, and institutions involved emphasize the prevention of disease and the health needs of the population as a whole. Public health activities change with changing technology and social values, but the goals remain the same: to reduce the amount of disease, premature death and disease-produced discomfort and disability in the population. Public health is thus a social institution, a discipline, and a practice.[1,85,225,313,325]

PUBLIC HEALTH IMPACT ASSESSMENT An analysis, evaluation, and assessment of the consequences and implications for public health of specific social or environmental initiatives or processes (e.g., construction of a power plant, housing developments and roads, legal status of immigrants). A combination of procedures, methods, and tools by which a policy, program, or project may be judged as to its potential effects on the health of a population and the distribution of those effects within the population. Considered as a major opportunity to *integrate health into all policies*, PHIA aims to influence the decision-making process, addressing all determinants of health, tackling inequities, and providing a new impetus for participation and empowerment in health.[70,326]

PUBLIC HEALTH MEDICINE The practice of public health by physicians. See SOCIAL MEDICINE.

PUNCH CARD A card on which data were stored by means of holes punched in specified positions. The position of the hole was the means of identifying the value of a variable. Punch cards were sorted mechanically or electrically to process and analyze data. They became obsolete in many areas by the mid-1980s, following the advent of computerized data processing. Hollerith cards were a commonly used variety of punch cards.

***P* VALUE** (probability)

1. The probability that a test statistic would be as extreme as observed or more extreme if the null hypothesis were true. The letter P stands for this probability. It is usually close to the probability that the difference observed or greater could have occurred by chance alone, i.e., under the NULL HYPOTHESIS. Investigators may arbitrarily set their own significance levels, but in most biomedical and epidemiological work, a study result whose P value is less than 5% ($P < 0.05$) or 1% ($P < 0.01$) is considered sufficiently unlikely to have occurred by chance to justify the designation "statistically significant."
2. More generally, the probability that a test statistic would be as extreme as or more extreme than observed if the TEST HYPOTHESIS were true. It is usually close to the probability that the deviation between what was observed and the hypothesized (test) value for the difference, or a greater deviation, could have occurred by chance alone. See also STATISTICAL SIGNIFICANCE.

QUADAS Quality Assessment of studies of Diagnostic Accuracy included in Systematic reviews. An evidence-based quality assessment tool to be used in systematic reviews of diagnostic accuracy studies. The checklist includes items that cover patient spectrum, reference standard, DISEASE PROGRESSION BIAS, verification bias, review bias, clinical review bias, incorporation bias, test execution, study withdrawals, and indeterminate results. It is presented together with guidelines for scoring each of the items included in the tool.[327] See also CONSORT; QUORUM; STARD; STROBE; TREND.

QALYs See QUALITY-ADJUSTED LIFE YEARS.

QUALITATIVE DATA

1. Observations or information characterized by measurement on a categorical scale, i.e., a dichotomous or nominal scale, or, if the categories are ordered, an ordinal scale. Examples are sex, hair color, death or survival, and nationality. See also MEASUREMENT SCALE.
2. Systematic nonnumerical observations by sociologists, anthropologists, etc., using approved methods such as participant observation or key informants. Qualitative data can enrich understanding of complex problems and help to explain why things happen.

QUALITATIVE RESEARCH Any type of research that employs nonnumeric information to explore individual or group characteristics, producing findings not arrived at by statistical procedures or other quantitative means. Examples include clinical case studies, narrative studies of behavior, ethnography, and organizational or social studies.[328]

QUALITY-ADJUSTED LIFE EXPECTANCY (QALE) A model for clinical decision making in which estimates of impairment or disability are included in the calculation of life expectancy.

QUALITY-ADJUSTED LIFE YEARS (QALYs) An adjustment of life expectancy that reduces the overall life expectancy by amounts that reflect the existence of chronic conditions causing impairment, disability, and/or handicap as assessed from health survey data, hospital discharge data, etc. In practice, numerical weights representing severity of residual disability are established by the judgment of patients and health professionals. Procedures for calculating QALYs, like those for calculating DALYs, begin with chronological age and multiply this by a "utility-weight" for the health state. A variety of techniques have been used, including STANDARD GAMBLE and TIME TRADE-OFF. See also DISABILITY-ADJUSTED LIFE YEARS.

QUALITY ASSURANCE System of procedures, checks, audits, and corrective actions to ensure that all research, testing, MONITORING, sampling, analysis, and other technical and reporting activities are of the highest achievable quality. The term is used in health services with the same meaning.

QUALITY CONTROL The supervision and control of all operations involved in a process, usually involving sampling and inspection, in order to detect and correct systematic or excessively random variations in quality.

QUALITY OF CARE A level of performance or accomplishment that characterizes the health care provided. Ultimately, measures of the quality of care always depend upon value judgments, but there are ingredients and determinants of quality that can be measured objectively. These ingredients and determinants were classified by Donabedian[329] into measures of structure (e.g., manpower, facilities), process (e.g., diagnostic and therapeutic procedures), and outcome (e.g., case fatality rates, disability rates, and levels of patient satisfaction with the service). See also HEALTH SERVICES RESEARCH.

QUALITY OF LIFE

1. The degree to which persons perceive themselves able to function physically, emotionally, mentally, and socially. Contrast HEALTH STATUS, which is an objective measurement. In a general sense, that which makes life worth living.
2. In a more "quantitative" sense, an estimate of remaining life free of impairment, disability, or handicap, as used in the expression QUALITY-ADJUSTED LIFE YEARS. Somewhere between these is an estimate of the utility of life; for instance, in clinical decision analysis, the utility of life that is impaired by a disabling degree of angina pectoris may be compared with that of a life that may be shorter in duration but free of disabling pain as a result of applying therapeutic procedures. Such trade-offs are part of clinical decision analysis. See also UTILITY.

QUOROM Quality of Reporting of Meta-analyses. A consensus checklist and a flow diagram to improve the quality of reports of META-ANALYSES of randomized clinical trials.[95,106,330] The checklist describes ways to present the abstract, introduction, methods, results, and discussion sections of a report of a meta-analysis. The flow diagram provides information about the numbers of trials identified, included, and excluded and the reasons for exclusion of trials. See also CONSORT; MOOSE; QUADAS; STARD; STROBE; TREND.

QUANGO A semipublic body partly or wholly supported by government funds and with some members appointed by the government but otherwise having the characteristics of a nongovernmental organization, i.e., a quasi-autonomous NGO, hence the name, originally slang. A term used mainly in Britain.

QUANTAL EFFECT (Syn: all-or-none effect) An effect that can be expressed only in binary form, e.g., as "occurring" or "not occurring."[200]

QUANTILES Divisions of a distribution into equal, ordered subgroups. Deciles are tenths; quartiles, quarters; quintiles, fifths; terciles, thirds; and centiles, hundredths.

QUANTITATIVE DATA Data in numerical quantities, such as continuous measurements or counts.

QUARANTINE

1. Restriction of the activities of well persons or animals who have been exposed to a case of communicable disease during its period of communicability (i.e., contacts) to prevent disease transmission during the incubation period if infection should occur.
   a. Absolute or complete quarantine: The limitation of freedom of movement of those exposed to a communicable disease for a period of time not longer than

the longest usual incubation period of that disease in such manner as to prevent effective contact with those not so exposed.

b. Modified quarantine: A selective, partial limitation of freedom of movement of contacts, commonly on the basis of known or presumed differences in susceptibility and related to the danger of disease transmission. It may be designed to meet particular situations. Examples are exclusion of children from school, exemption of immune persons from provisions applicable to susceptible persons, or restriction of military populations to the post or to quarters. It includes personal surveillance, the practice of close medical or other supervision of contacts in order to permit prompt recognition of infection or illness but without restricting movements; and segregation, the separation of some part of a group of persons or domestic animals from the others for special consideration, control, or observation—for example, removal of susceptible children to homes of immune persons or establishment of a sanitary boundary to protect uninfected from infected portions of a population.[52]

2. The word *quarantine* comes from the Italian *quaranta*, meaning forty, and refers to the 40 days arbitrarily (or empirically) believed to be an adequate isolation period, perhaps based on the biblical 40 days. The clinical distinction between isolation and quarantine is that isolation is the procedure for persons already sick, whereas quarantine is often applied to (apparently) healthy contacts. This has legal and ethical implications if apparently healthy persons must submit to restrictions upon their freedom to move at large in society. See also ISOLATION.

QUASI-EXPERIMENT A situation in which the investigator lacks full control over the allocation and/or timing of intervention but nonetheless conducts the study as if it were an experiment, allocating subjects to groups. Inability to allocate subjects randomly is a common situation that may be best described as a quasi-experiment. See also NATURAL EXPERIMENT.

QUESTIONNAIRE A predetermined set of questions used to collect data—clinical data, social status, occupational group, etc. This term is often applied to a self-completed survey instrument, as contrasted with an INTERVIEW SCHEDULE.

QUETELET'S INDEX See BODY MASS INDEX.

QUEUEING THEORY A mathematical discipline featuring models that analyze the flow of people through a service or their use of resources and that attempts to optimize utilization.

"QUICK AND DIRTY" METHOD A colloquial expression to refer to a method that yields a result rapidly but not necessarily with scientific rigor or validity. At least one variety, RAPID EPIDEMIOLOGICAL ASSESSMENT, has value and is not necessarily "dirty" (i.e., unreliable).

QUOTA SAMPLING A method by which the proportions in the sample in various subgroups (according to criteria such as age, sex, and social status of the individuals to be selected) are chosen to agree with the corresponding proportions in the population. The resulting sample may not be representative of characteristics that have not been taken into account.

QUOTIENT The result of the division of a numerator by a denominator.

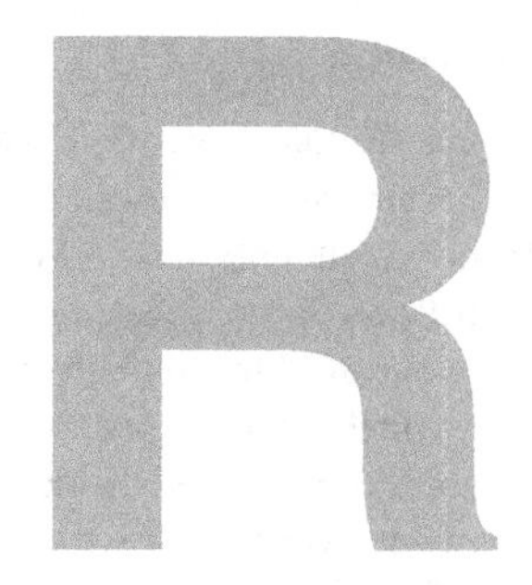

RACE

1. By historical and common usage, the group (*subspecies* in traditional scientific use) or a person who belongs to as a result of a mix of physical features such as skin color and hair texture, which reflect ancestry and geographical origins; as identified by others; or, increasingly, as self-identified. The importance of social factors in the creation and perpetuation of racial categories has led to broadening of the concept to include a common social and political heritage, making its use similar to ETHNICITY.[188]
2. In biology, a category used in the classification of organisms or a group of individuals within a species that are geographically, ecologically, physiologically, or chromosomally distinct from other members of the species.[331]

Biological classification of human races is difficult—and sometimes meaningless—because of significant genetic overlaps among population groups. Social scientists have challenged the biological definition of race, arguing that the concept of race most often reflects social and ideological conventions.[332] Economic, social, cultural, and behavioral differences are more important than biological differences in determining health status. However, race is a useful concept from the public health perspective because some diseases are strongly correlated with biological aspects of race; this may relate to gene-environment interaction or to the presence of specific genes, which may be due to environmental exposures of prior generations. Useful insights into human biology and genetics derive from analysis by racial group of large data sets such as the census and national health surveys. See also ETHNIC GROUP.

RADIX The size of the hypothetical BIRTH COHORT in a life table, commonly 1000 or 100,000.

RAHE-HOLMES SOCIAL READJUSTMENT RATING SCALE See LIFE EVENTS.

RANDOM (Syn: aleatory, stochastic) Governed by chance; not completely determined by measurable factors.

RANDOM ALLOCATION, RANDOMIZATION Allocation of individuals to groups in a CLINICAL TRIAL (e.g., intervention and control) by chance. It makes the trial a RANDOMIZED CONTROLLED TRIAL. It makes differences between the intervention and control groups random. Within the limits of chance variation (e.g., if the number of subjects is large), it yields groups similar at the start of an investigation and does so for both known and unknown variables (i.e., including measured and unmeasured determinants of the outcomes). No other methodological procedure can accomplish this. Randomization enables statistical procedures to account for uncertainty about unmeasured differences via standard errors, *P* values, and confidence intervals. It also ensures that personal judgment and views of the investigator do not influence allocation (e.g., of treatment).

Random allocation should not be confused with haphazard assignment: random allocation follows a predetermined plan that is usually devised with the aid of a computer program. Unsatisfactory (nonrandom) methods are allocation by alternation or date of birth, case record, day of the week, presenting or enrollment order. These methods, sometimes called "pseudorandomization," are not reliable in producing similar groups, prone to breakdown of ALLOCATION CONCEALMENT, and not accepted as appropriate allocation methods. See also BLOCKED RANDOMIZATION; CONFOUNDING BIAS; STRATIFIED RANDOMIZATION.

RANDOM-DIGIT DIALING A method for sampling people in telephone surveys in which telephone numbers are randomly dialed.

RANDOMIZATION, MENDELIAN See MENDELIAN RANDOMIZATION.

RANDOMIZED CONTROLLED TRIAL (RCT) An epidemiological experiment in which subjects in a population are randomly allocated into groups, usually called *study* and *control* groups, to receive or not to receive an experimental preventive or therapeutic procedure, maneuver, or intervention. The results are assessed by rigorous comparison of rates of disease, death, recovery, or other appropriate outcome in the study and control groups. RCTs are generally regarded as the most scientifically rigorous method of hypothesis testing available in epidemiology and medicine. Nonetheless, they may suffer serious lack of generalizability, due, for example, to the nonrepresentativeness of patients who are ethically and practically eligible, chosen, or consent to participate. A few authors refer to this method as "randomized control trial." See also COMMUNITY TRIAL; CLINICAL TRIAL; EXPERIMENTAL EPIDEMIOLOGY.

RANDOM SAMPLE A sample that is arrived at by selecting sample units such that each possible unit has a fixed and known or equal probability of selection. See also SAMPLE.

RANDOM VARIABLE

1. A variable whose distribution incorporates some element of chance, randomness, or unpredictability.
2. A variable that has or may be assigned a (possibly unknown) PROBABILITY DISTRIBUTION.

RANDOM WALK The path traversed by a particle that moves in steps, each step being determined by chance in regard to direction, magnitude, or both. The theory of random walks has many applications (e.g., to sequential sampling and to the migration of insects, including disease vectors).

RANGE OF DISTRIBUTION The difference between the largest and smallest values in a distribution.

RANK (v.) To arrange in a meaningful order or sequence (e.g., numerical order, degree of severity).

RANKING SCALE (Syn: ordinal scale) A scale that arrays the members of a group from high to low according to the magnitude of the observations, assigns numbers to the ranks, and neglects distances between members of the array. See also MEASUREMENT SCALE.

RAPID EPIDEMIOLOGICAL ASSESSMENT Methods that can be used to yield results as rapidly and efficiently as available resources permit; e.g., to assess health problems and evaluate health programs in developing countries or to delineate the health impact of a public health emergency, such as a disaster or an epidemic with unusual features.[333] See also DISASTER EPIDEMIOLOGY; TRIAGE.

RARE-DISEASE ASSUMPTION (Syn: rarity assumption) Reliance on the use of approximations, based on the assumption that the disease being studied is rare in the studied population. This assumption must be met for (1) prevalence to be approximately equal to the incidence rate multiplied by the average duration of disease (i.e., for the validity of the approximation $P = I \times D$); (2) the incidence proportion to be approximately equal to the incidence rate multiplied by the length of the follow-up period (i.e., for $IP = IR \times T$); and (3) for the odds ratio to be approximately equal to the incidence rate ratio or the risk ratio or cumulative incidence ratio (i.e., $OR \approx IRR$ or $OR \approx RR$) in some but not other case-control studies, depending on the method used to select controls. When the density sampling method is used to select controls, $OR = IRR$ regardless of the rarity or frequency of the disease. Decisions about "rarity" are rather arbitrary; the odds ratio will usually be within p% of the risk ratio if the risk does not exceed p% in any group being compared (e.g., if the risk is always below 5%, the odds ratio will generally be within 5% of the risk ratio and even closer to the rate ratio).[12]

RATE A measure of the frequency of occurrence of a phenomenon. In epidemiology, demography, and vital statistics, a rate is an expression of the frequency with which an event occurs in a defined population, usually in a specified period of time. Physical units other than time may be used for constructing rates, however; for example, in accident epidemiology, deaths per passenger-mile is a more meaningful way of comparing modes of transportation. The use of rates rather than raw numbers is essential for comparison of experience between populations at different times, different places, or among different classes of persons.

The components of a rate are the numerator, the denominator, the specified time in which events occur, and usually a multiplier, a power of 10, that converts the rate from an awkward fraction or decimal to a whole number.

In vital statistics,

$$\text{Rate} = \frac{\text{number of events in specified period}}{\text{average population during the period}} \times 10^n$$

In epidemiology, the denominator is usually person-time.

All rates are ratios, calculated by dividing a numerator (e.g., the number of deaths or newly occurring cases of a disease in a given period) by a denominator (e.g., the average population during that period). Some rates are proportions, where the numerator is contained within the denominator. Rate has several different usages in epidemiology:

1. As a wrong synonym for ratio, it refers to proportions as rates, as in the terms *cumulative incidence rate* or *survival rate. Proportion* and *ratio* are not synonyms for *rate*.
2. In other situations, *rate* refers only to ratios representing relative changes (actual or potential) in two quantities. This accords with the *Oxford English Dictionary,* which gives "relative amount of variation" among its definitions for *rate*.
3. Sometimes rate is further restricted to refer only to ratios representing changes over time. In this sense, the term *prevalence rate* is to be avoided, because PREVALENCE cannot (and does not need to) be expressed as a change in time; of course, different prevalence estimates may vary, change, and be compared. In contrast, the force of mortality and the force of morbidity (hazard rate) are proper rates, for they can be expressed as the number of cases developing per unit time divided by the total size of the population at risk.

RATE DIFFERENCE (RD) The absolute difference between two rates; for example, the difference in incidence rate between a population group exposed to a causal factor and a population group not exposed to the factor:

$$RD = I_e - I_u$$

where I_e = incidence rate among exposed and I_u = incidence rate among unexposed. In comparisons of exposed and unexposed groups, the term *excess rate* may be used as a synonym for *rate difference*.

RATE-ODDS RATIO See ODDS RATIO.

RATE RATIO The ratio of two rates; e.g., the rate in an exposed population divided by the rate in an unexposed population:

$$Rate\ ratio = \frac{I_e}{I_u}$$

where I_e is the incidence rate among the exposed and I_u is the incidence rate among the unexposed. See also RELATIVE RISK.

RATIO The value obtained by dividing one quantity by another. RATE, PROPORTION, and percentage are types of ratios. The numerator of a proportion is included in the population defined by the denominator, whereas in other types of ratios numerator and denominator are distinct quantities, neither being included in the other. The dimensionality of a ratio is obtained through algebraic cancellation, summation, etc., of the dimensionalities of its numerator and denominator terms. Both counted and measured values may be included in the numerator and in the denominator. There are no general restrictions on the dimensionalities or ranges of ratios, but there are in some types of ratios (e.g., proportion, prevalence). Ratios are sometimes expressed as percentages (e.g., standardized mortality ratio). In these cases, the value may exceed 100.

RATIO SCALE See MEASUREMENT SCALE.

RAW DATA The entire set of information that has been collected in a study before any cleaning, editing, or statistical manipulation begins.

REASON FOR ENCOUNTER (RFE) The statement of reason(s) why a person enters the health care system, representing that person's demand for care. The terms recorded by the health care provider clarify the reason for encounter without interpreting it in the form of a diagnosis.[258]

RECALL BIAS Systematic error due to differences in ACCURACY or completeness of recall to memory of past events or experiences.[12,14,31] For example, a mother whose child has died of leukemia may be more likely than the mother of a healthy living child to remember details of such past experiences as use of x-ray services when the child was in utero.

RECEIVER OPERATING CHARACTERISTIC (ROC) CURVE (Syn: relative operating characteristic curve) A graphic means for assessing the ability of a screening or diagnostic test to discriminate between persons with and without the target disorder. For an ordinal or continuous diagnostic test, the ROC curve depicts the plot of all pairs of sensitivity and 1-specificity (false-positive probability) over all possible or chosen cutoff values. The term *receiver operating characteristic* comes from psychometry, where the characteristic operating response of a receiver-individual to faint stimuli or nonstimuli was recorded. The term was first used in studies of radar during World War II.

RECESSIVE In genetics, a gene that is phenotypically manifest only when present in the homozygous state.[23,134,243]

RECOMMENDATIONS See GUIDELINES.

RECORD LINKAGE A method for bringing together the information contained in two or more records—e.g., in different sets of medical charts, and in vital records such as birth and death certificates—and a procedure to ensure that each individual is identified and counted only once. This procedure incorporates a unique identifying system such as a personal identification number and/or birth name(s) of the individual's mother.[334]

Record linkage makes it possible to relate significant health events that are remote from one another in time and place or to bring together records of different individuals (e.g., members of a family). The resulting information is generally stored and retrieved by a computer, which can be programmed to tabulate and analyze the data.

PRIVACY and CONFIDENTIALITY must both be respected in record linkage studies. This is usually accomplished by requiring an oath of secrecy from all who handle the records involved. Each person in the world creates a book of life. This book starts with birth and ends with death. Its pages are made of the records of the principal events during the LIFE COURSE. Record linkage is the name given to the process of assembling the pages of this book into a volume.[335]

RECRUDESCENCE Reactivation of infection. See also RELAPSE.

RECTANGULARIZATION OF MORTALITY The shape of survival curves as life expectancy increases: higher proportions of all who are born survive to old age and the graph becomes more "rectangular" in shape. Empirical observations in several countries have failed to demonstrate it, and the opposite was found in the United States, where the range of age at death was widening because of the impact of HIV disease and violence. See also COMPRESSION OF MORTALITY.

RECURRENCE The second episode of a disease occurring after a first episode was considered cured. For instance, in tuberculosis, molecular techniques have shown that some recurrences are due to reinfection by a different strain rather than relapse with the same strain that had caused the first episode.[336] Thus REINFECTION and RELAPSE are two different causes of disease recurrence.

RECURRENCE RISK Risk of a second episode (and of subsequent episodes) of a disease. It provides information on the heterogeneity of risk in the population; it is thus useful for etiological studies. Observable in many areas of epidemiology, it is particularly accessible in the study of perinatal events. High recurrence rates of pregnancy problems may result from interactions between genetic causes and persistent environmental causes. Patterns of recurrence risk provide clues about the relative importance of genetic, epigenetic, and environmental factors; e.g., through comparisons of recurring pregnancy problems in women who change their male partner and women who keep the same partner.[337]

RECURRENT DISEASE A bacteriologically confirmed disease episode needing retreatment after a patient was successfully treated or defaulted during a previous disease episode.[338] See also REINFECTION.

REDEFINING THE UNACCEPTABLE An expression to describe the history of public health. The public health advances when there is a combination of knowledge of the causes of public health problems, technical capability to deal with these causes, a sense of values that the health problems are important, and political will. It is the last of these that Vickers described as "redefining the unacceptable."[339]

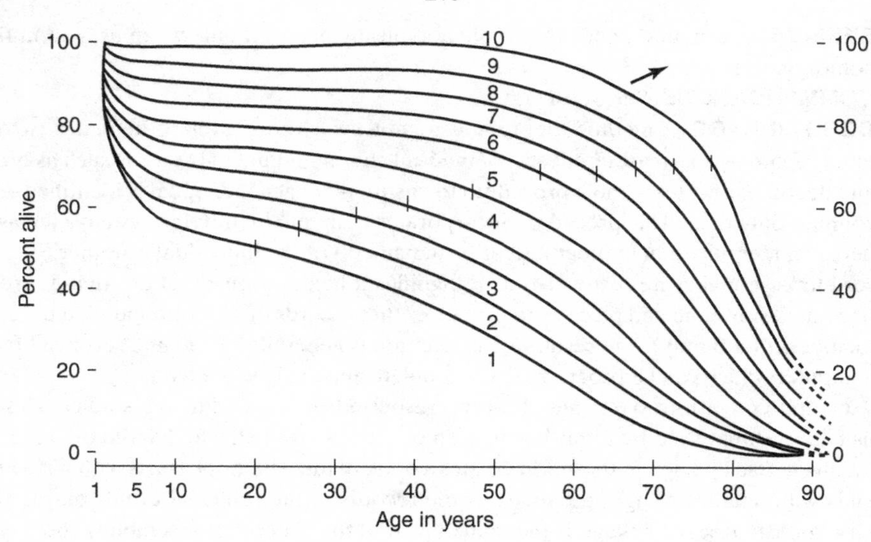

1. India, Male, 1901–1911. (Expectation of life at birth, 22.59 years)
2. Guatemala, Male, 1921. (25.59 years)
3. Mexico, Male, 1930. (33.02 years)
4. England and Wales, Male, 1861. (40.47 years)
5. Guatemala, Male, 1964. (48.51 years)
6. England and Wales, Male, 1921. (55.94 years)
7. Venezuela, Male, 1964. (63.74 years)
8. Netherlands, Male, 1947–49. (69.40 years)
9. Sweden, Male, 1964. (75.93 years)
10. Sweden, Female, 1974. (78.10 years)

Rectangularization of mortality. Survivorship curves by age and sex, selected countries, 1861–1974. Vertical bars show life expectancy at birth. From Basch PF. *Textbook of International Health*. New York: Oxford University Press, 1990. With permission.

REDUCTION (of data)

1. (Syn: "collapsing") Reducing the number of categories of a set of data to simplify analysis. An important application is aggregation of small numbers and/or small areas in published tables from a national census in order to preserve the CONFIDENTIALITY of these localities and their residents.
2. Formation of composite (derived) variables based on several originally collected variables, using methods ranging from simple indexes to factor analysis.
3. Summarizing data by means of classification schemes and arithmetical manipulations.

REDUCTIONISM The philosophical concept of scientific investigation that is based on studying component parts of a system; e.g., proceeding from organs to tissues, to cells, to molecules. The reductionist view is that the whole can be explained in terms of the functioning of its parts. The discovery of the DNA structure can be viewed as a triumph for reductionist approaches. While some reductionist approaches have been fruitful, they may favor rigid compartmentalizing and fragmentation of sciences and hence delay progress.

They may also favor MEDICALIZATION and GENETIZATION. Epidemiological studies that focus exclusively on individual RISK FACTORS are also a form of reductionism (not necessarily wrong or irrelevant), which tends to disregard contextual influences on health. Clinical and molecular epidemiology are practiced with both reductionist and INTEGRATIVE approaches.[6,10,61–63] See also TRANSDISCIPLINARITY.

REED-FROST MODEL A mathematical model of infectious disease transmission and herd immunity developed by Lowell Reed (1886–1966) and Wade Hampton Frost (1880–1938). The model gives the number of new cases, *C*, of an infectious disease that can be expected in a closed, freely mixing population of immunes and susceptibles in time period *t* to *t* + 1, with varying assumptions about the distribution of each in the population:

$$C_{t+1} = S_t[1-(1-p)_t{}^{c}]$$

where C_{t+1} is the number of cases between time *t* and *t* + 1, S_t is the number of susceptibles at time *t*, and *p* is the probability that any specified individual will have contact with any other specified individual in the population. Elaborations of the model provide the theoretical basis for IMMUNIZATION programs that control infectious diseases without necessarily achieving 100% immunization coverage.[340]

REFERENCE POPULATION The standard against which a population that is being studied can be compared.

REFINEMENT The process of identifying new subcategories of study variables for the purpose of more accurate or more detailed description of relationships. An example is refinement of the concept of serum cholesterol level into high-, low-, and very low density lipoproteins.

REGISTER, REGISTRY In epidemiology the term *register* is applied to the file of data concerning all cases of a particular disease or other health-relevant condition in a defined population such that the cases can be related to a population base. With this information, incidence rates can be calculated. If the cases are regularly followed up, information on remission, exacerbation, prevalence, and survival can also be obtained. The *register* is the actual document and the *registry* is the system of ongoing registration.

In most developed countries all births and deaths are recorded through birth and death registration systems. Results and summaries are then tabulated and published. Examples of registries that have epidemiological value include the following:

Cancer registries, which secure reports of cancer patients as soon as possible after first diagnosis. The principal sources for these reports are the hospitals serving the community, but a few cases are not reported until death.

Twin registries, which have provided the basis for studies attempting to differentiate genetic from environmental factors in the etiology of cancer and other conditions where both genetic and environmental factors may be contributing causes.

Birth defect registries, which seek to document anomalies that are apparent at or soon after birth. They suffer from incompleteness owing to the omission of stillbirths and of anomalies that do not declare their presence until later in life, such as certain forms of congenital heart lesion, mental deficiency, and neurological disorders.

Many types of register—e.g., disease-specific, treatment-specific, "at risk," local (hospital- or clinic-based)—are not population-based. Population-based registers are usually considered to be the most useful type for epidemiological purposes; clinic-based, disease-specific registers can be used as a source of cases for case-control studies.[341]

REGISTRATION The term *registration* implies something more than notification for the purpose of immediate action or to permit the counting of cases. A register requires that a permanent record be established, including identifying data. Cases may be followed up, and statistical tabulations may be prepared on both frequency and survival. In addition, the persons listed on a register may be subjects of special studies.

REGRESSAND In REGRESSION ANALYSIS, the variable whose mean values are studied in relation to regressors; the dependent variable.

REGRESSION

1. As used by Francis Galton (1822–1911), one of the founders of modern biology and biometry, in his book *Hereditary Genius* (1869), this meant the tendency of offspring of exceptional parents (unusually tall, unusually intelligent, etc.) to possess characteristics closer to the average for the general population. Hence "regression to the mean"; i.e., the tendency of individuals at the extremes to have values nearer to the mean on repeated measurement.
2. In statistics, the relation of mean values of a dependent or regressand variable to independent or regressor variables (covariates).
3. A synonym for REGRESSION ANALYSIS.

REGRESSION ANALYSIS Given data on a regressand (dependent variable) y and one or more regressors (covariates or independent variables) x_1, x_2, etc., regression analysis involves finding a mathematical model (within some restricted class of models) that adequately describes y as a function of the x's, or that predicts y from the x's. The most common form of model for an unbounded continuous y is a linear model; the logistic and proportional hazards models are the most common forms used when y is binary or a survival time, respectively.[20]

REGRESSION CURVE, LINE, SURFACE, PLANE Diagrammatic presentation of a REGRESSION MODEL as a curve on a graph, usually drawn with the regressor, x, as the abscissa and the predicted average of the dependent variable (regressand), y, as ordinate. In the case of LINEAR REGRESSION, the curve reduces to a line. A model with three variables (two regessors and one regressand) can be shown diagrammatically on a three-dimensional plot or stereogram; the result is a regression surface, which in the case of MULTIPLE LINEAR REGRESSION reduces to a plane.

REGRESSION MODEL A MATHEMATICAL MODEL for the relation of the average value of a variable (the REGRESSAND) to other variables (the REGRESSORS). See also REGRESSION ANALYSIS.

REGRESSOR In REGRESSION ANALYSIS, a variable used to predict the regressand (dependent) variable. An independent variable or regression covariate.

REINFECTION A second infection by the same agent or a second infection of an organ with a different agent or strain. In tuberculosis, DNA fingerprinting of *Mycobacterium tuberculosis* showed that some RECURRENCES are not treatment failures (i.e., they are not a RELAPSE).[342,343]

REINFORCING FACTORS See CAUSATION OF DISEASE, FACTORS IN.

RELAPSE

1. Return of a disease state after remission or apparent cure.
2. Insufficient bacteriological cure of a first episode. In tuberculosis the episode is caused by the same strain. In malaria, true relapses are caused by reactivation

of dormant liver stage parasites (HYPNOZOITES) found in *Plasmodium vivax* and P. ovale.[131] See also RECURRENCE.

RELATIONSHIP See ASSOCIATION.

RELATIVE EFFECT A ratio of rates, proportions, or other measures of an effect. For example, the incidence rate ratio, calculated as the incidence rate in the exposed divided by the incidence rate in the unexposed, is a measure of relative effect.[12]

RELATIVE EXCESS RISK (RER) A measure that can be used in comparisons of adverse reactions to drugs (or other exposures), based solely on the component of risk due to the exposure or drug under investigation, removing the risk due to background exposure experienced by all in the population:

$$RER = (R_1 - R_0) / (R_2 - R_0)$$

where R_1 is the rate in the study population. R_2 is the rate in the comparison group, and R_0 is the rate in the general population.[344]

RELATIVE ODDS See ODDS RATIO.

RELATIVE POVERTY LEVEL The amount of income a person, family, or group needs to purchase a relative amount of basic necessities of life; these basic necessities are identified relative to each society and economy. See also ABSOLUTE POVERTY LEVEL.

RELATIVE RISK (RR)

1. The ratio of the risk of an event among the exposed to the risk among the unexposed; this usage is synonymous with RISK RATIO.
2. The ratio of the incidence rate in the exposed to the incidence rate in the unexposed (i.e., the RATE RATIO). It is not synonymous with ODDS RATIO (OR). In some biostatistical articles, it has been used for the ratio of FORCES OF MORBIDITY. The use of *relative risk* for OR arises from the fact that for "rare" (infrequent) diseases, the two quantities may approximate one another. For common occurrences (e.g., neonatal mortality in infants under 1500-g birth weight), the approximations do not hold.
3. Let ARC be the absolute risk of events in the control group and ART the absolute risk of events in the treatment group; then RR = ARC / ART = 1 – RR reduction (RRR). Example: an RR of 0.7 equals an RRR of 0.3, i.e., a 30% reduction in the RR of the outcome in the treatment group compared with the control group. See also ABSOLUTE RISK (AR); ABSOLUTE RISK REDUCTION (ARR); CONTROL GROUP; CUMULATIVE INCIDENCE RATIO; RISK DIFFERENCE.

RELATIVE RISK REDUCTION (RRR)

1. The difference in EVENT RATES between two groups expressed as a proportion of the event rate in the untreated group. The RRR may be similar in populations with different risks. An estimate of the number of people spared the consequences of an exposure that has been eliminated or controlled. The amount by which a person's risk of disease is reduced by elimination or control of an exposure to risk.
2. Let ARC be the absolute risk of events in the control group and ART the absolute risk of events in the treatment group; then RRR = (ARC – ART) / ARC = 1 – Risk Ratio.[14,15] See also ABSOLUTE RISK (AR); ABSOLUTE RISK REDUCTION (ARR); NUMBER NEEDED TO TREAT (NNT).
3. The RRR, ARC, and NNT are related as follows: NNT × RRR × ARC = 1. This equation is used to assess plausible benefits of an intervention in populations and individuals with different levels of baseline risk.[298]

RELEVANCE

1. The importance for existing ideas or practices. The degree to which a study, program, policy, or organization should theoretically change or can actually influence knowledge, beliefs, ideas, attitudes, decisions, actions, policies, structures, procedures, techniques, or processes of all sorts (social, cultural, political, organizational, individual, medical, biological, etc.).
2. In epidemiology, a relevant study or program may be one that makes a practical or a theoretical contribution to the identification, characterization, understanding, or solution of a public health, environmental, social, clinical, biological, or technological problem. EPIDEMIOLOGICAL RESEARCH usually aims at having social, environmental, or public health relevance; epidemiological studies often also have clinical, biological, methodological, or technological relevance.
3. In clinical and epidemiological research, *relevance* is commonly used as a synonym of importance and of *significance*. Statistical significance is always distinguished from clinical and public health significance. A statistically significant effect (e.g., with a $P < 0.01$) may be found in a study with a large number of participants and yet lack clinical or public health significance (because the magnitude of the effect is small, for instance). Hence, statistical significance never equals *significance*, and *significance* encompasses more than statistical significance. Clinical studies usually aim at being clinically significant, important, or relevant for the care of patients. They are often mechanistically relevant; e.g., they produce knowledge on mechanisms of disease or of drug action. The health sciences scientific literature contains several thousand articles with the word *relevance* in the title and over 200,000 with *relevance* or *relevant* in the abstract. See also SIGNIFICANCE, CLINICAL; SIGNIFICANCE, PUBLIC HEALTH; SIGNIFICANCE, STATISTICAL.

RELIABILITY The degree of stability exhibited when a measurement is repeated under identical conditions. *Reliability* refers to the degree to which the results obtained by a measurement procedure can be replicated. Lack of reliability may arise from divergences between observers or instruments of measurement or instability of the attribute being measured. See also MEASUREMENT, TERMINOLOGY OF; OBSERVER VARIATION.

REMOTE SENSING The collection and interpretation of information at a distance from the phenomenon or object being observed, e.g., by aerial photography, satellite imaging. Remote sensing has provided valuable information about ecological zones hospitable to mosquitoes and other vectors, plankton blooms that can potentiate cholera outbreaks, etc.

REPEATABILITY (Syn: reproducibility) A test or measurement is repeatable if the results are identical or closely similar each time it is conducted. See also MEASUREMENT, TERMINOLOGY OF; RELIABILITY.

REPLACEMENT-LEVEL FERTILITY The level of fertility at which a cohort of women are having only enough daughters to replace themselves in the population. By definition, it is equal to a net reproduction rate of 1.00. The total fertility rate is also used as a measure of replacement level fertility. In the United States today, a total fertility rate of 2.12 is considered to be replacement level; it is higher than 2 because of mortality and because of a sex ratio greater than 1 at birth. The higher the female mortality rate, the higher is the replacement-level fertility. See also GROSS REPRODUCTION RATE.

REPLICATION The execution of an experiment or survey more than once so as to confirm the findings, increase PRECISION, and obtain a closer estimation of sampling error.

Exact replication should be distinguished from *consistency of results on replication*. Exact replication is often possible in the physical sciences, but in the biological and behavioral sciences, to which epidemiology belongs, consistency of results on replication is often the best that can be attained. Consistency of results on replication is perhaps the most important criterion in judgments of causality.

REPORTING BIAS Selective revealing or suppression of information (e.g., about past medical history, smoking, sexual experiences).

REPRESENTATIVE SAMPLE The term *representative* as it is commonly used is undefined in the statistical or mathematical sense; it means simply that the sample resembles the population in some way.[98] The use of probability sampling will not ensure that any single sample will be "representative" of the population in all possible respects. If, for example, it is found that the sample age distribution is quite different from that of the population, it is possible to make corrections for the known differences. A common fallacy lies in the unwarranted assumption that, if the sample resembles the population closely on those factors that have been checked, it is "totally representative" and that no difference exists between the sample and the universe or reference population.

Some confusion arises according to whether *representative* is regarded as meaning "selected by some process which gives all samples an equal chance of appearing to represent the population" or, alternatively, whether it means "typical in respect of certain characteristics, however chosen." On the whole, it seems best to confine the word *representative* to samples that turn out to be so, however chosen, rather than applying it to those chosen with the objective of being representative.[98] See also GENERAL POPULATION; VALIDITY, STUDY.

REPRESSION BIAS Failing to pursue a line of enquiry because the enquiry fails to conform to prevailing dominant social or research paradigms. It may lead to PUBLICATION BIAS. It undermines public health because it delays the discovery of scientific knowledge on health risks and compromises credibility in science and administrative processes for assessing and preventing exposure to risks. See also SUPPRESSION BIAS; SCIENTIFIC MISCONDUCT.

REPRODUCIBILITY See REPEATABILITY.

REPRODUCTIVE ISOLATION Absence of interbreeding between populations.

REPRODUCTIVE SUCCESS In population genetics, quantitatively, the proportion of offspring surviving long enough to reproduce.

REPROGRAMMING In GENETICS and EPIGENETICS, the erasure and reestablishment of DNA methylation during mammalian development. After fertilization, the paternal and maternal genomes are once again demethylated and remethylated. This reprogramming might be required for totipotency of the newly formed embryo and erasure of acquired epigenetic changes. See also EPIGENETIC INHERITANCE.

RESCUE BIAS A form of INTERPRETIVE BIAS that occurs in discounting data by finding selective faults in a study when the data are viewed unfavorably or by discounting faults when the data are viewed favorably. A deliberate attempt to evade evidence that contradicts expectation or interests.[34,259] See also AUXILIARY HYPOTHESIS BIAS.

RESEARCH A class of activities designed to develop or contribute to generalizable knowledge; generalizable knowledge consists of theories, principles, or relationships or the accumulation of information on which these are based that can be corroborated by acceptable scientific methods of observation, inference, and/or experiment (adapted from the COUNCIL FOR INTERNATIONAL ORGANIZATIONS OF THE MEDICAL SCIENCES, 1993).

When humans are the subjects of EPIDEMIOLOGICAL RESEARCH, ethical review is mandatory; however, there is a blurry boundary between research, which must undergo review, and common clinical or public health practice (e.g., surveillance and epidemic control), to which the same rules may not apply. See also INTEGRATIVE RESEARCH.

RESEARCH DESIGN The "architecture" of a study: its structure, specific details of the studied population, time frame, method, and procedures, including ethical considerations, all of which should be explicitly stated in a research protocol. Details of all aspects of research design are essential to anyone seeking to replicate a study, so there is a moral obligation to ensure that these details are in the public domain. They must be adhered to by all centers in a multicenter study.

RESEARCH ETHICS BOARD, COMMITTEE See INSTITUTIONAL REVIEW BOARD.

RESEARCH SUBJECT A person who is studied. Under some circumstances the word *subject* is perceived as demeaning, and other terms may be more socially acceptable, e.g., *study participant*, *volunteer*, or *patient*.

RESERVOIR OF INFECTION

1. Any person, animal, arthropod, plant, soil, or substance, or combination of these in which an infectious agent normally lives and multiplies, on which it depends primarily for survival, and where it reproduces itself in such a manner that it can be transmitted to a susceptible host.
2. The natural habitat of the infectious agent.

RESILIENCE A process of positive ADAPTATION in the face of adversity; e.g., intrinsic and extrinsic factors confer educational, emotional, and behavioral resilience to children.[16]

RESIDUAL CONFOUNDING Confounding that persists after unsuccessful attempts to adjust for it. Also referred to as *unmeasured confounding*, although the problem lies with unmeasured or poorly measured confounders. Main sources of residual confounding are insufficiently detailed information, improper categorization, and misclassification of one or more confounding variables. It is an outcome-specific concept.[82,253] See also ADJUSTMENT; CONFOUNDING BIAS; INVERSE PROBABILITY WEIGHTING; STANDARDIZATION.

RESOLUTION, RESOLVING POWER

1. The capacity of a system to distinguish between truly distinct things that are close together.
2. A component of a measuring instrument that helps determine PRECISION. The degree of refinement of the measuring process is commonly referred to as the "resolution" or the "resolving power of the system." See also POWER. The capability of distinguishing between things that are indeed separate or distinct from one another.

RESOURCE ALLOCATION The process of deciding how to distribute financial, material, and human resources among competing claimants for these resources. Resource allocation is an essential feature of all health planning everywhere.[345] Epidemiological evidence on need, demand, supply, and use of existing services is integral to the process, although factors such as political, commercial, and emotional considerations sometimes carry more weight than objective epidemiological evidence; ethical considerations should affect decisions about resource allocation.

RESPONSE BIAS Systematic error due to differences in characteristics between those who choose or volunteer to take part in a study and those who do not.

RESPONSE RATE The number of completed or returned survey instruments (questionnaires, interviews, etc.) divided by the total number of persons who would have been surveyed if all had participated. Usually expressed as a percentage. Nonresponse can have several causes, e.g., death, removal from the survey community, and refusal. See also BIAS; COMPLETION RATE; NONPARTICIPANTS.

RETROLECTIVE Pertaining to data gathered without planning for the needs of an investigation. See also PROLECTIVE, also a term suggested by A. R. Feinstein.[321,322] See also DIRECTIONALITY.

RETROSPECTIVE STUDY A research design used to test etiological hypotheses in which inferences about exposure to the putative causal factor(s) are derived from data relating to characteristics of the persons under study or to events or experiences in their past. The essential feature is that some of the persons under study have the disease or other outcome condition of interest, and their characteristics and past experiences are compared with those of other, unaffected persons. Persons who differ in the severity of the disease may also be compared. It is no longer considered a synonym for CASE-CONTROL STUDY.

RETROVIRUS This name is given to a family of RNA viruses characterized by the presence of an enzyme, reverse transcriptase, that enables transcription of RNA to DNA inside an affected cell. Thus retroviruses can make copies of themselves in host cells. The most important retrovirus is the human immunodeficiency virus (HIV); this makes copies of itself in host cells, such as T4 "helper" lymphocytes, and normal immune responses are disrupted.

REVERSE TRANSCRIPTION The process by which an RNA molecule is used as a template to make a single-stranded DNA copy.[243] This is the mode of action of the HUMAN IMMUNODEFICIENCY VIRUS when it attacks T4 helper lymphocytes, which maintain immune competence.

REVES Réseau Espérances de Vie en Santé ([International] Network on Health Expectancy and the Disability Process) (www.reves.net).

REVIEW BIAS In diagnostic accuracy studies, bias that occurs when the investigator knows the results of the new diagnostic test when the "gold standard" test is interpreted or when the investigator knows the results of the gold standard test when the new diagnostic test in interpreted.

REVIEW, SYSTEMATIC The application of strategies that limit bias in the assembly, critical appraisal, and synthesis of all relevant studies on a specific topic. META-ANALYSIS may be, but is not necessarily, used as part of this process. Systematic reviews focus on peer-reviewed publications about a specific health problem and use rigorous, standardized methods for selecting and assessing articles. A systematic review differs from a meta-analysis in not including a quantitative summary of the results.[106,280,286,327,330]

RIDIT A method of presenting observed values, e.g., health measurement scale scores of a group, relative to a reference population.[345] The average ridit for the group shows the probability that a member of the group differs from a member of the reference population. For example, if the average ridit for a group is 0.62, 62% of persons in the reference population have higher scores than a randomly chosen member of the group.

RIDIT ANALYSIS A method proposed by Bross (1958) for analyzing subjectively categorized or poorly recorded data. It consists of allocating scores relative to the identified distribution of the data based upon a transformation to the uniform distribution rather than the normal distribution.

RISK The probability that an event will occur, e.g., that an individual will become ill or die within a stated period of time or by a certain age. Also, a nontechnical term encompassing a variety of measures of the probability of a (generally) unfavorable outcome. See also PROBABILITY.

RISK ASSESSMENT

1. The qualitative or quantitative estimation of the likelihood of adverse effects that may result from exposure to specified health hazards or from the absence of beneficial influences. Risk assessment uses clinical, epidemiologic, toxicologic, environmental, and any other pertinent data.
2. The process of determining risks to health attributable to environmental or other hazards. The process consists of four steps:
   Hazard identification: Identifying the agent responsible for the health problem, its adverse effects, the target population, and the conditions of exposure.
   Risk characterization: Describing the potential health effects of the hazard, quantifying dose-effect and dose-response relationships.
   Exposure assessment: Quantifying exposure (dose) in a specified population based on measurement of emissions, environmental levels of toxic substances, BIOLOGICAL MONITORING, etc.
   Risk estimation: Combining risk characterization, dose-response relationships, and exposure estimates to quantify the risk level in a specific population. The end result is a qualitative and quantitative statement about the health effects expected and the proportion and number of affected people in a target population, including estimates of the uncertainties involved. The size of the exposed population must be known.

RISK-BENEFIT ANALYSIS The process of analyzing and comparing on a single scale the expected positive (benefits) and negative (risks, costs) results of an action or lack of an action.

RISK-BENEFIT RATIO The results of a risk-benefit analysis expressed as the ratio of risks to benefits.

RISK CHARACTERIZATION See RISK ASSESSMENT.

RISK DIFFERENCE (RD) (Syn: ABSOLUTE RISK REDUCTION) The absolute difference between two risks: one minus the other. See also RELATIVE RISK REDUCTION.

RISK ESTIMATION See RISK ASSESSMENT.

RISK EVALUATION See RISK MANAGEMENT.

RISK FACTOR (Syn: risk indicator)

1. An aspect of personal behavior or lifestyle, an environmental exposure, or an inborn or inherited characteristic that, on the basis of scientific evidence, is known to be associated with meaningful health-related condition(s). In the twentieth century MULTIPLE CAUSE era, a synonymous with DETERMINANT acting at the individual level.
2. An attribute or exposure that is associated with an increased probability of a specified outcome, such as the occurrence of a disease. Not necessarily a causal factor: it may be a RISK MARKER.
3. A determinant that can be modified by intervention, thereby reducing the probability of occurrence of disease or other outcomes. It may be referred to as a modifiable risk factor, and logically must be a cause of the disease.

The term *risk factor* became popular after its frequent use by T. R. Dawber and others in papers from the Framingham study.[346] The pursuit of risk factors has motivated the search for causes of chronic disease over the past half-century. Ambiguities in risk and in risk-related concepts, uncertainties inherent to the concept, and different legitimate meanings across cultures (even if within the same society) must be kept in mind in order to prevent MEDICALIZATION of life and IATROGENESIS.[124–128,136,142,240]

RISK MANAGEMENT The steps taken to alter (i.e., reduce) the levels of risk to which an individual or a population is subject. The managerial, decision-making, and active hazard control process to deal with environmental agents of disease, such as toxic substances, for which risk evaluation has indicated an unacceptably high level of risk. The process consists of three steps:

1. RISK EVALUATION: Comparison of calculated risks or public health impact of exposure to an environmental agent with the risks caused by other agents or societal factors and with the benefits associated with the agent as a basis for deciding what is an ACCEPTABLE RISK.
2. EXPOSURE CONTROL: Actions taken to keep exposure below an acceptable maximum limit.
3. RISK MONITORING: The process of measuring reduction in risk after exposure control actions have been taken in order to reassess risks and initiate further control measures if necessary.

RISK MARKER (Syn: risk indicator) An attribute that is associated with an increased probability of occurrence of a disease or other specified outcome and that can be used as an indicator of this increased risk. Not necessarily a causal factor. See also RISK FACTOR.

RISK MONITORING See RISK MANAGEMENT

RISK RATIO The ratio of two risks, usually exposed/not exposed.

ROBUSTNESS

1. A property of a statistical test or procedure that confers to it a certain degree of insensitiveness to departures from the assumptions from which it is derived (e.g., that the data are normally distributed).
2. The resistance of genes to manipulations supposed to lead to a predicted phenotype. Essentially due to the fundamental regulatory role of interactions among genes, and to a common redundancy of functions and regulatory mechanisms converging towards a specific goal.[207,347]

ROUNDING The process of eliminating surplus digits, taking the nearest whole number, multiple of 10, etc., as an approximation of the value of a measurement. See also DIGIT PREFERENCE.

RUBRIC Section or chapter heading. Used in epidemiology with reference to groups of diseases, e.g., in the INTERNATIONAL CLASSIFICATION OF DISEASE (ICD).

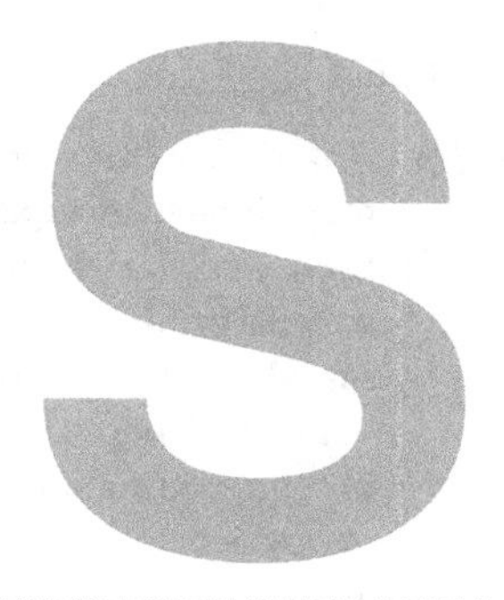

SAFETY FACTOR A multiplicative factor incorporated in risk assessments or safety standards to allow for unpredictable types of variation, such as variability from test animals to humans, random variation within an experiment, and person-to-person variability. Safety factors are often in the range of 10 to 1000 or even higher magnitudes.

SAFETY STANDARDS Under the requirements of the U.S. Occupational Safety and Health Act (OSHA, 1970), *occupational safety and health standard* means a standard that requires conditions, or the adoption of one or more practices, means, methods, operations, or processes, reasonably necessary or appropriate to provide safe or healthful employment and places of employment. Safety standards may be adopted by national consensus or established by federal regulation. These standards have been adopted in many other nations besides the United States, although some European and other countries have their own standards, which may be either more or less stringent than those in the United States.[266,299,300]

There are several varieties of safety standards:

1. OSHA-promulgated, mainly for carcinogens, also for cotton dust and lead. These are *Permissable Exposure Limits* (PELs).
2. National Institute of Occupational Safety and Health (NIOSH) recommendations, often lower limits, based on animal toxicity tests, empirical observations, epidemiologic investigations; these are *Recommended Exposure Limits* (RELs).
3. An older-established set of criteria has been set by the American Conference of Governmental Industrial Hygienists; these are *Threshhold Limit Values* (TLVs) that have replaced an earlier set of Maximum Allowable Concentrations (MACs).

SAMPLE A selected subset of a population. A sample may be random or nonrandom and may be representative or nonrepresentative. Several types of sample can be distinguished, including the following:

1. *Area sample* See AREA SAMPLING.
2. *Cluster sample* Each unit selected is a group of persons (all persons in a city block, a family, etc.) rather than an individual.
3. *Grab sample* (Syn: sample of convenience) These ill-defined terms describe samples selected by easily employed but basically nonprobabilistic (and probably biased) methods. "Man-in-the-street" surveys and a survey of blood pressure among volunteers who drop in at an examination booth in a public place are in this category. It is improper to generalize from the results of a survey based upon such a sample, for there is no way of knowing what sorts of BIAS may have been operating.

4. *Probability (random) sample* All individuals have a known chance of selection. They may all have an equal chance of being selected, or, if a stratified sampling method is used, the rate at which individuals from several subsets are sampled can be varied so as to produce greater representation of some classes than of others. A probability sample is created by assigning an identity (label, number) to all individuals in the "universe" population, e.g., by arranging them in alphabetical order and numbering in sequence, or simply assigning a number to each, or by grouping according to area of residence and numbering the groups. The next step is to select individuals (or groups) for study by a procedure such as use of a table of random numbers (or comparable procedure) to ensure that the chance of selection is known.
5. *Simple random sample* In this elementary kind of sample each person has an equal chance of being selected out of the entire population. One way of carrying out this procedure is to assign each person a number, starting with 1, 2, 3, and so on. Then numbers are selected at random, preferably from a table of random numbers, until the desired sample size is attained.
6. *Stratified random sample* This involves dividing the population into distinct subgroups according to some important characteristic, such as age or socioeconomic status, and selecting a random sample out of each subgroup. If the proportion of the sample drawn from each of the subgroups, or strata, is the same as the proportion of the total population contained in each stratum (e.g., age group 40–59 constitutes 20% of the population, and 20% of the sample comes from this age stratum), then all strata will be fairly represented with regard to numbers of persons in the sample.
7. *Systematic sample* The procedure of selecting according to some simple, systematic rule, such as all persons whose names begin with specified alphabetic letters, born on certain dates, or located at specified points on a master list. A systematic sample may lead to errors that invalidate generalizations. For example, persons' names more often begin with certain letters of the alphabet than with other letters, e.g., in English, A and S are common starting letters while Q and X are not, and are related to ethnic origin. A systematic alphabetical sample is therefore likely to be biased.

SAMPLE, EPSEM ("equal probability of selection method") A sample selected in such a manner that all the population units have the same probability of selection. A simple random sample is an EPSEM sample; a stratified sample is not unless the probability of selection is the same for all strata.

SAMPLE SIZE DETERMINATION The mathematical process of deciding, before a study begins, how many subjects should be studied. The factors to be taken into account include the incidence or prevalence of the condition being studied, the estimated or putative relationship among the variables in the study, the POWER that is desired, and the maximum allowable magnitude of TYPE I ERROR.

SAMPLING The process of selecting a number of subjects from all the subjects in a particular group, or "universe." Statistical inference based on sample results may be attributed only to the population sampled. Any extrapolation to a larger or different population involves judgments about population differences, along with any available data pertaining to the difference, and is not part of conventional statistical inference, although BAYESIAN STATISTICAL METHODS can incorporate these issues.

SAMPLING BIAS Systematic error due to the methods or procedures used to sample or select the study subjects, specimens, or items (e.g., scientific papers), including errors due to the study of a nonrandom sample of a population.

SAMPLING ERROR That part of the total estimation error caused by random influences on who or what is selected for study.

SAMPLING VARIATION Since the inclusion of individuals in a sample is partly determined by chance, the results of analysis in two or more samples will differ in part by chance. This is known as "sampling variation" or more precisely as "random sampling variation."

SANITARY CORDON See CORDON SANITAIRE.

SANTAYANA SYNDROME The neglect of what might be learned from the many blunders and errors contained in medical history.[348,349] A term coined and used by A.R. Feinstein in remembrance of a sentence from George Santayana (1863–1952), a Spanish and American philosopher and poet: "Those who cannot remember the past are condemned to repeat it."[350] See also INTERPRETIVE BIAS.

SARTWELL'S INCUBATION MODEL Philip Sartwell (1908–1999) found that the incubation periods for many communicable diseases tend to have a log-normal distribution, and that the "incubation" periods for certain cancers following certain well-defined external causes also tend to have a log-normal distribution.[351] This model is useful but should not be assumed to hold universally. See also INCUBATION PERIOD; LATENCY PERIOD.

SCALE A device or system for measuring equal portions. A logarithmic scale measures equal powers of 10. Many kinds of scale are used in medicine and epidemiology. From the French and Middle English *scale*, a ladder.

SCAN STATISTIC A test for detection of CLUSTERING over time. A technique used in surveillance epidemiology to detect an unusual rate of occurrence of a disease by comparing observed number of cases with the expected number on the basis of experience in a recent defined period.

SCATTER DIAGRAM, PLOT (Syn: scattergram) A graphic method of displaying the distribution of two variables in relation to each other. The values for one variable are measured on the horizontal axis and the values for the other on the vertical axis.

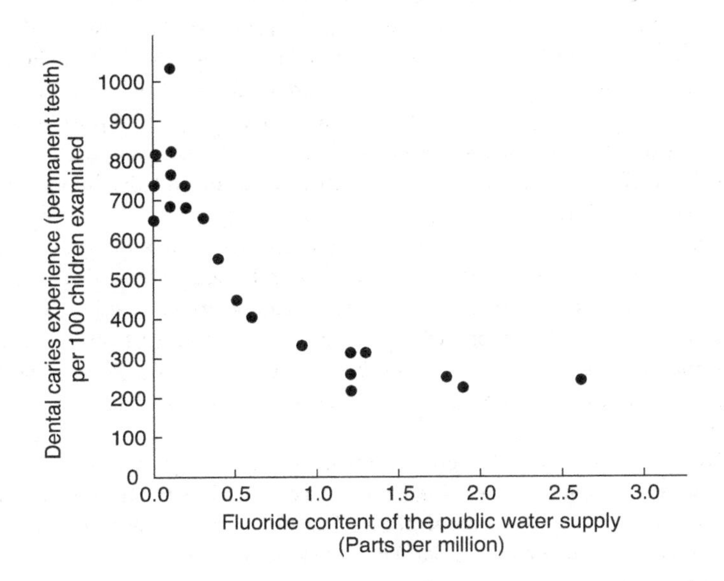

Scatter plot. Relationship between the number of dental caries in permanent teeth and fluoride content in the public water supply. From Lilienfeld and Stolley, 1994.

SCENARIO-BASED HEALTH RISK ASSESSMENT A variant of population health risk assessment in which the exposure input is not an actual measured or measurable exposure but a plausible, preferably model-generated scenario of future exposure. It is particularly relevant in using existing epidemiological knowledge to prepare plans for the future health impacts of anticipated environmental changes, such as climate change and stratospheric ozone depletion.

SCENARIO BUILDING A method of predicting the future that relies on a series of assumptions about alternative possibilities rather than on simple extrapolation of existing trends.[352] Trend lines for demographic composition, morbidity and mortality rates, etc., can then be modified by allowing for each assumption in turn, or combinations of assumptions. The method is claimed to lead to greater flexibility in long-range health planning than simple forecasting that relies only upon extrapolation of trends.

SCIENCE Systematic observation and experiment to explain and predict natural phenomena aimed at establishing, enlarging, or confirming knowledge. Science uses observations and/or experiments to make logical inferences, formulate and test hypotheses, and arrive at generalizable conclusions, expressed as testable laws and principles. Science advances through conjecture or intuition, hypothesis, refutation of deductions from hypotheses, and verification of hypotheses and theories by induction.[6,10,22,67,239,268,353] Occasionally science undergoes a paradigm shift as long-established principles and laws are overturned by new discoveries.[302]

A characteristic of vigorous science is ongoing tests of hypotheses and theories that are taken as "established" in order to detect failings. This activity stems from a point distinguishing science from other systems of knowledge: the idea that all knowledge of the real world is fallible at some level and must not be allowed to become completely unassailable dogma. See also EPISTEMIC COMMUNITIES; HYPOTHETICO-DEDUCTIVE METHOD; KNOWLEDGE CONSTRUCTION; SOCIOLOGY OF SCIENTIFIC KNOWLEDGE.

SCIENTIFIC MISCONDUCT A class of ethical violations in the conduct of research, generally taken to include falsification, fabrication, fraud, or plagiarism in the proposal, design, implementation, reporting, or review of research. May also include violation of the rights and dignity of participants in research, misuse of research funds, mistreatment of scientific colleagues (e.g., in peer review), and failure to report undesired findings.[37] See also PUBLICATION BIAS; REPPRESSION BIAS; SUPPRESSION BIAS.

SCIENTOMETRICS The measurement of scientific output and the impact of scientific findings (e.g., on public health policies).[40]

SCREENING Screening was defined in 1951 by the U.S. Commission on Chronic Illness as, "the presumptive identification of unrecognized disease or defect by the application of tests, examinations or other procedures which can be applied rapidly. Screening tests sort out apparently well persons who probably have a disease from those who probably do not. A screening test is not intended to be diagnostic. Persons with positive or suspicious findings must be referred to their physicians for diagnosis and necessary treatment."[354]

The initiative for screening usually comes from an agency or organization rather than from a patient with a complaint. Screening is usually concerned with chronic illness and aims to detect disease not yet under medical care. Screening may identify risk factors, genetic predisposition, and precursors, or early evidence of disease.

There are different types of medical screening, each with its own aim:

1. *Mass screening* usually means the screening of a whole population.

2. *Multiple* or *multiphasic screening* involves the use of a variety of screening tests on the same occasion or sequentially.
3. *Prescriptive screening* has as its aim the EARLY DETECTION in presumptively healthy individuals of specific diseases that can be controlled better if detected early in their natural history.[237] An example is the use of mammography to detect breast cancer.

The characteristics of a screening test must include ACCURACY, estimates of yield, PRECISION, reproducibility, sensitivity and specificity, and validity.[14,134,355] See also CASE FINDING; DETECTABLE PRECLINICAL PERIOD; PREVENTION.

SCREENING LEVEL The normal limit or cutoff point at which a screening test is regarded as positive.

SEASONAL VARIATION Change in physiological status or in disease occurrence that conforms to a regular seasonal pattern.

SECONDARY ATTACK RATE The number of cases of an infection that occur among contacts within the incubation period following exposure to a primary case in relation to the total number of exposed contacts; the denominator is restricted to susceptible contacts when these can be determined. The secondary attack rate is a measure of contagiousness and is useful in evaluating control measures. See also ATTACK RATE; BASIC REPRODUCTIVE RATE.

SECONDHAND TOBACCO SMOKE See INVOLUNTARY SMOKING; ENVIRONMENTAL TOBACCO SMOKE.

SECOND-LINE DRUGS (SLDS) See DRUG RESISTANCE, MULTIPLE.

SECTOR In the language used by UN agencies (WHO, UNICEF, etc.), a sector is a defined component of the body politic, such as the health sector, the education sector, the housing sector.

SECULAR TREND (Syn: temporal trend) Changes over a long period of time, generally years or decades. Examples include the decline of tuberculosis mortality and the rise, followed by a decline, in coronary heart disease mortality in many industrial countries in the past 50 years.

SEE Sociedad Española de Epidemiología (the Spanish Society of Epidemiology).

SEER Surveillance, Epidemiology and End Results (a program of the U.S. National Cancer Institute).

SER Society for Epidemiologic Research.

SELECTION In genetics, the force that brings about changes in the frequency of alleles and genotypes in populations through differential reproduction. In epidemiology, the process and procedure for choosing individuals for study, usually by an orderly means such as random allocation.

SELECTION BIAS

1. Bias of the estimated effect of an exposure on an outcome due to conditioning on a common effect of the exposure and the outcome (or of causes of the exposure and the outcome).[12,31,97,313] Example: the estimated effect of cigarette smoking on heart disease will be biased if study participants are volunteers and the decision to volunteer is affected by smoking status and by having a family history of heart disease.[356]
2. Distortions that result from procedures used to select subjects and from factors that influence participation in the study.[357] A distortion in the estimate of the effect due to the manner in which subjects are selected for the study. Systematic differences in past exposures and other characteristics between subjects who take part in a study and those who do not may or may not cause selection biases, depending on the study

aims and design. Examples of potential reasons for selection bias include surveys limited to volunteers or to persons present in a particular place at a particular time; studies based on disease survivors; hospital-based studies that cannot include patients who die before hospital admission due to acute illness or that do not include persons with mild conditions, which seldom require hospital care; case-control studies in which selection of cases and controls is differentially influenced by cost, distance, concomitant illnesses, access to diagnostic procedures, or other factors.[10,12,14] Selection biases may be related to CONFOUNDING and INFORMATION BIASES.[31] In CLINICAL TRIALS, two kinds of selection bias are especially relevant: sample selection bias or SAMPLING BIAS (systematic differences among participants and nonparticipants in trials) and ATTRITION BIAS (systematic differences due to selective loss of subjects, also known as follow-up bias).

Selection bias can virtually never be corrected by statistical analysis. It is a common and commonly overlooked problem, not just in epidemiological studies but also in clinical and basic biological studies. See also BERKSON'S BIAS; CONSENT BIAS; CONTROLS, HOSPITAL; INCEPTION COHORT.

SEMI-INDIVIDUAL DESIGN Individual-level studies (e.g., COHORT STUDIES, CROSS-SECTIONAL STUDIES, CASE-CONTROL STUDIES) in which outcome and covariates are measured at the individual level while exposure is characterized on the aggregate (or ecological) level. Used either because groups share the same exposure or because individual-level exposure measures are not available. Frequently used in environmental epidemiology to describe exposure to air, water, or soil pollutants. Not to be confused with ECOLOGICAL STUDIES.[107,358]

SEMIOLOGY (Syn: symptomatology)

1. In medicine, the study of signs and symptoms of disease. Their relevance to the practice of clinical medicine has long been recognized. They are important also to epidemiology-related activities like HEALTH SERVICES RESEARCH (e.g., when quality assurance programs monitor intervals from first symptom of disease to first consultation, diagnosis, and treatment). Symptoms and signs are also relevant to etiological research because they often reflect underlying pathophysiological processes that may alter levels of the exposures under study (e.g., when disease progression entails metabolic changes that alter exposure biomarkers). The analysis of the attribution of meaning to signs and symptoms is essential to understand the SICKNESS "CAREER"[124,128] and hence to PREVENTIVE MEDICINE, EARLY CLINICAL DETECTION, and clinical care. See also SYNDROME.
2. The study of signs, signals, and symbols, especially the relationship between written and spoken language.[359]

SENSITIVE PERIOD (Syn: critical period) A time during the development of a tissue, organ, or system when it can be permanently changed by harmful influences (e.g., undernutrition, hypoxia, stress). It often coincides with a period of rapid cell division and, for many tissues and systems, occurs before birth. The brain and liver are the main organs that remain plastic after birth.[45] The adverse (or protective) effects on health of exposures during a sensitive period may be apparent many years later. See also DEVELOPMENTAL ORIGINS HYPOTHESIS; PLASTICITY; PROGRAMMING; VULNERABILITY.

SENSITIVITY ANALYSIS A method to determine the ROBUSTNESS of an assessment by examining the extent to which results are affected by changes in methods, models, values of unmeasured variables, or assumptions.[360] The aim is to identify results that are most dependent on questionable or unsupported assumptions. See also INFLUENCE ANALYSIS; OUTLIERS.

SENSITIVITY AND SPECIFICITY (of a screening test, of a diagnostic test):

1. *Sensitivity* is the probability that a diseased person (case) in the population tested will be identified as diseased by the test (syn: true positive probability). Sensitivity is thus the probability of correctly diagnosing a case or the probability that any given case will be identified by the test (syn: true-positive rate).
2. *Specificity* is the probability that a person without the disease (noncase) will be correctly identified as nondiseased by the test. It is thus the probability of correctly identifying a nondiseased person with a test (syn: true-negative probability).

The relationships are shown in the following fourfold table, in which the letters *a, b, c,* and *d* represent the numbers in the table below.

Screening test results	True status		Total
	Diseased	Not diseased	
Positive	a	b	$a + b$
Negative	c	d	$c + d$
Total	$a + c$	$b + d$	$a + b + c + d$

a. Diseased individuals detected by the test (true positives)
b. Nondiseased individuals positive by the test (false positives)
c. Diseased individuals not detectable by the test (false negatives)
d. Nondiseased individuals negative by the test (true negatives)

$$\text{Sensitivity} = \frac{a}{a + c} \quad \text{Specificity} = \frac{d}{b + d}$$

$$\text{Predictive value of a positive test result} = \frac{a}{a + b}$$

$$\text{Predictive value of a negative test result} = \frac{d}{c + d}$$

$$\text{Accuracy} = \frac{a + d}{a + b + c + d}$$

The predictive value of a positive test result may be called the *yield*. See also LIKELIHOOD RATIO; PREDICTIVE VALUE.

SENSITIVITY TESTING A study of how the final outcome of an analysis changes as a function of varying one or more of the input parameters in a prescribed manner. See also SENSITIVITY ANALYSIS.

SENTINEL HEALTH EVENT A condition that can be used to assess the stability or change in health levels of a population, usually by monitoring mortality statistics. Thus, death due to acute head injury is a sentinel event for a class of severe traffic injury that may be reduced by such preventive measures as use of seat belts and crash helmets.

SENTINEL PHYSICIAN, SENTINEL PRACTICE In family medicine, a physician or practice that undertakes to maintain surveillance for and to report certain specific predetermined events, such as cases of certain communicable diseases or adverse drug reactions.

SENTINEL SURVEILLANCE Surveillance based on selected population samples chosen to represent the relevant experience of particular groups. This approach is useful in dealing with sensitive issues such as HIV/AIDS or when cooperation levels can be improved through participation of professional organizations, such as colleges or networks of family physicians, for the early detection of influenza epidemics. In sentinel surveillance, standard case definitions and protocols must be used to ensure VALIDITY of comparisons across time and sites despite lack of statistically valid sampling. Sentinel surveillance may include the use of animal sentinels to detect circulation of arboviruses. See also SURVEILLANCE.

SEQUENTIAL ANALYSIS A statistical method that allows an experiment to be ended as soon as an answer of the desired precision is obtained. Study and control subjects are randomly allocated in pairs or blocks. The result of the comparison of each pair of subjects, one treated and one control, is examined as soon as it becomes available and is added to all previous results.

SERENDIPITY The accidental (and happy) discovery of important new information. A well-known example is Fleming's discovery of the bactericidal properties of penicillin mold. In case-control studies aimed at testing a specific hypothesis (e.g., about the relationship between tobacco and cancer), questions on other aspects of lifestyle have serendipitously revealed statistically significant associations (e.g., between alcohol consumption and certain cancers).

SERIAL INTERVAL (Syn: generation time) The period of time between analogous phases of an infectious illness, in successive cases of a chain of infection, that is spread from person to person.

SEROEPIDEMIOLOGY Epidemiological study or activity based on serological testing of characteristic changes in the serum level of specific antibodies. Latent, subclinical infections and carrier states can thus be detected in addition to clinically overt cases.

SEROLOGY The branch of science dealing with the measurement and characterization of antibodies and other immunological substances in body fluids, particularly serum.

SET A defined group of events, objects, or data that is distinguishable from other groups.

SET THEORY Branch of mathematics and logic dealing with the characteristics and relationships of sets.

SEX RATIO The ratio of one sex to the other. Usually defined as the ratio of males to females (or of the rates observed in males and females).

SF36 Acronym for the 36-item questionnaire derived from the longer set of questions used in household interview surveys conducted by the U.S. National Center for Health Statistics. The SF36 questions measure eight multi-item variables: physical function, social function, role limitation, mental health, energy, vitality, pain, and general perception of health. The instrument has been widely adopted, although some authors have raised doubts about its validity.

SHARPS A jargon term for any sharp object used in a health care setting that is capable of penetrating the skin (e.g., hypodermic needles, scalpel blades, broken glass vials).

SHEA Society for Healthcare Epidemiology of America (www.shea-online.org).

"SHOE-LEATHER" EPIDEMIOLOGY Gathering information for epidemiological studies by direct inquiry among the people, e.g., walking from door to door and asking questions of every householder (wearing out shoe leather in the process).[27,313]

John Snow (1813–1858) did this when he was investigating the sources of water supply to households in the cholera epidemic in London in 1854; the method has been successfully used in many subsequent epidemic investigations. It is especially useful in investigations of sexually transmitted diseases. Much of the work of the Epidemic Intelligence Service (EIS) is based on shoe-leather epidemiology. EIS officers have a club tie displaying the sole of a shoe with a hole in it. See also NATURAL EXPERIMENT.

SHRINKAGE ESTIMATION (Syn: Stein estimation, penalized estimation) In statistics, a family of procedures to improve the overall accuracy of multiple estimates. This improvement is made by moving the estimates toward values judged or estimated to be more probable than most of the possible values for the parameters being estimated. The value chosen is often zero, whence the procedures make the estimates smaller, or "shrunk" toward zero. Most shrinkage methods are equivalent to EMPIRICAL-BAYES METHODS.

SIBLINGS Children borne by the same mother.

SIBSHIP All the brothers and sisters borne by the same mother.

SICKNESS See DISEASE.

SICKNESS "CAREER" The process of decisions made by and/or for a person as he or she becomes symptomatic, defined as sick, seeks informal and professional care, and becomes a patient. It takes place in specific settings, in interaction with other people who, in accordance with their assessment of the problem and taking into account their own needs and the opportunities for alternative courses of action, apply the social norms of their particular group and set expectations for behavior.[124–128] See also DISEASE LABEL; SEMIOLOGY.

SIDE EFFECT An effect, other than the intended one, produced by a preventive, diagnostic, or therapeutic procedure or regimen. Not necessarily harmful.

SIDESTREAM SMOKE Smoke from combusted tobacco products, usually cigarettes, that is not filtered through the cigarette or the smoker's respiratory system but directly enters the air, where its toxic and irritant effects on nonsmokers can lead to adverse health effects. See also ENVIRONMENTAL TOBACCO SMOKE; INVOLUNTARY SMOKING.

SIGNAL-TO-NOISE RATIO

1. In statistics and signal processing, the ratio of explained variation to unexplained (error) variation.
2. A jargon term for the relationship of pertinent findings to that which is extraneous or irrelevant or intrudes because measurement methods or other procedures are insufficiently sensitive.

SIGNIFICANCE, CLINICAL Importance, RELEVANCE, or meaning for the care of individuals, who may be—in clinical research—patients. A difference in effect size considered to be important (e.g., by a professional) in medical decisions regardless of the degree of statistical significance. Statistical significance can never be taken to equal clinical significance. For example, when large numbers of subjects are studied, some differences will be statistically significant even if their magnitude or size is small; hence they will be of little importance for patient care. Conversely, when small numbers of subjects are studied, some differences will not be statistically significant even if their magnitude is large; hence they may be of importance for patient care but not detected as such in the analysis.[12,14,31,62,63,75]

SIGNIFICANCE, PUBLIC HEALTH Importance, RELEVANCE, or meaning from a public health perspective; for example, an environmental factor may have public health significance or importance because of its impact on the BURDEN OF DISEASE in a given population. See also SIGNIFICANCE, CLINICAL.

SIGNIFICANCE, STATISTICAL

1. The probability of the observed or a larger value of a test statistic under the null hypothesis. Often equivalent to the probability of the observed or larger degree of association under the null hypothesis. This usage is synonymous with *P* VALUE.
2. A statistical property of an observation or an estimate that is unlikely to have occurred by chance alone. See also CHI-SQUARE TEST; SIGNIFICANCE, CLINICAL; SIGNIFICANCE, PUBLIC HEALTH; RELEVANCE.

SIGN TEST A DISTRIBUTION-FREE TEST that can be used in combining results of several studies. The test considers the direction of results of individual studies (i.e., whether the associations demonstrated are positive or negative).

SILENCING, GENE See GENE SILENCING.

SIMPSON'S PARADOX The possibility that a measure of association may reverse direction upon stratification by a third variable. In epidemiology, it has been presented as a form of confounding in which the presence of a confounding variable changes the direction of an association. This interpretation is narrower than Simpson's, however, for he used an example with pure association, with no causality or confounding implied. Simpson's paradox can occur in meta-analysis because the sum of the data or results from a number of different studies may be affected by confounding variables that have been excluded by design features from some studies but not others. Simpson's paradox is not really a paradox but rather an extreme manifestation of the fact that associations may change according to the level of stratification.[361] It is an extreme extreme violation of COLLAPSIBILITY, in which results of the data analysis in every mutually exclusive stratum or subgroup are the opposite of the crude results.[69,362] See also CONFOUNDING BIAS.

SIMULATION The use of a model system (e.g., a mathematical model or an animal model) to approximate the functioning or action of a real system; often used to study the properties of a real system. See also MONTE-CARLO STUDY.

SINGLE-PATIENT TRIAL See N-OF-ONE STUDY.

SITUATION ANALYSIS Study of a situation that may require improvement. This begins with a definition of the problem and an assessment or measurement of its extent, severity, causes, and impacts upon the community; it is followed by appraisal of interactions between the system and its environment and evaluations of performance.

SKEW DISTRIBUTION An older and less recommended term for an asymmetrical frequency distribution. If a unimodal distribution has a longer tail extending toward lower values of the variate, it is said to have negative skewness; in the contrary case, it is said to have positive skewness. An example is the LOG-NORMAL DISTRIBUTION.

SLDs (SECOND-LINE DRUGS) See DRUG RESISTANCE, MULTIPLE.

SLOW VIRUS Agent causing degenerative (often, neurological) diseases characterized by a long incubation period and a prolonged, slowly progressive course. Multiple sclerosis is possibly a slow virus disease. See also PRION.

SMALL FOR GESTATIONAL AGE (SGA) See BIRTH WEIGHT

SMOOTHING General term for methods of minimizing irregularities in a set of data. Examples include ROUNDING, KRIGING, and MOVING AVERAGES.

SNOWBALL SAMPLING A method of selecting for study the members of "hidden" populations, e.g., illicit drug users. Those initially identified are asked to name acquaintances who are added to the sample; these, in turn, are asked to name further acquaintances,

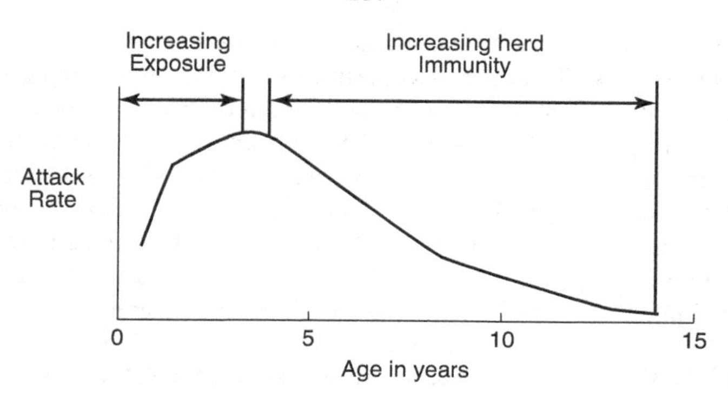

Skew diagram. Skew distribution of attack rate of measles in relation to age. From Lilienfeld and Stolley, 1994.

and so on until enough numbers are accumulated to give adequate power to the proposed study. The sample is, of course, not random. Compare CAPTURE-RECAPTURE METHOD.

SOCIAL CLASS A stratum in society composed of individuals and families of equal standing. A method of socially stratifying populations according to occupation, education, or income. See also LIFE COURSE; SOCIOECONOMIC CLASSIFICATION; CLASS.

SOCIAL DRIFT Downward social class mobility as a result of impaired health, sometimes due to reduced earning potential, mental disorders, or substance abuse. The "social drift hypothesis" also suggests that persons with poor mental health are more likely to move to neighborhoods with poor-quality environments.

SOCIAL EPIDEMIOLOGY A branch or subspecialty of epidemiology that studies the role of social structure and social factors in the production of health and disease in populations; it uses epidemiological principles, reasoning, and methods to study the social determinants and distribution of health states and events. An interface between epidemiology and the social sciences. It includes studies of personal and population health in the social context, behavior, social networks, and determinants of individual and population health such as ethnicity, socioeconomic status, social class, and housing conditions. It may use a LIFE COURSE approach. In intervention studies, it seeks to modify adverse factors and ameliorate determinants that can enhance good health.[137,363–365] See also CAUSES IN PUBLIC HEALTH SCIENCES; ETHNOEPIDEMIOLOGY. As mentioned above, this dictionary includes definitions for just a few branches of EPIDEMIOLOGY.

SOCIAL MARKETING The use of marketing theory, skills, and practice to achieve social change; to promote the general health or in other public health activities; to raise awareness and induce changes in behavior by individuals and groups aiming at enhancing their level of health.

SOCIAL MEDICINE The practice of medicine concerned with health and disease as a function of group living. Social medicine is concerned with the health of people in relation to their behavior in social groups; as such, it involves care of the individual patient as a member of a family and of other significant groups in everyday life. It is also concerned with the health of these groups and with that of the whole community. The "father of social medicine" was Johann Peter Frank (1745–1821), who described many features of this discipline in *System einer vollständigen medicinischen Polizey* (*A System of Complete Medical Police*, 1779). After the appointment of John Ryle (1889–1950) as the first professor of social medicine at the University of Oxford, this became the preferred term to describe academic departments dealing with this range of disciplines in the United Kingdom; in the 1970s, the preferred term became COMMUNITY MEDICINE. The Acheson Report (1988) advocated the term PUBLIC HEALTH MEDICINE, which was for some years adopted by the Faculty of Community Medicine of the UK Royal Colleges of Physicians and many British academic departments; it later became the Faculty of Public Health (FPH) (www.fphm.org.uk). The FPH is the standard setting body for specialists in public health in the United Kingdom; a joint Faculty of the three Royal Colleges of Physicians of the United Kingdom (London, Edinburgh, and Glasgow). See also COMMUNITY MEDICINE; PUBLIC HEALTH.

SOCIAL NETWORK INDEX A measure of the extent to which individuals or groups are connected to or isolated from others (e.g., family, friends, and work colleagues). Health status has been found to be positively associated with the extent of social networks.[366]

SOCIETAL RISK Probability of harm to the human population, including probability of adverse health effects to descendants and probability of disruption resulting from loss of services, such as industrial plant, loss of material goods, electricity.

SOCIOECONOMIC CLASSIFICATION Arrangement of persons into groups according to such characteristics as prior education, occupation, and income. Upon analysis, this usually reveals a strong connection with health-related characteristics, such as average length of life and risk of dying from certain specific causes.[137,363–367]

The oldest such classification that is epidemiologically useful is the registrar-general's (RG's) occupational classification, developed in 1911 by Stephenson, Registrar-General of England and Wales. This classified all occupations into five groups—the five "social classes." Social class III is often further subdivided into nonmanual and manual groups, as follows:

I	Professional occupations
II	Intermediate occupations
IIIN	Nonmanual skilled occupations
IIIM	Manual skilled occupations
IV	Partly skilled occupations
V	Unskilled occupations

This has proven to be a valuable epidemiological tool; social class is a reliable and consistent predictor of health experience and status.

There have been many attempts to develop more refined classifications; however, most refinements require the collection of more detailed information. For example, Hollingshead's scale requires details about education and income as well as occupation. In developing countries, where up to 90% of the population may be classified under "agriculturalist" or "pastoralist" (farming or herding), other types of classifications have been developed.

One's prestige in society and attitudes or values (e.g., setting a high value on getting a good education) are generally an integral part of social class or socioeconomic status. Attitudes toward health are often part of the set of values and may explain part of the observed difference in health between social classes.

SOCIOECONOMIC STATUS (SES) Descriptive term for a person's position in society, which may be expressed on an ORDINAL SCALE using such criteria as income, level of education attained, occupation, value of dwelling place, etc.

SOCIOLOGY OF EPIDEMIOLOGY The application of the scientific principles and methods of sociology to the science, discipline, and profession of epidemiology in order to improve understanding of the wider social causes and consequences of epidemiologists' professional and scientific organization, patterns of practice, ideas, knowledge, and cultures (e.g., institutional arrangements, academic norms, scientific discourses, defense of identity and epistemic authority). It also addresses the patterns of interaction of epidemiologists with other branches of science and professions (e.g., clinical medicine, public health, the other health, life and social sciences), and with social agents, organizations, and systems (e.g., the economic, political, and legal systems). The tradition of sociology *in* epidemiology is rich; the sociology *of* epidemiology is virtually uncharted (in the sense of not mapped neither surveyed) and unchartered (i.e., not furnished with a charter or constitution). See also EPIDEMIOLOGY, DEMARCATION OF; EPISTEMIC COMMUNITIES; KNOWLEDGE CONSTRUCTION.

SOCIOLOGY OF SCIENTIFIC KNOWLEDGE (SSK) An approach to the understanding of science that focuses on the social causes of the scientists' convictions, knowledge, and beliefs. It centers on *science as knowledge*, by contrast with the "constructivist approach," which is more interested on the constructive elements of scientific production (i.e., it considers *science as practice*). Both approaches tend to agree that the content of natural science is accessible by way of empirical sociological analysis and should be subjected to it; science is not to be investigated merely as a social institution; science's EPISTEMIC core is a matter of investigation in its own right and should not be studied only by philosophers of science.[268] See also EPISTEMIC COMMUNITIES; EPISTEMOLOGY; INTERPRETIVE BIAS; KNOWLEDGE CONSTRUCTION.

SOJOURN TIME (Syn: detectable preclinical period) The interval between detectability at screening and clinical presentation of a condition—i.e., the interval during which the condition is potentially detectable but not yet diagnosed.[368]

SOUNDEX CODE A sequence of letters used for recording names phonetically, especially in RECORD LINKAGE.

SOURCE OF INFECTION The person, animal, object, or substance from which an infectious agent passes to a host. Source of infection should be clearly distinguished from source of CONTAMINATION, such as overflow of a septic tank contaminating a water supply or an infected cook contaminating a salad.[52,57] See also RESERVOIR OF INFECTION.

SPEARMAN'S RANK CORRELATION See CORRELATION COEFFICIENT.

SPECIFICATION

1. The process of selecting a particular functional form or model for the relationships to be analyzed in a study.
2. The process of selecting variables for inclusion in the analysis of an effect or association. This process may lead to the identification of variables that are EFFECT MODIFIERS and CONFOUNDING VARIABLES. See also STRATIFICATION.

SPECIFICITY (OF A TEST) See SENSITIVITY AND SPECIFICITY.

SPECTRUM BIAS A problem that may affect a study of diagnostic accuracy when it fails to account for the variation or heterogeneity of the test performance across population subgroups. Failure to recognize and address such heterogeneity will lead to estimates of test performance that are not generalizable to the relevant clinical populations. Bias may occur when diagnostic test performance varies across patient subgroups and the study does not adequately include all subgroups.[62,63,321] For instance, overestimation of the sensitivity and specificity of the test will occur when the study includes a healthy group and a group with overt disease. Originally described as a BIAS,[369] the variation is no longer considered to necessarily create a bias; rather, the spectrum of patients is considered a clinically relevant piece of information to be reported accurately and analyzed appropriately (e.g., by stratification). The term *spectrum bias* would hence be less appropriate than *spectrum effect*, which reflects the inherent variation in test performance among population subgroups.[370] In interpreting results of a diagnostic study, assessing the spectrum of patients included will help determine whether results are generalizable to other populations of patients. See also WORKUP BIAS.

SPECTRUM OF DISEASE The full range of manifestations of a disease; e.g., from precursor states, to subclinical and mild cases, to florid and fulminating disease. The natural history of a disease from onset to resolution.[62,63,87] See also INCEPTION COHORT; INDUCTION PERIOD.

SPELL OF SICKNESS An episode of sickness with a well-defined onset and termination. As used in the monitoring or SURVEILLANCE of disease, the spell is often defined by the duration of absence from work or school. See also DISEASE; SICKNESS "CAREER."

SPLEEN RATE A term used in malaria epidemiology to define the frequency of enlarged spleens detected on survey of a population in which malaria is prevalent. In association with the HACKETT SPLEEN CLASSIFICATION, it summarizes the severity of malaria endemicity.

SPORADIC Occurring irregularly, haphazardly, from time to time, and generally infrequently (e.g., cases of certain infectious diseases).

SPOT MAP Map showing the geographic location of people with a specific attribute (e.g., cases of a disease or elderly persons living alone). The making of a spot map is a common procedure in the investigation of a localized outbreak of disease. Inferences from such a map depend on the assumption that the population at risk of developing the disease is fairly evenly distributed over the area or that at least the heterogeneities are known and can be considered in interpreting the map. A refinement is to indicate multiple cases at a single location by a series of short horizontal bars, as John Snow did to mark the location of cases of cholera in the epidemic in London in 1849; the method has been used by innumerable field epidemiologists ever since.

SPREADSHEET A computer matrix of columns and rows in which numerical entries can be made on screen, stored, systematically manipulated, and modified.

STABLE POPULATION A population that has constant fertility and mortality rates, no migration, and consequently a fixed age distribution and constant growth rate; a population with stable structure. See also STATIONARY POPULATION.

STANDARD Something that serves as a basis for comparison; a technical specification or written report drawn up by experts based on the consolidated results of scientific study, technology, and experience, aimed at optimum benefits and approved by a recognized and representative body.

STANDARD DEVIATION A measure of dispersion or variation. It is the most widely used measure of dispersion of a frequency distribution. It is equal to the positive square root of the VARIANCE. The mean tells where the values for a group are centered. The standard deviation is a summary of how widely dispersed the values are around this center.

STANDARD ERROR The standard deviation of an estimate. Used to calculate CONFIDENCE INTERVALS.

STANDARD GAMBLE See VON NEUMANN-MORGENSTERN STANDARD GAMBLE.

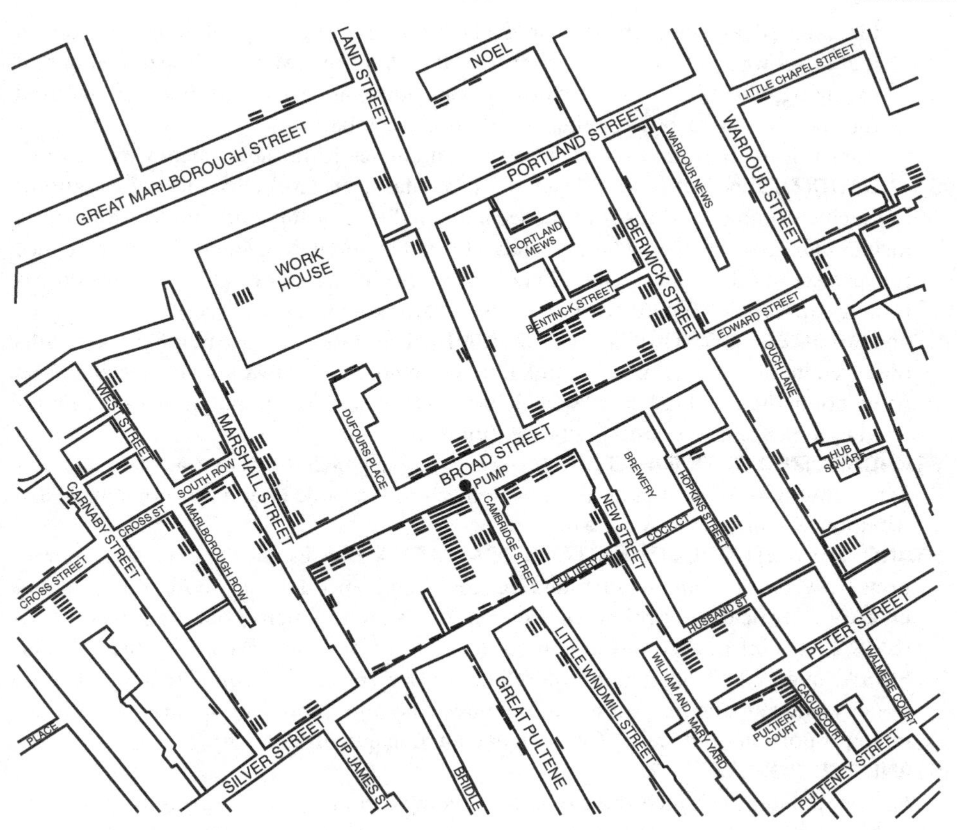

Spot map. From Snow J. *On the Mode of Communication of Cholera*. London: Churchill, 1855.

STANDARDIZATION A set of techniques, based on weighted averaging, used to remove as much as possible the effects of differences in age or other confounding variables in comparing two or more populations. The common method uses weighted averaging of rates specific for age, sex, or some other potential confounding variable(s) according to some specified distribution of these variables. There are two main methods, as follows:

Direct method: The specific rates in a study population are averaged, using as weights the distribution of a specified standard population. The directly standardized rate represents what the crude rate would have been in the study population if that population had the same distribution as the standard population with respect to the variable(s) for which the adjustment or standardization was carried out. INVERSE PROBABILITY WEIGHTING can be seen as a generalization.

Indirect method: This is used to compare study populations for which the specific rates are either statistically unstable or unknown. The specific rates in the standard population are averaged, using as weights the distribution of the study population. The ratio of the crude rate for the study population to the weighted average so obtained is the standardized mortality (or morbidity) ratio, or SMR. The indirectly standardized rate itself is the product of the SMR and the crude rate for the standard population, but this product is rarely used in etiological studies. A problem that arises with indirect standardization is that different SMRs are based on different weighting schemes (one for each study population) and so are not fully standardized for comparison to one another. As a result, comparisons of SMRs (or indirectly standardized rates) may remain partially confounded by the adjustment variables.[12]

STANDARDIZED INCIDENCE RATIO (Syn: standardized morbidity ratio) The ratio of the incident number of cases of a specified condition in the study population to the incident number that would be expected if the study population had the same incidence rate as a standard or other population for which the incidence rate is known; this ratio is usually expressed as a percentage. See also STANDARDIZATION (indirect).

STANDARDIZED MORTALITY RATIO (SMR) The ratio of the number of deaths observed in the study group or population to the number that would be expected if the study population had the same specific rates as the standard population. Often multiplied by 100. See also STANDARDIZATION (indirect).

STANDARDIZED RATE RATIO (SRR) A rate ratio in which the numerator and denominator rates have been standardized (weighted) to the same (standard) population distribution. See also STANDARDIZATION (direct).

STANDARD METROPOLITAN STATISTICAL AREA Because of the extensive interactions between a city and its surrounding areas, a unit encompassing both is needed as a base for statistical description. The concept of a standard metropolitan statistical area (SMSA) was introduced in the United States to furnish such a unit. To qualify as an SMSA, an area has to meet criteria related to size, social and economic integration of the city and surrounding county or counties, minimum population density, and minimum proportion of the labor force engaged in nonagricultural work.

STANDARD POPULATION

1. A population in which the age and sex composition is known precisely as a result of a census or by an arbitrary means (e.g., an imaginary population, the "standard million," in which age/sex composition is arbitrary). A standard population is used as a comparison group in the actuarial procedure of standardization of mortality rates.
2. A population used as the reference in STANDARDIZATION.

STARD Standards for Reporting of Diagnostic Accuracy. A consensus checklist and flow diagram aimed at improving the accuracy and completeness of reporting of studies of diagnostic accuracy.[95,371,372] See also CONSORT; MOOSE; STROBE; TREND.

STATIONARY POPULATION A stable population that has a zero growth rate with constant numbers of births and deaths each year.

STATISTICAL ERROR See ERROR.

STATISTICAL INFERENCE See INFERENCE.

STATISTICAL MODEL A MATHEMATICAL MODEL for distribution of samples or data.

STATISTICAL SIGNIFICANCE See SIGNIFICANCE, STATISTICAL.

STATISTICAL TEST A procedure intended to decide whether a statistical hypothesis (which may be about the distribution of one or more populations or variables or the size of an association or effect) should be rejected or not. Statistical tests may be parametric or nonparametric.

STATISTICS

1. The science of collecting, summarizing, and analyzing data. Data may or may be not subject to random variation.
2. The data themselves and summarizations of the data.

STEIN ESTIMATION See SHRINKAGE ESTIMATION

STEM-AND-LEAF DISPLAY A method of presenting numbers in a form resembling a histogram, with multiples of 10 along the "stem" and the integers forming the "leaves." See also BOX-AND-WHISKERS PLOT.

STOCHASTIC PROCESS A process (usually a temporal sequence) that incorporates some element of randomness.

STOPPING RULES In randomized controlled trials and other forms of systematic experiments, stopping rules are laid down in advance, specifying conditions or criteria under which the trial or experiment shall cease or be terminated. For example, in a RANDOMIZED CONTROLLED TRIAL, the unequivocal demonstration of superiority of one regimen over another is the most obvious reason for terminating the trial; a less frequent situation is the demonstration that a regimen causes harm to participants in the trial. The rule must be based on appropriate statistical tests to ensure that the empirically observed results are not due to chance.

STRATEGY

1. In public health, a set of essential measures (e.g., social, sanitary, environmental) proven to be effective or efficient to control a health problem.[168,317] A mid- and long-term plan to improve chances of success for adoption and implementation of HEALTHY PUBLIC POLICIES.
2. In preventive medicine, seminal work by Geoffrey Rose helped establish the important distinction between the "HIGH-RISK" STRATEGY and the "POPULATION" STRATEGY.[72] See also PREVENTION.
3. In game theory, a mathematical function.
4. In politics, the means that policymakers choose to attain desired ends. A course of action, an overall plan for achieving specified goals. See also POLICY; TACTICS.

STRATEGY, "HIGH-RISK" A clinically oriented approach to PREVENTIVE MEDICINE that focuses its efforts on needy individuals with the highest levels of the risk factor ('the deviant minority with high-risk status') and utilizes the established framework of medical services. "A targeted rescue operation for vulnerable individuals."[72] The aim is to help each person reduce the high level of exposure to a cause or to some intermediate variable. Main strengths of this strategy include that the intervention may be matched to the needs of the individual; it may avoid interference with those who are not at a special risk; it may be accommodated within the ethical and cultural values, organization, and economics, of the health care system; selectivity may increase the likelihood of a cost-effective use of resources. Main weaknesses of the high-risk strategy are that prevention may become medicalized; success may be palliative and temporary; the contribution to overall (population) control of a disease may be small; the preventive intervention may be behaviorally or culturally inadequate or unsustainable; it has a poor ability to predict which individuals will benefit from the intervention.[72]

STRATEGY, "POPULATION" A public health-oriented approach to preventive medicine and public health predicting that a shift in the population distribution of a risk factor will prevent more BURDEN OF DISEASE than targeting people at high risk. It starts with the recognition that the occurrence of common exposures and diseases reflects the functioning of society as a whole.[72] The approach is more relevant to decrease exposure to (1) certain environmental agents that individuals have little capacity to detect than to (2) risk factors that individuals may generally decide to avoid. Main strengths of this strategy include that it may be radical ("only the social and political approach confronts the root causes"); the societal effects of a distributional shift may be large; it may be more culturally appropriate and sustainable to seek a general change in behavioral norms and in the social values that facilitate their adoption than to attempt to individually change behaviors that are socially conditioned.[72] Main limitations of the population strategy are that it offers only a small benefit to each participating individual, which may be wiped out by a small risk; it requires major changes in the economics and mode of functioning of society, which often makes changes unlikely. Individuals generally prefer to pay as late as possible and to enjoy the benefits as soon as possible. Social benefits—which are often achieved through processes with the opposite timing of costs and benefits—may thus be scarcely attractive to the individual. Nevertheless, shared values and targets do exist at the community level.[19] See also COMMON GOOD.

STRATIFICATION The process of or result of separating a sample into several subsamples according to specified criteria, such as age groups, socioeconomic status, etc. The effect of confounding variables may be controlled by stratifying the analysis of results. For example, lung cancer is known to be associated with smoking. To examine the possible association between urban atmospheric pollution and lung cancer, controlling for smoking, the population may be divided into strata according to smoking status. The association between air pollution and cancer can then be appraised separately within each stratum. Stratification is used not only to control for confounding effects but also as a way of detecting modifying effects. In this example, stratification makes it possible to examine the effect of smoking on the association between atmospheric pollution and lung cancer. See also ADJUSTMENT; EFFECT MODIFICATION; STANDARDIZATION.

STRATIFIED RANDOMIZATION A randomization procedure in which strata are identified and subjects randomly allocated within each. This produces a situation intermediate between paired allocation and simple random allocation. See also RANDOM ALLOCATION; BLOCKED RANDOMIZATION.

STRENGTH OF AN ASSOCIATION See HILL'S CRITERIA OF CAUSATION; MEASURE OF ASSOCIATION.

STRESS The result of a process through which environmental demands challenge, strain, and exceed the adaptive capacity of a person or community, resulting in psychological, physiological, or clinical changes that place persons at risk for adverse health events. Distributions of stress depend on structural, interpersonal, cognitive, biological, and physical processes. Responses to stressors may favor survival and adaptation.

STROBE Strengthening the Reporting of Observational Studies in Epidemiology. An evidence-based and structured approach to reporting of analytical observational studies. Recommendations on what should be included in an accurate and complete report of cohort studies, case-control studies, and cross-sectional studies (www.cochrane.dk).[95,373] See also CONSORT; MOOSE; STARD; TREND.

STRUCTURED ABSTRACT An abstract or summary of a scientific article or report that is organized or structured in well-defined sections. A typical sequence of sections includes some or all of the following: "Objectives" or "Aims," "Design," "Setting," "Subjects," "Main outcome measures," "Results," and "Conclusions." The structured abstract is intended to be comprehensive and to provide a logical order for the presentation of a scientific communication. Structured abstracts are required by many journals.

STUDY BASE The persons or person-time in which the outcomes of interest are observed. The population experience actually captured ("harvested") by a study. In case-control studies, cases and controls should be representative of the same base experience.

Some authors, like Oli Miettinen (b.1936),[5] distinguish between primary and secondary bases; in the former, the population experience is defined in time and place; in the latter, the cases are defined before the study base is or can be defined. In a clinical trial, the base is the follow-up experience of the patients actually enrolled in the study.

STUDY DESIGN See RESEARCH DESIGN.

SUBCLINICAL DISEASE See DISEASE, SUBCLINICAL.

SUFFICIENT CAUSE A set of conditions, factors, or events sufficient to produce a given outcome. A complete causal mechanism that does not require the presence of any other determinant in order for an outcome, such as disease, to occur.[88] See also ASSOCIATION; CAUSALITY; CAUSATION OF DISEASE, FACTORS IN; COMPONENT CAUSES; DISEASES OF COMPLEX ETIOLOGY; EVANS'S POSTULATES; HILL'S CRITERIA OF CAUSATION; NECESSARY CAUSE.

SUMMATIVE RATING A rating scale based on measurements of individually scaled items that are monotonically related to an underlying attribute or attributes; the sum of the item scores is approximately linearly related to the attribute.

SUPERINFECTION Fresh infection in a host already infected with a parasite of the same species; a term mainly used in malaria epidemiology.

SUPPRESSION BIAS, OPPRESSION BIAS Bias that result when actions aimed at obstructing the conduct or publication of research produce a bias in the available evidence (e.g., on the relationships between exposures and outcomes). An organization, a group, or an individual whose priority interests are not consistent with those of public health can be obstructive. Suppression bias may lead to PUBLICATION BIAS. It undermines public health because it distorts and delays the discovery of scientific knowledge on health risks and compromises credibility in science and administrative processes for assessing and preventing exposure to hazards or risks. See also SCIENTIFIC MISCONDUCT.

SUPPRESSOR VARIABLE A variable that is causally related to the outcome of interest and, because it is associated with a causal variable, suppresses the study exposure's association with the outcome.[12] One variety of CONFOUNDING VARIABLE. For example, smoking can be a suppressor variable for pesticide-related Parkinson's disease.

SURVEILLANCE

1. Systematic and continuous collection, analysis, and interpretation of data, closely integrated with the timely and coherent dissemination of the results and assessment to those who have the right to know so that action can be taken. It is an essential feature of epidemiological and public health practice. The final phase in the surveillance chain is the application of information to health promotion and to disease prevention and control. A surveillance system includes a functional capacity for data collection, analysis, and dissemination linked to public health programs.[374] It is often distinguished from MONITORING by the notion that surveillance is continuous and ongoing, whereas monitoring tends to be more intermittent or episodic.
2. Continuous analysis, interpretation, and feedback of systematically collected data, generally using methods distinguished by their practicality, uniformity, and rapidity rather than by ACCURACY or completeness. By observing trends in time, place, and persons, changes can be observed or anticipated and appropriate action, including investigative or control measures, can be taken. Sources of data may relate directly to disease or to factors influencing disease. Thus they may include mortality and morbidity reports based on death certificates, hospital records, general practice sentinels, or notifications; laboratory diagnoses; outbreak reports; vaccine uptake and side effects; sickness absence records; changes in disease agents, vectors, or

reservoirs; serological surveillance through serum banks. The latter can also be seen as an example of BIOLOGICAL MONITORING.

SURVEY An investigation in which information is systematically collected but the experimental method is not used. A population survey may be conducted by face-to-face inquiry, self-completed questionnaires, telephone, postal service, or in some other way. Each method has its advantages and disadvantages. For instance, a face-to-face (interview) survey may be a better way than a self-completed questionnaire to collect information on attitudes or feelings, but it is more costly. Existing medical or other records may contain accurate information, but not about a representative sample of the population.

The information that is gathered in a survey is usually complex enough to require editing (for ACCURACY, completeness, etc.), coding, data entry, and processing and analysis, nearly always now by computer. The generalizability of results depends upon the extent to which the surveyed population is representative. The term *survey* is sometimes used in a narrow sense to refer specifically to a FIELD SURVEY.

SURVEY INSTRUMENT The interview schedule, questionnaire, medical examination record form, etc., used in a survey.

SURVIVAL ANALYSIS A class of statistical procedures for estimating the SURVIVAL FUNCTION and making inferences about the effects on it of treatments, prognostic factors, exposures, and other covariates. The PROPORTIONAL HAZARDS MODEL and the KAPLAN-MEIER ESTIMATE are examples of tools for survival analysis.

SURVIVAL CURVE A curve that starts at 100% of the study population and shows the percentage of the population still surviving at successive times for as long as information is available. May be applied not only to survival as such but also to the persistence of freedom from a disease or complication or some other endpoint.

SURVIVAL FUNCTION (Syn: survival distribution) A function of time, usually denoted by $S(t)$, that starts with a population 100% well at a particular time and provides the percentage of the population still well at later times. Survival functions may be applied to any discrete event; for example, disease incidence or relapse, death, or recovery after onset of disease (in which case the population is initially 100% diseased, and the "survival" function gives the percentage still diseased). See also KAPLAN-MEIER ESTIMATE.

SURVIVAL PROPORTION The proportion of a closed population at risk for a disease that does not become diseased during a specified interval, i.e., 1 minus the INCIDENCE PROPORTION.[12]

SURVIVAL RATE (Syn: cumulative survival rate, survival proportion) The proportion of survivors in a group (e.g., of patients studied and followed over a specified period). The proportion of persons in a specified group alive at the beginning of the time interval (e.g., a 5-year period) who survive to the end of the interval. It is equal to 1 minus the CUMULATIVE DEATH RATE. May be studied by current or cohort LIFE TABLE methods.

SURVIVAL RATIO The probability of surviving between one age and another; when computed for age groups, the ratios correspond to those of the person-years-lived function of a life table.

SURVIVAL, RELATIVE Adjustment of survival rate for independent cause(s) of death. Multiple regression models of relative survival take into account the mortality from all other causes in each area, permitting better comparisons of survival within and between populations with different life expectancies.[375]

SURVIVORSHIP STUDY Use of a cohort LIFE TABLE to provide the probability that an event, such as death, will occur in successive intervals of time after diagnosis and, conversely, the probability of surviving each interval. The multiplication of these probabilities of survival for each time interval for those alive at the beginning of that interval yields a cumulative probability of surviving for the total period of study.

SUSCEPTIBILITY

1. Vulnerability; lack of resistance to disease; the dynamic state of being more likely or liable to be harmed by a health determinant.
2. The condition or status of having one of two interacting causes already and therefore being susceptible to the effect of the other.[12]
3. A process occurring over time during which host factors (both inherited and learned or otherwise acquired and embodied) increase the likelihood that an exposure will produce disease. Susceptibility to positive influences and beneficial outcomes also exists.[16,124,128] Sometimes used as a synonym for VULNERABILITY.

In many living organisms, including humans, a clinically and epidemiologically meaningful increase in susceptibility to disease cannot be assumed only on the basis of mechanistic studies (since, for instance, studies often lack design characteristics required to estimate baseline risk and risk differences, and because significant changes in phenotype are prevented by ROBUSTNESS, redundancy, and compensatory mechanisms).[207,347,376–378] Assessment of the biological, clinical, and epidemiological COHERENCE of research findings helps to prevent overestimates of susceptibility to disease. See also LIFE COURSE; NONMALEFICENCE; SENSITIVE PERIOD.

SUSCEPTIBLE VARIABLE A variable that is potentially confounding in that it is subsequent, not antecedent, to the variable whose effect is being studied. It may or may not be an intermediate variable as well; if it is, special tools such as MARGINAL STRUCTURAL MODELS must be used to adjust for its confounding effects.

SUSTAINABILITY The ability to continue economic, social, cultural, and environmental aspects of human society and the nonhuman environment. The Brundtland Commission, led by the former Norwegian Prime Minister Gro Harlem Brundtland, defined sustainable development as development that "meets the needs of the present without compromising the ability of future generations to meet their own needs." Common principles in action programs to achieve sustainable development, sustainability, or sustainable prosperity include dealing transparently and systemically with risk, uncertainty, and irreversibility; ensuring appropriate valuation, appreciation, and restoration of nature; integration of environmental, social, human, and economic goals in policies and activities; equal opportunity; community participation; conservation of biodiversity and ecological integrity; intergenerational equity; commitment to best practices; no net loss of human capital and natural capital; good governance. To varying degrees all these principles are relevant to EPIDEMIOLOGY.[111,136–138]

SYMBIOSIS The biological association of two or more species to their mutual benefit.

SYNDROME A complex of signs and symptoms that tend to occur together, often characterizing a disease.

SYNERGISM, SYNERGY (Opposite: ANTAGONISM)

1. One of two types of *effect modification* or INTERACTION: the EFFECT MODIFIER enhances the effect of the putatively causal variable. Under an additive model, a situation in which the combined effect of two or more factors is greater than the sum of their solitary effects.
2. In BIOASSAY, two factors act synergistically if there are persons who will get the disease when exposed to both factors but not when exposed to either alone.

Under this definition and definition 2 of ANTAGONISM, two factors may act synergistically in some persons and antagonistically in others.

SYSTEMATIC ERROR See BIAS.

SYSTEMATIC REVIEW See REVIEW, SYSTEMATIC.

SYSTEMS ANALYSIS

1. The examination of various elements of a system with a view to ascertaining whether the proposed solution to a problem will fit into the system and, in turn, effect an overall improvement in the system.
2. The analysis of an activity in order to determine precisely what is required of the system, how this can best be accomplished, and in what ways the computer can be useful.
3. Any formal analysis whose purpose is to suggest a course of action by systematically examining the objectives, costs, effectiveness, and risks of alternative policies or strategies and designing additional ones if those examined are found wanting. It is an approach to or way of looking at complex problems of choice under uncertainty; it is not yet considered to be a method.

T

TACTICS The detailed directions and instructions designed to achieve an aim or target. See STRATEGY.

TARGET An aspired outcome that is explicitly stated. What a health policy or program will achieve by a specified date; for example, reduced unwanted pregnancy rates, lower teenage smoking rates, enhanced QALYs. Usually but not necessarily expressed in quantitative terms.

TARGET POPULATION

1. The collection of individuals, items, measurements, etc., about which inferences are desired. The term is sometimes used to indicate the population or group from which a sample or study population is drawn and sometimes to denote a reference population about which inferences are desired.
2. The group to which inference from the study is directed.
3. The group of persons for whom an intervention is planned.

TAXON (plural, taxa) The general term for a group or entity; e.g., a species or family in a taxonomy.

TAXONOMY A systematic classification into related groups.

TAXONOMY OF DISEASE The orderly CLASSIFICATION of diseases into appropriate categories on the basis of relationships among them, with the application of names. See also NOSOGRAPHY, NOSOLOGY.

TCDD 2,3,7,8-tetrachlorodibenzo-p-dioxin. The strongest agonist of the arylhydrocarbon receptor (AhR). A NONGENOTOXIC human carcinogen.[219] A by-product of the manufacture of polychlorinated phenols that is generated through waste incineration. Both epidemiological evidence and mechanistic studies have indicated a relationship between TCDD exposure and the occurrence of some cancers. Many XENOBIOTIC metabolizing enzymes are induced through TCDD-mediated AhR activity. To assess the clinical and epidemiological impact of compounds like dioxins and other persistent organic pollutants (POPs) is one of the challenges faced by MOLECULAR EPIDEMIOLOGY, ENVIRONMENTAL EPIDEMIOLOGY, and related approaches. See also BIOLOGICAL MONITORING.

***T*-DISTRIBUTION, *T*-TEST** The *t*-distribution is the distribution of a quotient of independent random variables, the numerator of which is a standardized normal variate and the denominator of which is the positive square root of the quotient of a chi-square distributed variate and its number of degrees of freedom. The *t*-test uses a statistic that, under the null hypothesis, has the *t*-distribution to test whether two means differ significantly, or to test linear regression or correlation coefficients. The *t*-distribution and the *t*-test were developed by W. S. Gossett, who wrote under the pseudonym "Student," as his employment precluded individual publication.

TEPHINET Training Programs in Epidemiology and Public Health Interventions Network (www.tephinet.org). A professional alliance of field epidemiology training programs (FETPs) located in some 30 countries around the world.

TERATOGEN A substance that produces abnormalities in the embryo or fetus by disturbing maternal homeostasis or acting directly on the fetus in utero.

TEST OF SIGNIFICANCE See *P* VALUE; SIGNIFICANCE, STATISTICAL.

TEST HYPOTHESIS In statistics, the hypothesis subject to a statistical test, such as a significance test. A test hypothesis may concern any possible value for the measure under study; e.g., it test whether a risk ratio is 0.5, 1, 2, 4, or any other value of interest. The NULL HYPOTHESIS is a special case of test hypothesis.

THE 3 BY 5 TARGET (Syn: the 3 by 5 initiative) A target set by WHO of providing antiretroviral therapy (ART) to 3 million people in resource-limited countries by the end of the year 2005. www.who.int/3by5/en.

THEORETICAL EPIDEMIOLOGY

1. The discipline of how to study the occurrence of phenomena of interest in the health field;[5] epidemiological methodology.
2. The development of mathematical and statistical models to explain different aspects of the occurrence of a variety of diseases. With some infectious diseases, for instance, models have been generated to elucidate the reasons for epidemics and to predict the behavior of the disease as a reaction to given control measures. See also MECHANISTIC EPIDEMIOLOGY; MODEL.

THERAPEUTIC TRIAL See CLINICAL TRIAL; RANDOMIZED CONTROLLED TRIAL.

THRESHOLD DOSE The dose above which effects occur.

THRESHOLD LIMIT VALUE See SAFETY STANDARDS.

THRESHOLD PHENOMENA Events or changes that occur only after a certain level of a characteristic is reached.

THRIFTY PHENOTYPE A term coined by D. J. P. Barker to describe the hypothesis that insulin resistance and type 2 diabetes originate through undernutrition in the womb.

THRIFTY PHENOTYPE HYPOTHESIS The hypothesis proposing that an undernourished baby becomes thrifty. It maintains high levels of sugar in the bloodstream to benefit the brain but less sugar in muscles. Muscle growth may be "traded off" to protect the brain. Once adopted, this thrifty behavior becomes permanent and, combined with adiposity in later life, leads to type 2 diabetes. See also "BRAIN SPARING"; DEVELOPMENTAL ORIGINS HYPOTHESIS.

TIME CLUSTER See CLUSTERING.

TIME ORDER The only necessary PROPERTY OF CAUSE: a cause must always precede an effect. Conceptually obvious as it may seem, assessment of the TEMPORAL RELATIONSHIP relies heavily on an often complex and subtle assessment of tests and designs.

TIME-PLACE CLUSTER See CLUSTERING.

TIME SERIES A single-group research design in which measurements are made at several different times, thereby allowing trends to be detected. An interrupted time series features several measurements both before and after an intervention and is usually more valid than a simple pretest-posttest design. A multiple time series involves several groups, including a control group.

TIME TRADE-OFF A method of determining UTILITY in which members of a panel express preferences either for normal life expectancy in a defined suboptimal health state or reduced life expectancy in good health.[379] The magnitude of reduced life expectancy is varied until there is EQUIPOISE between the choices.

"TIME WILL TELL" BIAS A form of INTERPRETIVE BIAS that occurs because different scientists need different amounts of confirmatory evidence. Certainly the position that more evidence is necessary before making a judgment indicates a judicious attitude that is central to scientific scepticism.[34] See also CONSISTENCY; PRECAUTIONARY PRINCIPLE; REPLICATION.

TOLERANCE In toxicology and pharmacology, the adaptive state characterized by diminished effects of a particular dose of a substance.

TORT A legal term for the harmful consequence of an act. Such acts are tried in courts of law, and damages are awarded if wrong or harm is demonstrated. A "toxic tort" is a lawsuit centered around a claim for harm due to a toxic chemical. Epidemiologists sometimes have to testify in legal cases involving tort.

TOTAL FERTILITY RATE (TFR) The average number of children that would be born per woman if all women lived to the end of their childbearing years and bore children according to a given set of age-specific fertility rates. It is computed by summing the age-specific fertility rates for all ages and multiplying by the interval into which the ages are grouped. The TFR is an important fertility measure, providing the most accurate answer to the question "How many children does a woman have on average?"

TOWNSEND SCORE An index of social deprivation developed by the British social scientist Peter Townsend (b.1928), used mainly in the United Kingdom; based on numbers economically active but unemployed, households with no car, households not owner-occupied, households overcrowded. The Townsend score uses readily available census data and can be used to rank administratively defined jurisdictions. See also JARMAN SCORE; OVERCROWDING.[380]

TOXICOLOGY The scientific discipline involving the study of actual or potential danger presented by the harmful effects of chemicals (poisons) on living organisms and ecosystems; of the relationship of such harmful effects to exposure; and of the mechanisms of action, diagnosis, prevention, and treatment of intoxications.[200] Toxicology has an increasingly broad interface with epidemiology.

TRACER DISEASE METHOD Tracer or indicator conditions are easily diagnosed, reasonably frequent illnesses or health states whose outcomes are believed to be affected by health care and that, taken in aggregate, should reflect the gamut of patients and health problems encountered in a medical practice.[381] The extent to which the recorded care of these conditions concurs with preset standards of care is used as an index of the quality of care delivered. However, it should first be shown that the preset standards contribute to a favorable outcome. See also SENTINEL HEALTH EVENT.

TRANSCRIPTION Copying of a strand of DNA to generate a complementary strand of RNA.

TRANSDISCIPLINARITY The philosophical concept of scholarly inquiry that ignores conventional boundaries among ways of thinking about and solving problems.[382] It is based on recognition of the complexity of many problems confronting humans and seeks to mobilize all pertinent scholarly disciplines: physical, biological, social and behavioral sciences, ethics, moral philosophy, communication sciences, economics, politics, and the humanities. Many problems in public health have required transdisciplinary analyses and solutions. Epidemiology thus has a long tradition of transdisciplinary analysis of complex problems, of INTEGRATIVE RESEARCH (i.e., research that integrates multiple disciplines and levels of analysis), and of multidimensional intervention on the population and individual DETERMINANTS on health. The ecological impact of global climate change—which includes the epidemiological impact—is a most current and relevant example of the important contributions of epidemiology to transdisciplinary research.[138] Sometimes it may be practically opposed to—but it is not an antonym of—REDUCTIONISM.

TRANSMISSION OF INFECTION Transmission of infectious agents. Any mechanism by which an infectious agent is spread from a source or reservoir to another person. These mechanisms are defined as follows:

1. Direct transmission. Direct and essentially immediate transfer of infectious agents to a receptive portal of entry through which human or animal infection may take place. This may be by direct contact such as touching, kissing, biting, or sexual intercourse or by the direct projection (droplet spread) of droplet spray onto the conjunctiva or the mucous membranes of the eyes, nose, or mouth. It may also be by direct exposure of susceptible tissue to an agent in soil, compost, or decaying vegetable matter or by the bite of a rabid animal. Transplacental transmission is another form of direct transmission.
2. Indirect transmission. *Vehicle-borne:* Contaminated inanimate material or objects (fomites) such as toys, handkerchiefs, soiled clothes, bedding, cooking or eating utensils, and surgical instruments or dressings (indirect contact); water, food, milk; biological products including blood, serum, plasma, tissues, or organs; or any substance serving as an intermediate means by which an infectious agent is transported and introduced into a susceptible host through a suitable portal of entry. The agent may or may not have multiplied or developed in or on the vehicle before being transmitted.

Vector-borne: (a) *Mechanical:* Includes simple mechanical carriage by a crawling or flying insect through soiling of its feet or proboscis or by passage of organisms through its gastrointestinal tract. This does not require multiplication or development of the organism. (b) *Biological:* Propagation (multiplication), cyclic development, or a combination of these (cyclopropagative) is required before the arthropod can transmit the infective form of the agent to humans. An incubation period (extrinsic) is required following infection before the arthropod becomes infective. The infectious agent may be passed vertically to succeeding generations (transovarian transmission); transstadial transmission is its passage from one stage of the life cycle to another, as nymph to adult. Transmission may be by saliva during biting or by regurgitation or deposition on the skin of feces or other material capable of penetrating subsequently through the bite wound or through an area of trauma from scratching or rubbing. Transmission by an infected nonvertebrate host must be differentiated for epidemiological purposes from simple mechanical carriage by a vector in the role of a vehicle. An arthropod in either role is termed a *vector*.

Airborne: The dissemination of microbial aerosols to a portal of entry, usually the respiratory tract. Microbial aerosols are suspensions in the air of particles consisting partially or wholly of microorganisms. Particles in the range of 1 to 5 μm are easily drawn into the alveoli of the lungs and may be retained there. They may remain suspended in the air for long periods.

Airborne transmission includes:

Droplet nuclei: residues that result from evaporation of fluid from droplets emitted by an infected host. Droplet nuclei also may be created purposely by a variety of atomizing devices, or accidentally, as in microbiology laboratories or in abattoirs, rendering plants, or autopsy rooms. They usually remain suspended in the air for long periods.

Dust: The small particles of widely varying size that may arise from soil (fungus spores) or from clothes, bedding, or contaminated floors.

See also ACQUAINTANCE NETWORK; AIRBORNE INFECTION; CARRIER; COMMON VEHICLE SPREAD; CONTACT; CONTAMINATION; DROPLET NUCLEI.

TRANSMISSION PARAMETER (r) In infectious disease epidemiology, the proportion of total possible contacts between infectious cases and susceptibles that lead to new infections.

TRANSOVARIAL TRANSMISSION See VECTOR-BORNE INFECTION.

TRANSPORT HOST See PARATENIC HOST.

TRANSVECTION An EPIGENETIC phenomenon that results from an interaction between an allele on one chromosome and the corresponding allele on the homologous chromosome. It can lead to either gene activation or repression. See also EPIGENETIC INHERITANCE.

TRAP, DEMOGRAPHIC See DEMOGRAPHIC ENTRAPMENT.

TREND A long-term movement in an ordered series (e.g., a time series). An essential feature is that the movement, while possibly irregular in the short term, shows movement consistently in the same direction over a long term. Also used loosely to refer to an association that is consistent in several samples or strata but is not statistically significant.

TREND (STATEMENT) A proposal for an structured approach to reporting and evaluating studies of behavioral and public health interventions that use nonrandomized designs.[95,383] See also CONSORT; QUADAS, QUOROM; STARD; STROBE.

TREND LINE The line that best fits the distribution of a set of values plotted on two axes.

TRIAGE The process of selecting for care or treatment those of highest priority or, when resources are limited, those thought most likely to benefit. From the French *trier*, to separate, choose. See also RAPID EPIDEMIOLOGICAL ASSESSMENT.

TRIAL See CLINICAL TRIAL.

TRIAL PROFILE See CONSORT.

"TRIMMING" (data trimming) The practice, which can be akin to a form of scientific fraud or misrepresentation, of excluding from analysis observations or measurements that lie outside the range the investigator expects; the grounds for exclusion are that these outlying observations would distort the results. Data trimming is permissible only when rules written in advance in the research protocol specify circumstances in which it may be done. Even then it should be done with caution, and openly. See also OUTLIERS.

TRIPLE BLIND STUDY A study in which subjects, observers, and analysts are blinded as to which subjects received what interventions. See also BLIND(ED) STUDY.

TROHOC STUDY A retrospective CASE-CONTROL STUDY. The term, proposed by A. R. Feinstein,[322] is the inversion of "cohort"; its use is rare.

TRUE-POSITIVE RATE See SENSITIVITY AND SPECIFICITY.

TRUE-NEGATIVE RATE See SENSITIVITY AND SPECIFICITY.

TUBERCULOSIS A chronic disease since Neolithic times, afflicting an estimated 0.2% of the world's population, caused by *Mycobacterium tuberculosis*.[384] It merits mention in this dictionary because it continues to present an epidemiological challenge.[385] The tuberculin skin test, which has long been a simple, cheap means of screening, is less efficient in populations that have been vaccinated with bacille Calmette-Guérin (BCG) and in which there are large numbers of immunocompromised persons infected with HIV.

TUKEY'S METHOD See MULTIPLE COMPARISON TECHNIQUES.

TWIN STUDY Method of detecting genetic etiology in human disease. The basic premise of twin studies is that monozygotic twins, being formed by the division of a single fertilized ovum, carry identical genes, while dizygotic twins, being formed by the fertilization of two ova by two different spermatozoa, are genetically no more similar than two siblings born after separate pregnancies.

TWO-BY-TWO TABLE See TWO-WAY TABLE.

TWO-TAIL TEST A statistical significance test based on the assumption that deviation from the TEST HYPOTHESIS in either direction is of interest. See also ONE-TAIL TEST.

TWO-WAY TABLE A contingency table for categorical variables. A table with *r* rows and *c* columns in which the entry in each cell represents the frequency for each outcome. Such a table is called an r-by-c table (e.g., a 3-by-4 table). If r = 2 and c = 2 then it is called a two-by-two table.

TYPE I ERROR See ERROR, TYPE I.

TYPE II ERROR See ERROR, TYPE II.

TYPE III ERROR See ERROR, TYPE III.

"TYPHOID MARY" A slang expression for an individual who unwittingly transmits infection to others. The original Typhoid Mary, Mary Mallon, was an itinerant cook and an infamous carrier of typhoid in New York City and environs early in the twentieth century.

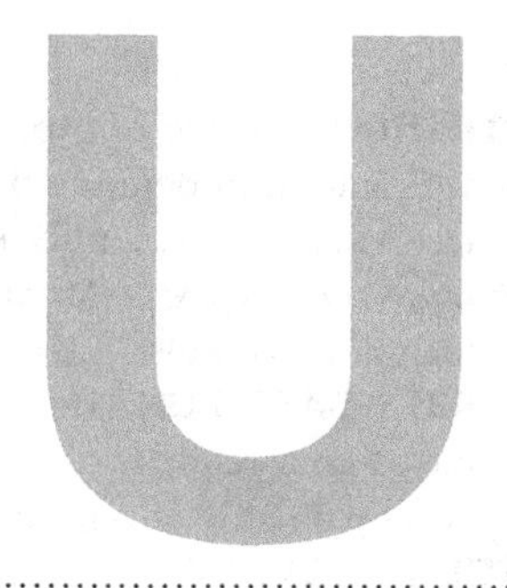

UICC Union Internationale Contre le Cancer (International Union Against Cancer) (www.uicc.org).

UIP Universal Immunisation Program (www.who.int/immunization).

UN United Nations (www.un.org).

UNAIDS Joint United Nations Programme on HIV/AIDS (www.unaids.org).

UNBIASED ESTIMATOR An estimator that, for all sample sizes, has an expected value equal to the parameter being estimated. If an estimator tends to be unbiased as sample size increases, it is referred to as asymptotically unbiased.

UNDERLYING CAUSE OF DEATH The disease or injury that initiated the train of events leading directly to death, or the circumstances of the accident or violence that produced the fatal injury. See DEATH CERTIFICATE.

UNDERREPORTING Failure to identify and/or count all cases, leading to reduction of the numerator in a rate. See also ERROR.

UNDP United Nations Development Programme (www.undp.org).

UNEP United Nations Environmental Programme (www.unep.org).

UNFPA United Nations Population Fund (www.unfpa.org).

UNHCR United Nations High Commission for Refugees (www.unhcr.org).

UNICEF United Nations Children's Fund (www.unicef.org).

UNIVERSAL PRECAUTIONS Procedures to be followed when health workers anticipate the possibility of infection by a patient who may harbor a highly contagious, dangerous pathogen. Universal precautions may include segregation of the patient in a private room; use of gloves, gown, mask, Perspex shield (eye protection); and rigorous attention to ensuring that no blood or other body fluid from such a patient can come into contact with the skin or mucous membranes of the health care worker. See also NEEDLE STICK and BARRIER NURSING.

UNIVERSE, UNIVERSE POPULATION The entire population from which a sample is selected for study. The term is seldom used and is preferably avoided outside of theoretical discussions.

UNMEASURED CONFOUNDING See RESIDUAL CONFOUNDING.

UNOBTRUSIVE MEASURES A set of methods for assessing behavior without actually asking people how they behave or examining them physically to determine the effects of their behavior.[386]

USPHS United States Public Health Service (www.usphs.gov).

UTILITY The value of a particular health state, usually expressed on a scale from 0 to 1; it is used in defining QUALITY-ADJUSTED LIFE YEARS (QALYs) and HEALTH-ADJUSTED LIFE EXPECTANCY. Utility is determined from preferences expressed by an individuals in a VON NEUMANN–MORGENSTERN STANDARD GAMBLE, TIME TRADE-OFF, or other related technique. See also COST-UTILITY ANALYSIS.

UTILITY-BASED UNITS In the context of QUALITY-ADJUSTED LIFE YEARS (QALYs), utility-based units relate to a person's level of well-being estimated on the basis of the total life years gained from a procedure or intervention.

UTILITY, CLINICAL Risks and benefits associated with the introduction of a screening or diagnostic test into clinical practice.[14,62,193,210–213,355,387] See also SIGNIFICANCE, CLINICAL.

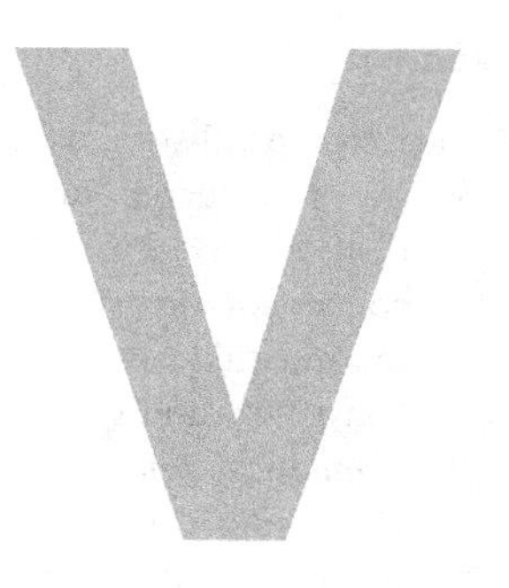

VACCINATION Strictly speaking, *vaccination* refers to inoculation (from Latin *in oculus*, into a bud) with vaccinia virus against smallpox. Nowadays the word is broadly used synonymously with procedures for IMMUNIZATION against all infectious disease. The original use of the word was confined to vaccination against smallpox. This was the first method of preventing a lethal disease by immunizing humans. It was introduced by Edward Jenner (1749–1823) and described by him in *An Inquiry into the Cause and Effects of the Variolae Vaccinae* (1798). Jenner's discovery led directly to the worldwide eradication of smallpox.

VACCINE Immunobiological substance used for active immunization by introducing into the body a live modified, attenuated, or killed inactivated infectious organism or its toxin. The vaccine is capable of stimulating an immune response by the host, who is thus rendered resistant to infection. The word *vaccine* was originally applied to the serum from a cow infected with vaccinia virus (cowpox; from Latin *vacca*, "cow"); it is now used of all immunizing agents.

VACCINE EFFICACY (Syn: protective efficacy) Mathematically, this is defined as the proportion of persons in the placebo group of a vaccine trial who would not have become ill if they had received the vaccine; alternatively, it is the percentage reduction of cases among vaccinated individuals.

VALIDATION The process of establishing that a method is sound.

VALIDITY Relative absence of BIAS or systematic error. Contrast with PRECISION, the relative lack of random error.[12,20,31,97] As a principle, internal validity must take precedence over precision. In the health, life, and social sciences, the term is often accompanied by a qualifying word or phrase. See also ACCURACY; RELIABILITY; REPEATABILITY; VALIDITY, STUDY; CONFOUNDING BIAS; SELECTION BIAS.

VALIDITY, ANALYTICAL The ability of a test to correctly identify a property or characteristic in a specimen. This term encompasses both "analytical sensitivity" and "analytical specificity."

VALIDITY, CLINICAL The ability of a test to correctly identify a person who does or does not have the disease of interest.[62,63,134,321] This term encompasses both "clinical sensitivity" and "clinical specificity."

VALIDITY, INTERNAL See VALIDITY, STUDY.

VALIDITY, EXTERNAL See VALIDITY, STUDY.

VALIDITY, MEASUREMENT An expression of the degree to which a measurement measures what it purports to measure. See also MEASUREMENT, TERMINOLOGY OF. Several varieties are distinguished, including construct validity, content validity, and criterion validity (concurrent and predictive validity).

1. *Construct validity:* The extent to which the measurement corresponds to theoretical concepts (constructs) concerning the phenomenon under study. For example, if, on theoretical grounds, the phenomenon should change with age, a measurement with construct validity would reflect such a change.
2. *Content validity:* The extent to which the measurement incorporates the domain of the phenomenon under study. For example, a measurement of functional health status should embrace activities of daily living: occupational, family, and social functioning, etc.
3. *Criterion validity:* The extent to which the measurement correlates with an external criterion of the phenomenon under study. Two aspects of criterion validity can be distinguished:
   a. *Concurrent validity:* The measurement and the criterion refer to the same point in time. An example is a visual inspection of a wound for evidence of infection validated against bacteriological examination of a specimen taken at the same time.
   b. *Predictive validity:* The measurement's validity is expressed in terms of its ability to predict the criterion. An example is an academic aptitude test that is validated against subsequent academic performance.

VALIDITY, STUDY The degree to which the inferences drawn from a study are warranted when account is taken of the study methods and the characteristics of the participants in the study.

Two fundamental types of study validity must be distinguished:

1. INTERNAL VALIDITY The degree to which a study is free from BIAS or systematic error. Relative lack of bias. Contrast with PRECISION, the relative lack of random error. The soundness of the study design, conduct, and analysis in answering the question that it posed for the study participants. Internal validity depends on methods and on substantive knowledge. More specifically, it depends on methods used to select the study subjects, collect information, and conduct analyses. For instance, the index and comparison groups must be selected and compared in such a manner that the observed differences between their effect on the outcome variables under study may, apart from sampling error, be attributed only to the hypothesized effect under investigation. Internal validity also depends on subject-matter knowledge; e.g., the application of equipotent doses of drugs in some clinical trials, the choice of valid windows of exposure in longitudinal studies, or the planning of valid intervals and procedures for outcome detection. Internal validity is a prerequisite for external validity.
2. EXTERNAL VALIDITY (Syn: generalizability) The degree to which results of a study may apply, be relevant, or be generalized to populations or groups that did not participate in the study. A study is externally valid, or generalizable, if it allows unbiased inferences regarding some other specific target population beyond the subjects in the study. Hence it concerns the capacity to make fair inferences to an external population that did not participate in the study. In etiological research, such inferences to an external population are not merely statistical in nature: they must be rigorously based on all available knowledge that is relevant for the study hypotheses.

Conclusions about the external and internal validity of a study both require wisdom to apply judgment strictly based on knowledge of the subject matter and of methodology; methodological knowledge may be slightly more important in judging internal validity, whereas substantive knowledge on the subject may be somewhat more relevant in judging external validity; however, these nuances must not obscure the need to integrate the two types of knowledge. [20,93,181]

These epidemiological definitions of internal and external validity do not correspond exactly to some definitions found in the sociological literature. See also CRITICAL APPRAISAL; EVIDENCE-BASED MEDICINE; FEASIBILITY; GENERALIZABILITY.

VALUES

1. In the health, life, and social sciences, what we believe in, what we hold dear about the way we live. Values influence the behavior of persons, groups, communities, cultures.. They are strong influences on the health of individuals and populations (scientists are here included).[85,104,128,184–187]
2. Concepts used to explain how and why things matter. Values are involved wherever we distinguish between things good and bad, better or worse. Values are pervasive in human activities, including epidemiological research and public health.[36]
3. In statistics, the magnitudes of measurements, statistics, or parameters.

VARIABLE Any quantity that varies. Any attribute, phenomenon, or event that can have different values.

VARIABLE, ANTECEDENT A variable that causally precedes the association or outcome under study. See also EXPLANATORY VARIABLE.

VARIABLE, CONFOUNDING See CONFOUNDING VARIABLE.

VARIABLE, CONTROL Independent variable other than the "hypothetical causal variable" that has a potential effect on the outcome variable and is subject to control by analysis.

VARIABLE, DEPENDENT See DEPENDENT VARIABLE.

VARIABLE, DISTORTER A CONFOUNDING VARIABLE that diminishes, masks, or reverses the association under study.

VARIABLE, EXPERIENTIAL See INDEPENDENT VARIABLE.

VARIABLE, INDEPENDENT See INDEPENDENT VARIABLE.

VARIABLE, INTERVENING See INTERMEDIATE VARIABLE.

VARIABLE, MANIFESTATIONAL See DEPENDENT VARIABLE.

VARIABLE, PASSENGER See PASSENGER VARIABLE.

VARIABLE, UNCONTROLLED A (potentially) confounding variable that has not been brought under control by design or analysis. See CONFOUNDING VARIABLE; RESIDUAL CONFOUNDING.

VARIANCE A measure of the variation shown by a set of observations, defined by the sum of the squares of deviation from the mean, divided by the number of DEGREES OF FREEDOM in the set of observations.

VARIATE See RANDOM VARIABLE.

VECTOR

1. In infectious disease epidemiology, an insect or any living carrier that transports an infectious agent from an infected individual or its wastes to a susceptible individual or its food or immediate surroundings. The organism may or may not pass through a developmental cycle within the vector.
2. In statistics, an ordered set (list) of numbers representing the values of an ordered set of variables (which is a vector of variables).

VECTOR-BORNE INFECTION Several classes of vector-borne infections are recognized, each with epidemiological features determined by the interaction between the infectious agent and the human host on the one hand and the vector on the other. Therefore environmental factors, such as climatic and seasonal variations, influence the epidemiological pattern by virtue of their effects on the vector and its habits.

The terms used to describe specific features of vector-borne infections are as follows:

1. BIOLOGICAL TRANSMISSION: Transmission of the infectious agent to susceptible host by the bite of a blood-feeding (arthropod) vector, as in malaria, or by other inoculation, as in *Schistosoma* infection.
2. EXTRINSIC INCUBATION PERIOD: Time necessary after acquisition of infection by the (arthropod) vector for the infectious agent to multiply or develop sufficiently that it can be transmitted by the vector to a vertebrate host.
3. HIBERNATION: A possible mechanism by which the infected vector survives adverse cold weather by becoming dormant.
4. INAPPARENT INFECTION: Response to infection without developing overt signs of illness. If this is accompanied by viremia or bacteremia in a high proportion of infected animals or persons, the receptor species is well suited as an epidemiologically important host in the transmission cycle.
5. MECHANICAL TRANSMISSION: Transport of the infectious agent between hosts by arthropod vectors with contaminated mouthparts, antennae, or limbs. There is no multiplication of the infectious agent in the vector.
6. OVERWINTERING: Persistence of the infectious microorganism in the vector for extended periods, such as the cooler winter months, during which the vector has no opportunity to be reinfected or to infect a vertebrate host. Overwintering is an important concept in the epidemiology of vector-borne diseases, since the annual recrudescence of viral activity after periods (winter, dry season) adverse to continual transmission depends on a mechanism for local survival of an infectious microorganism or its reintroduction from outside the endemic area. To some extent, the risk of a summertime epidemic may be determined by the relative success of microorganism survival in the local winter reservoir. Since overwinter survival may in turn depend upon the level of activity of the microorganism during the preceding summer and autumn, outbreaks sometimes occur for 2 or more successive years.
7. TRANSOVARIAL INFECTION (Syn: transovarial transmission): Transmission of the infectious microorganism from the affected female arthropod to her progeny.

VECTOR SPACE The entire collection of possible values for a VECTOR (ordered list) of variables.

VEHICLE OF INFECTION TRANSMISSION The mode of transmission of an infectious agent from its reservoir to a susceptible host. This can be person-to-person, via food, vector-borne, etc.

VENN DIAGRAM A pictorial presentation of the extent to which two or more quantities or concepts overlap.

VERBAL "AUTOPSY" A procedure for gathering information that may make it possible to determine the cause of death in situations where the deceased has not been medically attended. It is based on the assumption that most common and important causes of death have distinct symptom complexes that can be recognized, remembered, and reported by lay respondents. It is promoted as a useful way of enhancing the quality of mortality statistics in developing countries.[388]

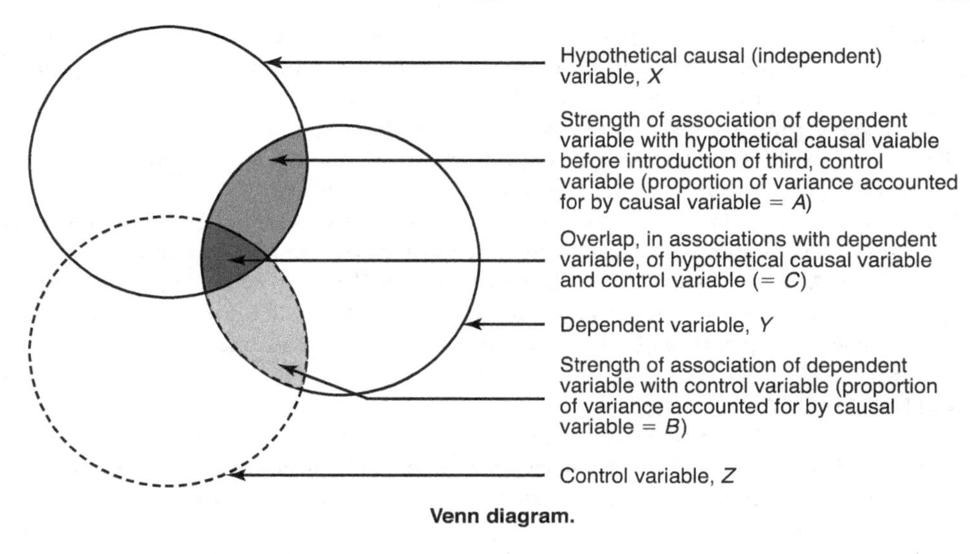

Venn diagram.

Venn diagram. From Susser MW.[22]

VERIFICATION The process aimed at converting speculative ideas and hypotheses into facts. It usually results either in the rejection of false hypotheses by deduction (see DEDUCTIVE LOGIC) or the acceptance and consensus by induction (see INDUCTIVE LOGIC). A most illustrative case history is William Harvey's confirmation of his hypothesis of the circulation of the blood, now universally recognized. In its broadest sense, verification is a summary of a process of CAUSAL INFERENCE.

VERIFICATION BIAS In studies evaluating screening and diagnostic tests, this bias occurs when some patients with negative test results are not evaluated with the "gold standard" test. Sensitivity can be overestimated and specificity underestimated; however, the final bias depends on the variables associated with receiving or not receiving the gold standard. When the gold standard is invasive, clinicians will tend to perform it on patients whose experimental test results increase the probability of disease and to refrain from performing it in those whose experimental test results decrease the probability of disease.[14,31,327] See also QUADAS; WORKUP BIAS.

VERTICAL TRANSMISSION (Syn: intergenerational transmission) The transmission of infection from one generation to the next, especially of HIV infection from mother to infant prenatally, during delivery, or in the postnatal period via breast milk.

VIOLENCE Harm caused by the use of force. Harm takes the form of traumatic injury or death. Epidemiologically, two main varieties, unintentional and intentional violence, can be distinguished; the former occurs mainly in traffic and industry, the latter mainly in warfare and in domestic settings.

VIRGIN POPULATION A population that has never been exposed to a particular infectious agent.

VIRULENCE The degree of pathogenicity; the disease-evoking power of a microorganism in a given host. Numerically expressed as the ratio of the number of cases of overt infection to the total number infected as determined by immunoassay. When death is the only criterion of severity, this is the case-fatality rate.

VIRUS A microorganism composed of a piece of genetic material (RNA or DNA) surrounded by a protein coat. To replicate, a virus must infect a living cell: viruses can reproduce only by entering a host cell and using the translational system of the cell to initiate the synthesis of viral proteins and to undergo replication.

VITAL RECORDS Certificates of birth, death, marriage, and divorce required for legal and demographic purposes. Literally, records "to do with living."

VITAL STATISTICS Systematically tabulated information concerning births, marriages, divorces, separations, and deaths based on registrations of these vital events.

VON NEUMANN–MORGENSTERN STANDARD GAMBLE Procedure used to assess the risk a seriously ill person is prepared to take when the trade-off is between potentially enhanced quality of life and a finite possibility that the treatment regimen will be fatal.[389]

VULNERABILITY

1. A position of relative disadvantage; e.g., owing to impaired nutrition, cognition, or social position. The extent to which a person, population, or ecosystem is unable or unlikely to respond to threats. May be used as a synonym for SUSCEPTIBILITY See ALSO ROBUSTNESS.
2. A process of negative adaptation in the face of adversity (Opposite: RESILIENCE).

VULNERABLE POPULATION A population at risk of coercion, abuse, exploitation, discrimination, imposition of unjust burdens of risk, and poorer health outcomes by reason of diminished competence or decision-making capacity, lack of power or social standing, fragile health, deprivation, or limited access to basic needs, including public health and medical care. Similar acts may be construed to be coercive in a vulnerable population which would not be so in other, well-situated populations. Includes children, institutionalized persons, the frail, and those with mental disorders as well as those on the lower sectors of societies.[37]

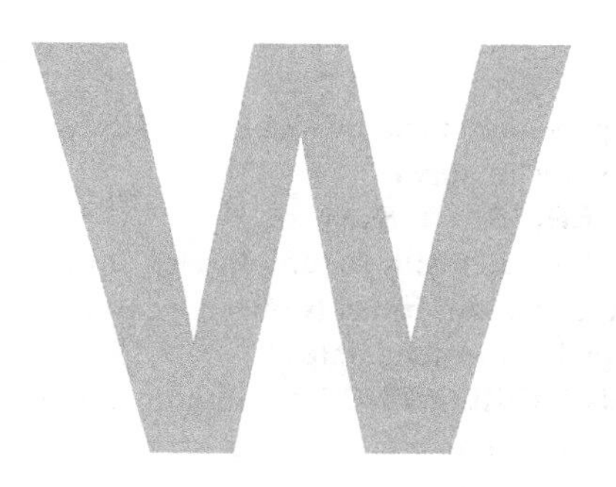

WASHOUT PHASE That stage in a study, especially a therapeutic trial, when symptomatic treatment is withdrawn so that its effects disappear and the subject's characteristics return to their baseline state.[14,330] An effective washout phase is essential in a CROSSOVER EXPERIMENT.

WEB OF CAUSATION (Syn: causal web). In epidemiology and public health, a popular METAPHOR for the theory of sequential and linked multiple causes of diseases and other health states (MULTIPLE CAUSE THEORY). The term appears in several monographs on epidemiology published in the early 1960s[169] and was probably first published in 1959 by Dawber et al.[390] and in 1960 by Brian MacMahon (1923–2007) et al.[391] Originally deployed mainly for an epidemiology practised at the individual level of organization (although not necessarily confined to it), the metaphor can be extended to incorporate a sequence of multiple dimensions.[89] See also ASSOCIATION; CAUSAL DIAGRAMS; DISEASES OF COMPLEX ETIOLOGY; ECOEPIDEMIOLOGY; MULTILEVEL ANALYSIS; MULTIPLE CAUSATION; PROBABILITY OF CAUSATION.

WEIBULL MODEL Dose-response model of the form

$$P(d) = 1 - \exp(-bd^m)$$

where $P(d)$ is the probability of response due to a continuous dose rate d; b and m are constants. The model is useful for extrapolating from high- to low-dose exposures—e.g., animal to human or occupational to environmental. Also used to model SURVIVAL PROPORTIONS.

WEIGHTED AVERAGE A value determined by assigning weights to individual measurements or estimates. Each value is assigned a nonnegative coefficient (weight); the sum of the products of each value by its weight divided by the sum of the weights is the weighted average.

WEIGHTED SAMPLE A sample that is not strictly proportional to the distribution of classes in the universe population. A weighted sample has been adjusted to include larger proportions of some than other parts of the UNIVERSE population because those parts accorded greater "weight" would otherwise not have sufficient numbers in the sample to lead to generalizable conclusions or because they are considered to be more important, more interesting, more worthy of detailed study, etc.

WER *Weekly Epidemiological Record* An instrument for the rapid and accurate dissemination of epidemiological information on cases and outbreaks of diseases under the International Health Regulations and on other communicable diseases of public health importance, including emerging or reemerging infections. Published by the WHO (www.who.int/wer).

WESTERN BLOT See BLOT.

WHA World Health Assembly. The supreme decision-making body for the World Health Organization. It meets once a year and is attended by delegations from all of WHO's over 190 member states.

"WHISTLE-BLOWING" Informing authorities or the media when fraud or misrepresentation of research results or any other form of wrongdoing is suspected.

WHO World Health Organization (www.who.int).

WILD TYPE The normal, nonaltered sequence of a gene; the opposite is a mutated sequence.

WONCA World Organization of National Colleges, Academies, and Academic Associations of General Practitioners/Family Physicians, the World Organization of Family Doctors.[257] See also INTERNATIONAL CLASSIFICATION OF PRIMARY CARE, SECOND EDITION REVISED (ICPC-2-R).

WOOLF-HALDANE CORRECTION A modification of the observed data that permits statistical analysis when cell(s) in a table have a value of zero. An increment close to zero (e.g., 0.5) is added to all the cells to enable computation of the stratum-specific odds ratio and other quantities.[97] Now largely obsolete owing to the availability of packaged software for methods that require no such correction (e.g., FISHER'S EXACT TEST and the MANTEL-HAENSZEL ODDS RATIO).

WORKUP BIAS Bias due to incorrectly or incompletely diagnosed cases being more numerous in one group than another in a study in which comparison is made between groups. Usually this happens because patients with a positive screening-level test receive a more thorough workup with diagnostic ("GOLD STANDARD") tests than those whose screening-level test was negative.[63,327,369] It is a form of VERIFICATION BIAS. See also SPECTRUM BIAS.

WORM COUNT A method of surveillance of helminth infection of the gut that depends upon counts of worms, or cysts or ova, in quantitatively titrated samples of feces. Other terms to describe this form of surveillance are *egg count, cyst count*, and *parasite count*.

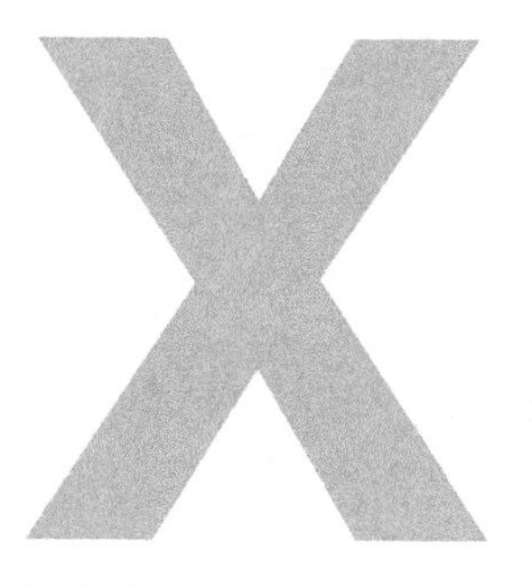

X CHROMOSOME INACTIVATION (Syn: lyonization) A process by which one of the two copies of the X chromosome present in female mammals is inactivated by packaging in repressive heterochromatin. X-inactivation occurs so that the female, with two X chromosomes, does not have twice as many X chromosome gene products as the male, which only has a single copy of the X chromosome. See also EPIGENETIC INHERITANCE.

XDR (EXTENSIVELY DRUG-RESISTANT TUBERCULOSIS) See DRUG-RESISTANT TUBERCULOSIS, EXTENSIVELY.

XENOBIOTIC

1. A chemical compound that is foreign to a biological or an ecological system. A substance, typically a synthetic chemical, that is foreign to the body. Examples include many synthetic pesticides and their derivatives, food additives, or persistent toxic substances such as dioxins and polychlorinated biphenyls (PCBs).[219] See also CARCINOGEN.
2. (Syn: commensal, symbiosis) Pertaining to an association of two animal species, usually insects, in the absence of a dependency relationship, as opposed to parasitism. Contrast ENDOBIOTIC. See also COMMENSAL.

XENODIAGNOSIS Detection of a (human) pathogenic organism by allowing a noninfected vector (e.g., mosquito) to consume infected material and then examining this vector for evidence of the pathogen.

X-LINKED (Syn: sex-linked) Heritable characteristic transmitted by a gene located on the X chromosome.

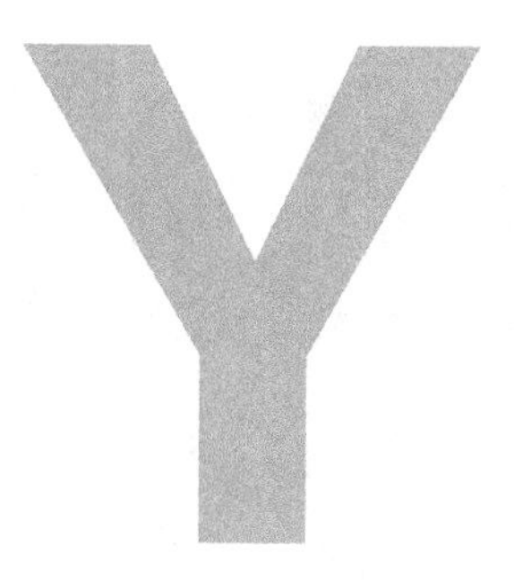

YATES'S CORRECTION An adjustment proposed by Yates (1934) in the chi-square calculation for a 2 × 2 table that brings the distribution based on discontinuous frequencies closer to the continuous chi-square distribution from which the published tables for testing chi-squares are derived.

YEARS OF POTENTIAL LIFE LOST (YPLL) See POTENTIAL YEARS OF LIFE LOST.

YIELD The number or proportion of cases of a condition accurately identified by a screening test.

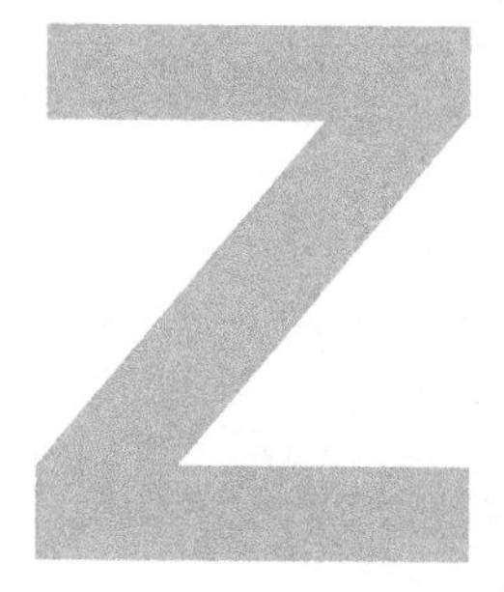

ZELEN DESIGN (Syn: prerandomization design, post-randomized consent) A modified double-blind RANDOMIZED CONTROLLED TRIAL design proposed by Marvin Zelen (b. 1927).[392] The essential feature of the Zelen design is randomization before informed consent procedures, which are claimed to be needed only for the group allocated to receive the experimental regimen. Many ethicists disagree, holding that it is necessary to obtain the INFORMED CONSENT of all participants regardless of the group to which they are allocated.

ZERO POPULATION GROWTH The status of a population in which there is no net increase of numbers; the number of births (plus immigrants) equals the number of deaths (plus emigrants).

ZERO REPORTING Reporting of the absence of cases of a disease under surveillance; this ensures that participants have not merely forgotten to report.

ZERO-SUM GAME A situation in which one participant can "gain" only at the expense of or to the detriment of another.

ZERO-TIME SHIFT The selection of a starting point for the measurement of survival following the detection of disease. It denotes the movement "backward" (toward the starting point of a disease) of time between onset and detection that may accompany use of a screening procedure.

ZOONOSIS An infection or infectious disease transmissible under natural conditions from vertebrate animals to humans. Examples include rabies and plague. May be enzootic or epizootic.

Z SCORE Score expressed as a deviation from the mean value in standard deviation units; the term is used in analyzing continuous variables, such as heights and weights, of a sample, to express results of behavioral tests, etc. The use of Z scores has been criticized for reducing interpretability and comparability of results from different studies or populations.

Bibliography

This bibliography complements the references mentioned in the text, which can be found after this section (page 273).

Dictionaries, glossaries, general reference works

For many types of English and subject dictionaries: Oxford Reference Online: www.oxfordreference.com

Abercrombie N, Hill S, Turner BS, eds. *The Penguin Dictionary of Sociology*. 4th ed. London: Penguin, 2000.

Allaby M. *Dictionary of the Environment*. Southampton, England: London Press, 1975.

Armitage P, Colton T, eds. *Encyclopedia of Biostatistics*. 2nd ed. Chichester, New York, Weinheim: Wiley, 2005.

Bander EJ, Wallach JJ. *Medical Legal Dictionary*. Dobbs Ferry, NY: Oceana, 1970.

Bannock MRG, Baxter RE, Davis E. *The Penguin Dictionary of Economics*. 7th ed. London: Penguin, 2003.

Breslow L, ed. *Encyclopedia of Public Health*. New York: Macmillan, 2002.

Campbell RJ, ed. *Campbell's Psychiatric Dictionary*. 8th ed. New York: Oxford University Press, 2004.

Detels R, McEwen J, Beaglehole T, Tanaka H, eds. *Oxford Textbook of Public Health*. 4th ed. Oxford, UK: Oxford University Press, 2002.

Everitt BS. *The Cambridge Dictionary of Statistics*. 3rd ed. Cambridge, UK: Cambridge University Press, 2006.

Farmer R, Miller D, Lawrenson R. *Lecture Notes on Epidemiology and Public Health Medicine*. Oxford: Blackwell, 1996.

Florey C du V, editor. *EPILEX. A Multilingual Lexicon of Epidemiological Terms*. v. 3.0.1; 2006. http://www.personal.dundee.ac.uk/~cdvflore/Epilex06.htm

Forbis P, Bartolucci S. *Stedman's Medical Eponyms*. 2nd ed. Baltimore: Williams & Wilkins, 2004.

Froom J. An International Glossary for Primary Care. *J Fam Pract* 1981; 13:673–681.

Goldstein AS. *Dictionary of Health Care Administration*. Rockville, MD: Aspen, 1989.

Gunton T, ed. *The Penguin Dictionary of Information Technology*. London: Penguin Books, 1994.

International Programme on Chemical Safety (IPCS). *Glossary of Terms on Chemical Safety for Use in IPCS Publications*. Geneva: WHO, 1989.

Jammal A, Allard R, Loslier G, eds. *Dictionnaire d'Épidémiologie*. Ste-Hyacinthe, Maloine, Paris: Edisem, 1988.

King RC, Stansfield WD, Mulligan PK. *A Dictionary of Genetics*. 7th ed. New York: Oxford University Press, 2006.

Kohn GC, ed. *Encyclopedia of Plague and Pestilence*. New York: Facts on File, 2007.

Landau SI, ed. *International Dictionary of Medicine and Biology*. New York: Wiley, 1986.

Leclerk A, Papoz L, Bréart G, Lellouch J. *Dictionnaire d' épidémiologie*. Paris: Frison-Roche, 1990.

Lewalle P, ed. *Joint OECD/IPCS Project on the Harmonization of Hazard/Risk Assessment Terminology: Annotated List of Selected Key Terms Used in Risk Assessment*. Paris: OECD, 1998 (mimeographed).

Meadows AJ, Gordon M, Singleton A. *A Dictionary of New Information Technology*. London: Century, 1982.

Meinert CL. *Clinical Trials Dictionary*. Baltimore: Johns Hopkins Center for Clinical Trials, 1996.

Millar D, et al. *The Cambridge Dictionary of Scientists*. 2nd ed. Cambridge, UK: Cambridge University Press, 2002.

Morton LG, ed. *Garrison & Morton's Medical Bibliography*. 4th ed. London: Gower, 1983.

Oxford English Dictionary. 2nd ed. on CD-ROM. Oxford, New York, Melbourne: Oxford University Press, 2000.

Pressat R. *Dictionnaire de Démographie (The Dictionary of Demography)*. English translation edited by Christopher Wilson. Oxford, UK: Blackwell, 1985.

Segen JC, ed. *Dictionary of Modern Medicine*. Camforth, UK, and Park Ridge, NJ: Parthenon, 1992.

Seldon A, Pennance FG, eds. *Everyman's Dictionary of Economics*. London: Dent, 1973.

Simpson JA, Weiner ESC, eds. *The Compact Oxford English Dictionary* (OED). 2nd ed. Oxford and New York: Oxford University Press, 1991.

Skinner HA. *The Origin of Medical Terms.* 2nd ed. Baltimore, MD: Williams & Wilkins, 1961.

Sohm ED, ed. *Glossary of Evaluation Terms*. Geneva: United Nations, 1978.

Stedman's Medical Dictionary. 27th ed. Baltimore, MD: Lippincott Williams & Wilkins, 2000.

Thériault Y, Beauregard E, Charuest M. *Statistics and Surveys Vocabulary;* Terminology Bulletin No. 208. Ottawa: Secretary of State, 1992.

Toma B, Bénet JJ, Dufour B, Eloit M, et al. *Glossaire d'Épidémiologie Animale*. Maisons-Alfort, France: Editions du Point Vétérinaire, 1991.

US House of Representatives, 94th Congress. *A Discursive Dictionary of Health Care.* Washington, DC: USGPO, 1976.

Vogt WP. *Dictionary of Statistics and Methodology: A Nontechnical Guide for the Social Sciences*. 3rd ed. Newbury Park, London: Sage, 2005.

van de Walle E. *Multilingual Demographic Dictionary*. English section. 2nd ed. Liège, Belgium: Ordina, 1982.

Wolañski N. *Glossary of Terms for Human Ecology*. Warsaw: Commission for Human Ecology of the International Union of Anthropological and Ethnological Sciences, 1990.

Wolman BB, ed. *Dictionary of Behavioral Science*. New York: Van Nostrand, 1973.

World Bank. *A Glossary of Population Terminology*. Washington, DC: World Bank, 1985.

Epidemiology, biostatistics, public health, preventive medicine

Abramson JH. *Survey Methods in Community Medicine*. 4th ed. London: Churchill Livingstone, 1990.

Abramson JH, Abramson ZH. *Making Sense of Data. A Self-Instruction Manual of the Interpretation of Epidemiological Data*. 3rd ed. New York: Oxford University Press, 2001.

Adami HO, Hunter D, Trichopoulos D, eds. *Textbook of Cancer Epidemiology*. 2nd. ed. New York: Oxford University Press, 2008.

Armenian HK, Shapiro S. *Epidemiology and Health Services*. New York: Oxford University Press, 1997.

Armitage P, Berry G, Matthews JNS. *Statistical Methods in Medical Research*. 4th ed. Oxford: Blackwell, 2002.

Babbie E. *The Pactice of Social Research*. 10th ed. Belmont, CA: Thompson/Wadsworth, 2004.

Bailar III JC, Mosteller F. *Medical Uses of Statistics*. 2nd ed. Waltham, MA: New England Journal of Medicine Books, 1992.

Baker D, Nieuwenhuijsen M, eds. *Environmental Epidemiology: Study Methods and Applications*. Oxford, UK: Oxford University Press, 2008.

Barker DJP, Cooper C, Rose G. *Epidemiology in Medical Practice*. 5th ed. New York: Churchill Livingstone, 1998.

Bayer R, Gostin LO, Jennings B, Steinbock B. *Public Health Ethics. Theory, Policy, and Practice*. New York: Oxford University Press, 2006.

Beaglehole R. *Global Public Health. A New Era*. New York: Oxford University Press, 2003.

Beaglehole R, Bonita R. *Public Health at the Crossroads: Achievements and Prospects*. 2nd ed. Cambridge, UK: Cambridge University Press, 2004.

Berridge V. *Marketing Health*. New York: Oxford University Press, 2007.

Bland JM. *An Introduction to Medical Statistics*. 3rd ed. New York: Oxford University Press, 2000.

Bland JM, Peacock J. *Statistical Questions in Evidence-Based Medicine*. New York: Oxford University Press, 2000.

Breslow NE, Day NE. *Statistical Methods in Cancer Research*. Vol 1. *The Analysis of Case-Control Data*. Lyon: IARC, 1980. Vol. 2. *The Design and Analysis of Cohort Studies*. Lyon: IARC, 1987.

Browson RC, Baker EA, Lee TL, Gillespie KN. *Evidence-Based Public Health*. New York: Oxford University Press, 2002.

Coggon D, Rose G, Barker DJP. *Epidemiology for the Uninitiated*. 5th ed. London: British Medical Journal Publications, 2003.

Committee on Environmental Epidemiology, Commission on Life Sciences, National Research Council. *Environmental Epidemiology*. Washington, DC: National Academy Press, 1991 (Vol 1) and 1995 (Vol 2).

Coughlin SS, Beauchamp TL. *Ethics and Epidemiolgy*. New York: Oxford University Press, 1996.

Dawson-Saunders B, Trapp RG. *Basic and Clinical Biostatistics*. 2nd ed. Norwalk, CT: Appleton & Lange, 1994.

Elliott P, Cuzick J, English D, Stern R. *Geographical and Environmental Epidemiology: Methods for Small-Area Studies*. New York: Oxford University Press, 1996.

Elston RC, Olson JM, Palmer L, eds. *Biostatistical Genetics and Genetic Epidemiology*. New York: Wiley, 2002.

Elwood M. *Critical Appraisal of Epidemiological Studies and Clinical Trials*. 3rd ed. Oxford, New York, Melbourne: Oxford University Press, 2007.

Exworthy M, Stuart M, Blane D, Marmot M. *Tackling Health Inequalities Since the Acheson Inquiry*. Bristol, UK: The Joseph Rowntree Foundation & The Policy Press, 2003.

Fleiss JL. *Statistical Methods for Rates and Proportions*. 2nd ed. New York: Wiley, 1981.

Friedman GD. *Primer of Epidemiology*. 4th ed. New York: McGraw-Hill, 1994.

Friedman LM, Furberg CD, DeMets DL. *Fundamentals of Clinical Trials*. 3rd ed. New York: Springer-Verlag, 1998.

Goodman KW. *Ethics and Evidence-Based Medicine: Fallibility and Responsibility in Clinical Science*. Cambridge, UK: Cambridge University Press, 2002.

Gordis L. *Epidemiology*. 3rd ed. Amsterdam: Elsevier, 2004.

Gore SM, Altman DG. *Statistics in Practice*. London: British Medical Journal Publications, 1982.

Green A. *An Introduction to Health Planning for Developing Health Systems*. New York: Oxford University Press, 2007.

Greenberg RS, Daniels SR, Flanders WD, Eley JW, Boring JR. *Medical Epidemiology*. 3rd ed. New York: McGraw-Hill, 2001.

Haddix AC, Teutsch SM, Corso PS. *Prevention effectiveness. A Guide to Decision Analysis and Economic Evaluation*. 2nd ed. New York: Oxford University Press, 2002.

Hartzema AG, Porta M, Tilson HH, eds. *Pharmacoepidemiology: An Introduction*. 3rd ed. Cincinnati, OH: Harvey Whitney Books, 1998.

Hasselhorn HM, Toomingas A, Lagerström M, eds. *Occupational Health for Health Care Workers. A Practical Guide*. New York: Elsevier, 1999.

Hill A, Griffiths S. *Public Health and Primary care*. New York: Oxford University Press, 2007.

Holford TR. *Multivariate Methods in Epidemiology*. New York: Oxford University Press, 2002.

Hosmer DW, Lemeshow S. *Applied Logistic Regression*. 2nd ed. New York: Wiley, 2000.

Hudson TW, Reinhart MA, Rose SD, Stewart GK, eds. *Clinical Preventive Medicine: Health Promotion and Disease Prevention*. Boston: Little, Brown, 1988.

Hulka BS, Wilcosky TC, Griffith J, eds. *Biological Markers in Epidemiology*. New York: Oxford University Press, 1990.

Hulley SB, Cummings SR, Browner WS, Grady DG, Newman TB. *Designing Clinical Research*. 3rd ed. Philadelphia: Lippincott, Williams & Wilkins, 2006.

Jenicek M. *Epidemiology: The Logic of Modern Medicine*. Montreal: Epimed, 1995.

Kalbfleisch JD, Prentice RL. *The Statistical Analysis of Failure Time Data*. 2nd ed. New York: Wiley, 2002.

Kawachi I, Kennedy BP. *The Health of Nations. Why Inequality is Harmful to your Health*. New York: The New York Press, 2002.

Kawachi I, Wamala S. *Globalization and Health*. New York: Oxford University Press, 2006.

Kelsey JL, Thompson WD, Evans AS. *Methods in Observational Epidemiology*. 2nd ed. New York: Oxford University Press, 1996.

Kahn HA, Sempos CT. *Statistical Methods in Epidemiology*. New York: Oxford University Press, 1989.

Keating C. *Richard Doll. A Revolutionary Doctor*. New York: Oxford University Press, 2008.

Kerr C, Taylor R, Heard G, eds. *Handbook of Public Health Methods*. New York: McGraw Hill, 1998.

Kleinbaum DG, Klein M. *Logistic Regression. A Self-Learning Text*. 2nd ed. New York: Springer, 2002.

Kleinbaum DG, Kupper LL, Muller KE, Nizam A. *Applied Regression Analysis and Multivariable Methods*. 3rd ed. Pacific Grove, CA: Duxbury, 1998.

Kleinbaum DG, Sullivan KM, Barker ND. *ActivEpi Companion Textbook. ActivEpi CD-ROM*. New York: Springer, 2003.

Kleinbaum DG, Sullivan KM, Barker ND. *A Pocket Guide to Epidemiology*. New York: Springer, 2007.

Kogevinas M, Pearce N, Susser M, Boffetta P, eds. *Social Inequalities and Cancer*. IARC Scientific Publications no. 138. Lyon, France: International Agency for Research on Cancer, 1997.

Lairson DR, Aday LA, Balkrishnan R, Begley AC. *Evaluating the Healthcare System: Effectiveness, Efficiency and Equity*. 3rd ed Ann Arbor, MI: Health Administration Press, 2004.

Lang T, Barling D, Caraher M. *Food, Health and Policy*. New York: Oxford University Press, 2008.

Lasky T, ed. *Epidemiologic Principles and Food Safety*. New York: Oxford University Press, 2007.

Levy BS, Sidel VW. *Terrorism and Public Health*. New York: Oxford University Press, 2002.

Lilienfeld DE, Stolley PD. *Foundations of Epidemiology*. 3rd ed. New York: Oxford University Press, 1994.

Loue S. *Case Studies in Forensic Epidemiology*. Dordrecht: Kluwer, 2002.

MacMahon B, Trichopoulos D. *Epidemiology: Principles and Methods*. 2nd ed. Boston: Little, Brown, 1996.

Margetts B, Nelson M. *Design Concepts in Nutritional Epidemiology*. 2nd ed. New York: Oxford University Press, 1997.

Meinert CL. *Clinical Trials: Design, Conduct and Analysis*. New York: Oxford University Press, 1986.

McDowell I. *Measuring Health: A Guide to Rating Scales and Questionnaires*. 3rd ed. New York: Oxford University Press, 2006.

McMichael AJ. *Human Frontiers, Environments and Diseases. Past Patterns, Uncertain Futures*. Cambridge, UK: Cambridge University Press, 2001.

Murphy EA. *A Companion to Medical Statistics*. Baltimore, MD: Johns Hopkins Press, 1985.

Nelson KE, Williams CM, Graham NMH. *Infectious Diseases Epidemiology. Theory and Practice*. Gaithersburg, MD: Editorial Kathy Litzenberg, 2001.

Nieuwenhuijsen MJ. *Exposure Assessment in Occupational and Environmental Epidemiology*. Oxford, UK: Oxford University Press, 2003.

Norell S. *Workbook of Epidemiology*. New York: Oxford University Press, 1995.

Oleske DM, ed. *Epidemiology and the Delivery of Health Care Services*. Dordrecht: Kluwer, 2001.

Olsen J, Saracci R, Trichopoulos D. *Teaching Epidemiology. A Guide for Teachers in Epidemiology, Public Health and Clinical Medicine*. 2nd ed. New York: Oxford University Press, 2001.

Pencheon D, Guest C, Melzer D, Gray M, eds. *Oxford Handbook of Public Health Practice*. 2nd ed. Oxford, UK: Oxford University Press, 2006.

Pfeiffer DU, Robinson TP, Stevenson M, Stevens KB, Rogers DJ, Clements ACA, eds. *Spatial Analysis in Epidemiology*. New York: Oxford University Press, 2008.

Pickles A, Maughan B, Wadsworth M, eds. *Epidemiological Methods in Life Course Research*. New York: Oxford University Press, 2007.

Prince M, Stewart R, Ford T, Hotof M, eds. *Practical Psyquiatric Epidemiology*. New York: Oxford University Press, 2003.

Rhodes R, Battin MP, Silvers A, eds. *Medicine and Social Justice. Essays on the Distribution of Health Care*. New York: Oxford University Press, 2002.

Robertson L. *Injury Epidemiology. Research and Control Strategies*. 3rd ed. New York: Oxford University Press, 2007.

Robins J, Hernán M, eds. *Causal Inference*. New York: Chapman & Hall/CRC, 2009

Schlesselman JJ, Stolley PD. *Case-Control Studies. Design, Conduct, Analysis*. New York: Oxford University Press, 1982.

Schottenfeld D, Fraumeni JF, eds. *Cancer Epidemiology and Prevention*. 3rd ed. New York: Oxford University Press, 2006.

Siegrist J, Marmot M. *Social Inequalities in Health*. New York: Oxford University Press, 2006.

Spasoff RA. *Epidemiologic Methods for Health Policy*. New York: Oxford University Press, 1999.

Staquet MJ, Hays RD, Fayers PM, eds. *Quality of Life Assessment in Clinical Trials*. Oxford, New York, Melbourne: Oxford University Press, 1998.

Steenland K, ed. *Case Studies in Occupational Epidemiology*. New York: Oxford University Press, 1993.

Streiner DL, Norman GR. *Health Measurement Scales. A Practical Guide to their Development and Use*. 3rd ed. New York: Oxford University Press, 2003.

Susser MW. *Epidemiology, Health and Society: Selected Papers*. New York: Oxford University Press, 1987.

Susser MW, Watson W, Hopper K. *Sociology in Medicine*. 3rd ed. New York: Oxford University Press, 1985.

Teutsch SM, Churchill RE, eds. *Principles and Practice of Public Health Surveillance*. 2nd ed. New York: Oxford University Press, 2000.

Thomas DC. *Statistical Methods in Genetic Epidemiology*. New York: Oxford University Press, 2004.

Thomas JC, Weber DJ. *Epidemiologic Methods for the Study of Infectious Diseases*. New York: Oxford University Press, 2001.

Toniolo P, Boffetta P, Shuker DEG, et al., eds. *Application of Biomarkers in Cancer Epidemiology*. IARC Scientific Publications no. 142. Lyon, France: International Agency for Research on Cancer, 1999.

Valente TW. *Evaluating Helath Promotion Programs*. New York: Oxford University Press, 2002.

Walker AM. *Observation and Inference. An Introduction to the Methods of Epidemiology*. Baltimore: Williams & Wilkins, 1991.

Weiss NS. *Clinical Epidemiology: The Study of the Outcome of Illness*. 3rd ed. New York: Oxford University Press, 2006.

White E, Saracci R, Armstrong BK. *Principles of Exposure Measurement in Epidemiology*. 2nd ed. Oxford, UK: Oxford University Press, 2008.

Willett W. *Nutritional Epidemiology*. 2nd ed. New York: Oxford University Press, 1998.

World Health Organization. *The World Health Report 2000. Health Systems: Improving Performance*. Geneva: World Health Organization, 2000.

History of epidemiology, logic and philosophy of science, social studies of science

Ashton J, ed. *The Epidemiological Imagination*. Buckingham and Philadelphia: Open University Press, 1994.

Buck C, Llopis A, Nájera E, Terris M, eds. *The Challenge of Epidemiology: Issues and Selected Readings* [Spanish edition: *El desafío de la epidemiología. Problemas y lecturas seleccionadas*]. Washington, DC: Pan American Health Organization, 1988.

Bulger RE, Heitman E, Reiser SJ, eds. *The Ethical Dimensions of the Biological Sciences*. 2nd ed. Cambridge, UK: Cambridge University Press, 2002.

Daniels N, Kennedy B, Kawachi I. *Is inequality bad for our health?*. Boston: Beacon Press, 2000.

Evans AS. *Causation and Disease: A Chronological Journey*. New York: Plenum, 1993.

The James Lind Library. www.jameslindlibrary.org.

Jenicek M, Hitchcock DL. *Evidence-Based Practice. Logic and Critical Thinking in Medicine*. Chicago: American Medical Association (AMA Press), 2005.

Jenicek M. *A Physician's Self-Paced Guide to Critical Thinking*. Chicago: American Medical Association (AMA Press), 2006.

Knorr-Cetina K. *The Manufacture of Knowledge: An Essay on the Constructivist and Contextual Nature of Science*. Oxford, UK: Pergamon Press, 1981.

Knorr-Cetina K. *Epistemic Cultures: How the Sciences Make Knowledge*. Cambridge, MA: Harvard University Press, 1999.

Pickering A, ed. *Science as Practice and Culture*. Chicago: University of Chicago Press, 1992.

Silverman WA. *Human Experimentation: A Guided Step into the Unknown*. Oxford, New York, Tokyo: Oxford University Press, 1985.

White KL, Frenk J, Ordóñez C, et al., eds. *Health Services Research: An Anthology*. Washington, DC: Pan American Health Organization, 1992.

*This bibliography complements the references mentioned in the text, which can be found after this section.

References

1. Last JM. *A Dictionary of Public Health*. Oxford, UK: Oxford University Press, 2007.
2. Soanes C, Stevenson A. *The Oxford Dictionary of English*. 2nd ed rev. Oxford, UK: Oxford University Press, 2005.
3. Lock S, Last JM, Dunea G. *The Oxford Companion to Medicine*. Oxford, UK: Oxford University Press, 2001.
4. Amsterdamska O. Demarcating epidemiology. *Sci Technol Human Values* 2005; 30:17–51.
5. Miettinen OS. *Theoretical Epidemiology. Principles of Occurrence Research in Medicine*. New York: Wiley, 1985.
6. Greenland S, ed. *Evolution of Epidemiologic Ideas. Annotated Readings on Concepts and Methods*. Chestnut Hill, MA: Epidemiology Resources, 1987.
7. Susser M. Epidemiology in the United States after World War II. The evolution of technique. *Epidemiol Rev* 1985; 7:147–177.
8. Almeida-Filho N. *La ciencia tímida. Ensayos de deconstrucción de la epidemiología*. Buenos Aires: Lugar, 2000.
9. Bhopal R. *Concepts of Epidemiology. An Integrated Introduction to the Ideas, Theories, Principles and Methods of Epidemiology*. Oxford, UK: Oxford University Press, 2002.
10. Morabia A. *A History of Epidemiologic Methods and Concepts*. Basel: Birkhäuser/Springer, 2004. http://www.epidemiology.ch/history
11. Holland WW, Olsen J, du V Florey C. *The Development of Modern Epidemiology. Personal Reports from Those Who Were There*. New York: Oxford University Press, 2007.
12. Rothman KJ, Greenland S, Lash TL, eds. *Modern Epidemiology*. 3rd ed. Philadelphia: Lippincott-Raven, 2008.
13. UNICEF. www.unicef.org/sowc96/define.htm
14. Haynes RB, Sackett DL, Guyatt GH, Tugwell P. *Clinical Epidemiology. How to Do Clinical Practice Research*. 3rd. ed. Philadelphia: Lippincott, Williams & Wilkins, 2006.
15. Barratt A, Wyer PC, Hatala R, et al. Tips for learners of evidence-based medicine: 1. Relative risk reduction, absolute risk reduction and number needed to treat. *Can Med Assoc J* 2004; 171:353–358.
16. Kuh D, Ben-Shlomo Y, Lynch J, Hallqvist J, Power C. Life course epidemiology. *J Epidemiol Community Health* 2003; 57:778–783.
17. Katz S, Ford AB, Moskowitz RW, et al. Studies of illness in the aged: The index of ADL, a standardized measure of biological function. *JAMA* 1963; 185:914–919.
18. McLaren L, Hawe P. Ecological perspectives in health research. *J Epidemiol Community Health* 2005; 59:6–14.

19. Marinker M, ed. *From Compliance to Concordance: Toward Shared Goals in Medicine Taking*. London: The Royal Pharmaceutical Society of Great Britain, 1997.
20. Greenland S. Modeling and variable selection in epidemiologic analysis. *Am J Public Health* 1989; 79:340–349.
21. UNICEF. http://www.unicef.org/sowc96/define.htm
22. Susser MW. *Causal Thinking in the Health Sciences*. New York: Oxford University Press; 1973.
23. Calafell F, Malats N. Glossary. Basic molecular genetics for epidemiologists. *J Epidemiol Community Health* 2003; 57:398–400. Malats N, Calafell F. Basic glossary on genetic epidemiology. *J Epidemiol Community Health* 2003; 57:480–482. Malats N, Calafell F. Advanced glossary on genetic epidemiology. *J Epidemiol Community Health* 2003; 57:562–564.
24. Van der Weele TJ, Robins JM. Four types of effect modification. A classification based on directed acyclic graphs. *Epidemiology* 2007; 18:561–568.
25. Palese P, Young JF. Variation of influenza A, B, and C viruses. *Science* 1982; 215: 1468–1473.
26. Hargrove J, Nguyen HB. Bench-to-bedside review: Outcome predictions for critically ill patients in the emergency department. *Crit Care* 2005; 9:376–383.
27. Brownson RC, Petitti DB, eds. *Applied Epidemiology. Theory to Practice*. 2nd ed. New York: Oxford University Press, 2006.
28. Armitage P, Doll R. The age distribution of cancer and a multi-stage theory of carcinogenesis. *Br J Cancer* 1954; 8:1–12 (Reprinted: *Int J Epidemiol* 2004; 33:1174–1179).
29. Greenland S, Robins JM. Conceptual problems in the definition and interpretation of attributable fractions. *Am J Epidemiol* 1988; 128:1185–1197.
30. Steenland K, Armstrong B. An overview of methods for calculating the burden of disease due to specific risk factors. *Epidemiology* 2006; 17:512–519. *Erratum in: Epidemiology* 2007; 18:184.
31. Szklo M, Nieto FJ. *Epidemiology: Beyond the Basics*. 2nd. ed. Boston: Jones and Bartlett, 2007.
32. Jüni P, Egger M. Empirical evidence of attrition bias in clinical trials. *Int J Epidemiol* 2005; 34:87–88.
33. Robinson KA, Dennison CR, Wayman DM, et al. Systematic review identifies number of strategies important for retaining study participants. *J Clin Epidemiol* 2007; 60: 757–765.
34. Kaptchuk TJ. Effect of interpretive bias on research evidence. *BMJ* 2003; 326:1453–1455
35. Etzioni RD, Kadane JB. Bayesian statistical methods in public health and medicine. *Annu Rev Public Health* 1995; 16:23–41.
36. Weed DL, McKeown RE. Ethics in epidemiology and public health. I. Technical terms. *J Epidemiol Community Health* 2001; 55:855–857.
37. McKeown RE, Weed DL. Ethics in epidemiology and public health II. Applied terms. *J Epidemiol Community Health* 2002; 56:739–741.
38. Berkson J. Limitations of the application of fourfold table analysis to hospital data. *Biometrics Bull* 1946; 2:47–53.
39. *History and Development of the ICD*. ICD-10. Vol. 2. Geneva: WHO, 1993.
40. Garfield E. Citation indexes for science. A new dimension in documentation through association of ideas. *Science* 1955;122:108–11. Reprinted in: *Int J Epidemiol* 2006; 35:1123–1127. See also www.garfield.library.upenn.edu.

41. Porta M, Fernandez E, Bolúmar F. The "bibliographic impact factor" and the still uncharted sociology of epidemiology. *Int J Epidemiol* 2006; 35:1130–1135.
42. Pike MC, Krailo MD, Henderson BE, et al. "Hormonal" risk factors, "breast tissue age" and the age-incidence of breast cancer. *Nature* 1983; 303:767–770.
43. Khoury MJ, Little J, Gwinn M, Ioannidis JP. On the synthesis and interpretation of consistent but weak gene-disease associations in the era of genome-wide association studies. *Int J Epidemiol* 2007; 36:439–445.
44. Tukey J. *Exploratory Data Analysis*. Reading, MA: Addison-Wesley, 1977.
45. Barker DJP. Developmental origins of adult health and disease. *J Epidemiol Community Health* 2004; 58:114–115.
46. Burden of Disease Unit, Harvard School of Public Health. www.hsph.harvard.edu/organizations/bdu.
47. World Health Organization. Burden of Disease Project. www.who.int/healthinfo/bodproject/en.
48. World Health Organization. Environmental Burden of Disease Series. www.who.int/quantifying_ehimpacts/national/en/index.html.
49. Soskolne CL, Andruchow JE, Racioppi F. *Developing, Conducting and Disseminating Epidemiological Research: From Theory to Practice*. (In English, Russian and Azeri). United Nations Development Programme (Azerbaijan), World Health Organization (European Centre for Environment and Health (Rome, Italy), and the University of Alberta (Edmonton, Canada), 2007.
50. Wittes JT, Colton T, Sidel VW. Capture-recapture methods for assessing the completeness of ascertainment when using multiple information sources. *J Chronic Dis* 1974; 27:25–36.
51. Hook EB, Regal RR. Capture-recapture methods in epidemiology. Methods and limitations. *Epidemiol Rev* 1998; 17:243–264.
52. Chin J, ed. *Control of Communicable Disease Manual*. 17th ed. Washington, DC: American Public Health Association, 2000.
53. Kupper LL, McMichael AJ, Spirtas R. A hybrid epidemiologic study design useful in estimating relative risk. *J Am Stat Assoc* 1975; 70:524–528.
54. Rosenbaum PR. The case-only odds ratio as a causal parameter. *Biometrics* 2004; 60: 233–240.
55. Gillespie IA, O'Brien SJ, Frost JA, et. al. A Case-case comparison of campylobacter coli and campylobacter jejuni infection: A toll for generating hypotheses. *Emerg Infect Dis* 2002; 8:937–942.
56. McCarthy N, Giesecke J. Case-case comparison to study causation of common infectious diseases. *Int J Epidemiol* 1999; 28:764–768.
57. Giesecke J. *Modern Infectious Disease Epidemiology*. New York: Arnold, 2002.
58. Maclure M, Mittleman MA. Should we use a case-crossover design? *Annu Rev Public Health* 2000; 21:193–221.
59. Hyams KC. Developing case definitions for symptom-based conditions; the problem of specificity. *Epidemiol Rev* 1998; 20:148–156.
60. Khoury MJ, Flanders WD. Nontraditional epidemiologic approaches in the analysis of gene-environment interactions: case-control studies with no controls! *Am J Epidemiol* 1996; 144:207–213.
61. Vandenbroucke JP. Clinical investigation. In: Lock S, Last JM, Dunea G. *The Oxford Companion to Medicine*. Oxford, UK: Oxford University Press, 2001.

62. Fletcher RH, Fletcher SW. *Clinical Epidemiology—The Essentials*. 4th. ed. Philadelphia: Lippincott Williams & Wilkins, 2005.
63. Sackett DL, Haynes RB, Guyatt GH, Tugwell P. *Clinical Epidemiology: A Basic Science for Clinical Medicine*. 2nd ed. Boston: Little, Brown, 1991.
64. Zaffanella LE, Savitz DA, Greenland S, et al. The residential case-specular method to study wire codes, magnetic fields and disease. *Epidemiology* 1998; 9:16–20.
65. Suissa S. The case-time-control design. *Epidemiology* 1995; 6:248–253.
66. Rothman KJ, ed. *Causal Inference*. Chestnut Hill, MA: Epidemiology Resources, 1988.
67. Susser MW. What is a cause and how do we know one? *Am J Epidemiol* 1991; 133: 635–648.
68. Greenland S, Pearl J, Robins JM. Causal diagrams for epidemiologic research. *Epidemiology* 1999; 10:37–48.
69. Hernández-Díaz S, Schisterman EF, Hernán MA. The birth weight "paradox" uncovered? *Am J Epidemiol* 2006; 164:1115–1120.
70. Joffe M, Mindell J. Complex causal process diagrams for analyzing the health impacts of policy interventions. *Am J Public Health* 2006; 96:473–479.
71. Susser MW. Glossary: causality in public health science. *J Epidemiol Community Health* 2001; 55:376–378.
72. Rose GA. *The Strategy of Preventive Medicine*. Oxford, UK: Oxford University Press, 1992. (Annotated version edited by Khaw KT, Marmot M. Oxford, UK: Oxford University Press, 2007).
73. Kuller I. Circular epidemiology. *Am J Epidemiol* 1999; 150:897–903.
74. Walton D. *The Oxford Companion to Philosophy*. Oxford, UK: Oxford University Press, 2005.
75. Feinstein AR. *Clinimetrics*. New Haven, CT: Yale University Press, 1987.
76. McKean E, ed. *The New Oxford American Dictionary*. 2nd ed. Oxford, UK: Oxford University Press, 2005.
77. Blackburn S. *The Oxford Dictionary of Philosophy*. 2nd ed. Oxford, UK: Oxford University Press, 2005.
78. Scott J, Marshall G. *A Dictionary of Sociology*. Oxford, UK: Oxford University Press, 2005.
79. Sackett DL. Bias in analytic research. *J Chronic Dis* 1979; 32:51–63.
80. Porta M. Epidemiologic plausibility. *Am J Epidemiol* 1999; 150:217–218.
81. Samet JM, Muñoz A. Evolution of the cohort study. *Epidemiol Rev* 1998; 20:1–14.
82. Greenland S. Quantifying biases in causal models: classical confounding vs. collider-stratification bias. *Epidemiology* 2003; 14:300–306.
83. Bjornsson HT, Fallin MD, Feinberg AP. An integrated epigenetic and genetic approach to common human disease. *Trends Genet* 2004; 20:350–358.
84. London: HMSO, 1915; 1946, etc.
85. Anand S, Peter F, Sen A. *Public Health, Ethics, and Equity*. Oxford, UK: Oxford University Press, 2005.
86. Sen A. *Development as Freedom*. New York: Random House, 1999.
87. Morris JN. The uses of epidemiology. *Br Med J* 1955; 2:395–401.
88. Hoffmann K, Heidemann C, Weikert C, Schulze MB, Boeing H. Estimating the proportion of disease due to classes of sufficient causes. *Am J Epidemiol* 2006; 163:76–83.
89. Diez Roux AV. A glossary for multilevel analysis. *J Epidemiol Community Health* 2002; 56:588–594.
90. Colman AM. *A Dictionary of Psychology*. Oxford, UK: Oxford University Press, 2006.

91. Rubin DB. Causal inference using potential outcomes: design, modeling, decisions. *J Am Stat Assoc* 2005; 100:322–331.
92. Porta M. In: Hartzema AG, Porta M, Tilson HH, eds. *Pharmacoepidemiology: An Introduction.* 3rd ed. Cincinatti, OH: Harvey Whitney Books, 1998. pp. 1–28.
93. Hernán MA, Hernández-Díaz S, Werler MM, Mitchell AA. Causal knowledge as a prerequisite for confounding evaluation: an application to birth defects epidemiology. *Am J Epidemiol* 2002; 155:176–184.
94. Kane RL, Wang J, Garrard J. Reporting in randomized clinical trials improved after adoption of the CONSORT statement. *J Clin Epidemiol* 2007; 60:241–249.
95. Sanderson S, Tatt ID, Higgins JPT. Tools for assessing quality and susceptibility to bias in observational studies in epidemiology: a systematic review and annotated bibliography. *Int J Epidemiol* 2007; 36:666–676.
96. Pan American Health Organization. OSP, CE7, W-15. Washington, DC: PAHO, 1949.
97. Kleinbaum DG, Kupper LL, Morgenstern H. *Epidemiologic Research. Principles and Quantitative Methods.* Belmont, CA: Lifetime Learning Publications, 1982.
98. Kendall MG, Buckland WR. *A Dictionary of Statistical Terms.* 4th ed. London: Longman, 1982.
99. Dobson A. *The Oxford Dictionary of Statistical Terms.* Oxford, UK: Oxford University Press, 2003.
100. Jefferson TO, deMicheli V, Mugford M. *Elementary Economic Evaluation in Health Care.* London: BMJ Books, 1996.
101. Van der Weele TJ, Hernán MA. From counterfactuals to sufficient component causes and vice versa. *Eur J Epidemiol* 2006, 21:855–858.
102. Pearl J. *Causality.* New York: Cambridge University Press, 2000.
103. Clayton D, Hill M. *Statistical Models in Epidemiology.* Oxford, UK: Oxford University Press, 1993.
104. Marinker M, ed. *Constructive Conversations about Health. Policy and Values.* Oxford, UK, & Seattle, WA: Radcliffe Publishing, 2006.
105. Anonymous. Cross design synthesis: a new strategy for studying medical outcomes? [editorial]. *Lancet* 1992; 340:944–946.
106. Greenland S. Quantitative methods in the review of epidemiologic literature. *Epidemiol Rev* 1987; 9:1–30.
107. Greenland S, Robins J. Ecologic studies–Biases, misconceptions and counter-examples. *Am J Epidemiol* 1994; 139:747–771.
108. Janes CR, Stall R, Gifford SM, eds. *Anthropology and Epidemiology. Interdisciplinary Approaches to the Study of Health and Disease.* Dordrecht: Reidel, 1986.
109. Alderson M: *An Introduction to Epidemiology.* 2nd ed. London: Macmillan, 1983.
110. Li G, Baker S, Langlois J, et al. Are female drivers safer? An application of the decomposition method. *Epidemiology* 1998; 9:379–384.
111. McMichael AJ. Prisoners of the proximate: Loosening the constraints on epidemiology in an age of change. *Am J Epidemiol* 1999; 149:887–897.
112. Kuh D, Ben-Shlomo Y, eds. *A Life Course Approach to Chronic Disease Epidemiology.* 2nd ed. Oxford, UK: Oxford University Press, 2004.
113. De Stavola BL, Nitsch D, Silva ID, et al. Statistical issues in life course epidemiology. *Am J Epidemiol* 2006; 163:84–96.
114. Barker DJP. *Fetal and Infant Origins of Adult Disease.* London: British Medical Journal Publications, 1992.

115. Barker DJP. *Fetal Origins of Cardiovascular and Lung Disease*. New York: Marcel Dekker, 2001.
116. Feinberg AP. Phenotypic plasticity and the epigenetics of human disease. *Nature* 2007, 447:433–440.
117. Ozanne SE, Constancia M. Mechanisms of disease: the developmental origins of disease and the role of the epigenotype. *Nat Clin Pract Endocrinol Metab* 2007; 3:539–546.
118. Dolinoy DC, Huang D, Jirtle RL. Maternal nutrient supplementation counteracts bisphenol A–induced DNA hypomethylation in early development. *Proc Natl Acad Sci USA* 2007; 104:13056–13061.
119. Curtis VA. Dirt, disgust and disease: a natural history of hygiene. *J Epidemiol Community Health* 2007; 61:660–664.
120. Blalock HM. *Causal Inference in Non-experimental Research*. Chapel Hill, NC: University of North Carolina Press, 1964. Blalock HM Jr, ed. *Causal Models in the Social Sciences*. 2nd. ed. New York: Aldine, 1985. Blalock HM Jr, ed. *Causal Models in Experimental Designs*. Piscataway, NJ: Aldine Transaction, 2007.
121. Kramer MS, Boivin JF. Towards an "unconfounded" classification of epidemiologic research design. *J Chronic Dis* 1987; 40:683–688.
122. Arnesen T, Nord E. The value of DALY life: problems with ethics and validity of disability adjusted life years. *BMJ* 1999; 319:1423–1425.
123. Mathers CD, Robine JM, Wilkins R. Health expectancy indicators. Recommendations for terminology. In: Mathers CD, Robine JM, McCallum J, eds. *Proceedings of Seventh Meeting of the International Network on Health Expectancy (REVES)*. Canberra: Australian Institute of Health and Welfare, 1994.
124. Twaddle AC. Sickness and sickness career: Some implications. In: Eisenberg L, Kleinman A, eds. *The Relevance of Social Science for Medicine*. Dordrecht: Reidel, 1981. pp. 111–133.
125. Kleinman A. *The Illness Narratives. Suffering, Healing, and the Human Condition*. New York: Basic Books, 1988.
126. Coe RM. *Sociology of Medicine*. New York: McGraw-Hill, 1970. pp. 89–115.
127. Eisenberg L. The subjective in medicine. *Perspect Biol Med* 1983; 1:40–48.
128. Kleinman A, Eisenberg L, Good B. Culture, illness and care. Clinical lessons from anthropologic and cross-cultural research. *Ann Intern Med* 1978; 88:251–258..
129. Gunning-Schepers L. The health benefits of prevention: a simulation approach. *Health Policy* 1989; 12:1–255.
130. Aldrich T, Griffith J. *Environmental Epidemiology and Risk Assessment*. New York: Van Nostrand Reinhold, 1993.
131. United States National Center for Infectious Diseases, Division of Parasitic Diseases, 2004. www.cdc.gov/malaria/glossary.htm
132. American Lung Association (www.lungusa.org).
133. Raviglione MC, Smith IM. XDR tuberculosis–implications for global public health. *N Engl J Med* 2007; 356:656–659.
134. Khoury MJ, Burke W, Thomson EJ. *Genetics and Public Health in the 21st Century. Using Genetic Information to Improve Health and Prevent Disease*. New York: Oxford University Press, 2000.
135. Eimerl TS. Organized curiosity. *J Coll Gen Pract* 1960; 3:246–252.
136. Susser MW. Does risk factor epidemiology put epidemiology at risk? Peering into the future. *J Epidemiol Community Health* 1998; 52:608–611.

137. Krieger N. A glossary for social epidemiology. *J Epidemiol Community Health* 2001; 55:693–700.
138. Martens P, McMichael AJ, eds. Environmental change, climate and health. Cambridge, UK: Cambridge University Press, 2003.
139. Bosch X, ed. *Archie Cochrane: Back to the Front*. Barcelona: Institut Català d'Oncologia, 2004.
140. Cochrane AL. *Effectiveness and Efficiency; Random Reflections on Health Services*. London: Nuffield Provincial Hospitals Trust, 1972.
141. Palmer S, Torgerson DJ. Economic notes: definitions of efficiency. *BMJ* 1999; 318:1136.
142. Krieger N. Embodiment: a conceptual glossary for epidemiology. *J Epidemiol Community Health* 2005; 59:350–355.
143. Everett M. The social life of genes: privacy, property and the new genetics. *Soc Sci Med* 2003; 56:53–65.
144. Hall E. Spaces and networks of genetic knowledge making: the "geneticisation" of heart disease. *Health Place* 2004; 10:311–318.
145. Banta JE. Treating the traveler. A brief guide to emporiatrics. *Postgrad Med* 1973; 53:53–58.
146. Everitt BS. *Statistics in the Medical Sciences*. Cambridge, UK: Cambridge University Press, 1995.
147. Cohen JE. *How Many People Can the Earth Support?* New York: Norton, 1995. p. 13.
148. Herbst AL, Ulfelder H, Poskanzer DC. Adenocarcinoma of the vagina: Association of maternal stilbestrol therapy with tumor appearance in young women. *N Engl J Med* 1971; 284:878–881.
149. Centers for Disease Control: *Pneumocystis* pneumonia–Los Angeles. *MMWR* 1981; 30:250–252.
150. European Centre for Disease Prevention and Control (ECDC). Epidemic intelligence. www.ecdc.eu.int/Activities/Epidemic_Intelligence.html
151. World Health Organization. Epidemic and Pandemic Alert and Response (EPR). www.who.int/csr/alertresponse/epidemicintelligence/en/index.html
152. Stolley PD, Lasky T. *Investigating Disease Patterns. The Science of Epidemiology*. New York: Scientific American Library, 1995.
153. Hecker JFK. *Der Grossen Volkskrankheiten des Mittelalters (Epidemics of the Middle Ages)*. Berlin: Enslin, 1865 (English translation published by the Sydenham Society, London, 1883).
154. Creighton C. *A History of Epidemics in Britain*. Cambridge, UK: Cambridge University Press, 1891–1994 (2 Vols).
155. McNeill W. *Plagues and Peoples*. New York: Doubleday, 1976.
156. McKeown T. *The Origins of Human Disease*. Oxford: Blackwell, 1988.
157. Pusey WA. *The History and Epidemiology of Syphilis*. Springfield, IL: Thomas, 1933.
158. Dubos R, Dubos J. *The White Plague; Tuberculosis, Man and Society*. Boston: Little, Brown, 1952.
159. Paul JR. *A History of Poliomyelitis*. New Haven, CT: Yale University Press, 1971.
160. Zinsser H. *Rats, Lice and History*. Boston: Little, Brown, 1935.
161. Grmek MD. *Les Maladies à L'Aube de la Civilisation Occidentale*. Paris: Payot, 1983.
162. Omran AR. The epidemiologic transition; a theory of the epidemiology of population change. *Milbank Mem Fund Q* 1971; 49:509–538. Reprinted: *Bull WHO* 2001; 79:161–170.

163. Mackenbach JP. The epidemiologic transition theory. *J Epidemiol Community Health* 1994; 48:329–332.
164. Trichopoulos D. Accomplishments and prospects of epidemiology. *Prev Med* 1996; 25:4–6.
165. MacMahon B. Strengths and limitations of epidemiology. In: *The National Research Council in 1979.* Washington, DC: National Academy of Sciences, 1979.
166. Shy CM. The failure of academic epidemiology: witness for the prosecution. *Am J Epidemiol* 1997; 145:479–484.
167. Wing S. Limits of epidemiology. *Med Global Surv* 1994; 1:74–86.
168. Samet JM. Epidemiology and policy: The pump handle meets the new millennium. *Epidemiol Rev* 2000; 22:145–154.
169. Krieger N. Epidemiology and the web of causation: Has anyone seen the spider? *Soc Sci Med* 1994; 39:887–903.
170. Vandenbroucke JP. Is "The causes of cancer" a miasma theory for the end of the twentieth century? *Int J Epidemiol* 1988; 17:708–709.
171. Jablonka E. Epigenetic epidemiology. *Int J Epidemiol* 2004; 33:929–935.
172. Feinberg AP, Tycko B. The history of cancer epigenetics. *Nat Rev Cancer* 2004; 4:143–153.
173. Jaenisch R, Bird A. Epigenetic regulation of gene expression: how the genome integrates intrinsic and environmental signals. *Nat Genet* 2003; 33(Suppl):245–254.
174. Vercelli D. Genetics, epigenetics, and the environment: switching, buffering, releasing. *J Allergy Clin Immunol* 2004; 113:381–386.
175. Herman JG, Baylin SB. Gene silencing in cancer in association with promoter hypermethylation. *N Engl J Med* 2003; 349:2042–2054.
176. Jirtle RL, Skinner MK. Environmental epigenomics and disease susceptibility. *Nat Rev Genet* 2007; 8:253–262.
177. Ting AH, McGarvey KM, Baylin SB. The cancer epigenome–components and functional correlates. *Genes Dev* 2006; 20:3215–3231.
178. Knorr-Cetina K. Epistemic cultures. In: Restivo S, ed. *Science, Technology, and Society. An Encyclopedia.* Oxford, UK: Oxford University Press, 2005.
179. Carpiano RM, Daley DM. A guide and glossary on postpositivist theory building for population health. *J Epidemiol Community Health* 2006; 60:564–570.
180. Buck C. Popper's philosophy for epidemiologists. *Int J Epidemiol* 1975; 4:159–168.
181. Miettinen OS. Epidemiology: quo vadis? *Eur J Epidemiol* 2004; 19:713–718.
182. Bolúmar F, Porta M. Epidemiologic methods: beyond clinical medicine, beyond epidemiology. *Eur J Epidemiol* 2004; 19:733–735
183. Schwartz S, Carpenter KM. The right answer to the wrong question: consequences of type III error for public health research. *Am J Public Health* 1999; 89:1175–1180.
184. Bankowski Z, Bryant JH, Last JM, eds. *Ethics and Epidemiology: International Guidelines*. Geneva: CIOMS/WHO, 1991.
185. Fayerweather WE, Higginson J, Beauchamp TL, eds. *Ethics in Epidemiology*. New York: Pergamon Press, 1991.
186. International Epidemiological Association. Good Epidemiological Practice (GEP). Proper conduct in epidemiologic research. www.dundee.ac.uk/iea/GEP07.htm.
187. American College of Epidemiology. Ethics guidelines. *Ann Epidemiol* 2000; 10(Suppl 1): S1–S103.
188. Bhopal R. Glossary of terms relating to ethnicity and race: for reflection and debate. J Epidemiol Community Health 2004; 58:441–445.

189. Tajima K, Sonoda S. Ethnoepidemiology, a new paradigm for studying cancer risk factors and prevention strategy. In: Tajima K, Sonoda S, eds. *Ethnoepidemiology of Cancer*. Tokyo: Japan Scientific Societies Press, 1996.
190. Evans AS. Causation and disease: The Henle-Koch postulates revisited. *Yale J Biol Med* 1976; 49:175–195.
191. Straus S, Richardson WS, Glasziou P, Haynes RB. *Evidenced Based Medicine: How to Practice and Teach EBM.* 3rd ed. London: Churchill-Livingstone, 2005.
192. Ransohoff DF. Rules of evidence for cancer molecular-marker discovery and validation. *Nat Rev Cancer* 2004; 4:309–314.
193. Ransohoff DF. How to improve reliability and efficiency of research about molecular markers: roles of phases, guidelines, and study design. *J Clin Epidemiol* 2007; 60: 1205–1219.
194. Brownson RC, Gurney JG, Land G. Evidence-based decision making in public health. *J Public Health Manage Pract* 1999; 5:86–97.
195. Rychetnik L, Frommer M, Hawe P, Shiell A. Criteria for evaluating evidence on public health interventions. *J Epidemiol Community Health* 2002; 56:119–127.
196. Rychetnik L, Hawe P, Waters E, et al. A glossary for evidence based public health. *J Epidemiol Community Health* 2004; 58:538–545.
197. Rodríguez-Artalejo F. La salud pública basada en la evidencia. *Gac Sanit* 1997; 11: 201–203.
198. Kramer JM. The rising pandemic of mental disorders and associated chronic diseases and disabilities. *Acta Psychiatr Scand* 1980; 62 (Suppl 285):382–397.
199. Murray CJL Quantifying the burden of disease: the technical basis of quality-adjusted life years. *Bull WHO* 1994, 72:429–445.
200. Duffus JH, ed, for the International Union of Pure and Applied Chemistry. Glossary for chemists of terms used in toxicology (IUPAC recommendations, 1993). *Pure Appl Chem* 1993; 65:2003–2122.
201. Kazandjian VA. The extremal quotient in small area variation analysis. *Health Serv Res* 1989; 24:665–684.
202. ICD-10. Vol 1: *Report of the International Conference for the Tenth Revision of the International Classification of Diseases*. Geneva: WHO, 1993. pp. 9–28.
203. Farr W. *Vital Statistics. A Memorial Volume of Selections from the Reports and Writings of William Farr*. Edited by Noel Humphries. London: Stanford, 1985.
204. Gregg MB, ed. *Field Epidemiology*. 2nd ed. New York: Oxford University Press, 2002.
205. Goodman RA, Munson JW, Dammers K, et al. Forensic epidemiology: Law at the intersection of public health and criminal investigations. *J Law Med Ethics* 2003; 31:684–700. www.publichealthlaw.info.
206. Egger M, Smith GD, Schneider M, Minder C. Bias in meta-analysis detected by a simple, graphical test. *BMJ* 1997; 315:629–634.
207. Morange M. *The Misunderstood Gene*. Cambridge, MA: Harvard University Press, 2001.
208. Coping with complexity [editorial]. *Nature* 2006; 441:383–384.
209. ENCODE Project Consortium. Identification and analysis of functional elements in 1% of the human genome by the ENCODE pilot project. *Nature* 2007; 447:799–816.
210. Khoury MJ, Beaty TH, Cohen BH. *Fundamentals of Genetic Epidemiology*. New York: Oxford University Press, 1993.
211. Adelman DE. The false promise of the genomics revolution for environmental law. *Harvard Environ Law Rev* 2005; 29:117–177.

212. Davey Smith G, Ebrahim S, Lewis S, et al. Genetic epidemiology and public health: hope, hype, and future prospects. *Lancet* 2005; 366:1484–1498.
213. Vineis P, Schulte P, McMichael AJ. Misconceptions about the use of genetic tests in populations. *Lancet* 2001; 357:709–712.
214. Vainio H. Genetic biomarkers and occupational epidemiology—recollections, reflections and reconsiderations. *Scand J Work Environ Health* 2004; 30:1–3.
215. Caporaso NE. Why have we failed to find the low penetrance genetic constituents of common cancers? *Cancer Epidemiol Biomarkers Prev* 2002; 11:1544–1549.
216. Shostak S. Locating gene-environment interaction: at the intersections of genetics and public health. *Soc Sci Med* 2003; 56:2327–2342.
217. Porta M. The genome sequence is a jazz score. *Int J Epidemiol* 2003; 32:29–31.
218. Poirier MC. Chemical-induced DNA damage and human cancer risk. *Nat Rev Cancer* 2004; 4:630–637.
219. Luch A. Nature and nurture–lessons from chemical carcinogenesis. *Nat Rev Cancer* 2005; 5:113–125.
220. www.gis.com.
221. De Maio FG. Income inequality measures. *J Epidemiol Community Health* 2007; 61:849–852.
222. McDonald CJ, Overhage JM. Guidelines you can follow and can trust: an ideal and an example. *JAMA* 1994; 271:872–873.
223. A framework for health promotion policy: a discussion document. *Health Promotion* 1986; 1:335–340.
224. Stokes J III, Noren JJ, Shindell S. Definition of terms and concepts applicable to clinical preventive medicine. *J Community Health* 1982; 8:33–41.
225. Last JM. *Public Health and Human Ecology*. 2nd ed. Stamford, CT: Appleton & Lange, 1997.
226. Becker MH, ed. *The Health Belief Model and Personal Health Behavior*. Thorofare, NJ: Slack, 1974.
227. Robine JM, Mathers CD, Bucquet D. Distinguishing health expectancies and health-adjusted life expectancies. *Am J Public Health* 1993; 83:797–798.
228. World Health Organization. *Ottawa Charter for Health Promotion*. Geneva: WHO, 1986.
229. Milio N. *Public Health in the Market: Facing Managed Care, Lean Government, and Health Disparities*. Ann Arbor, MI: The University of Michigan Press, 2000.
230. McMichael AJ, Spirtas R, Kupper LL. An epidemiologic study of mortality within a cohort of rubber workers, 1964–72. *J Occup Med* 1974; 16:458–464.
231. Mehrez A, Gafni A. Quality adjusted life years, utility theory and healthy years equivalents *Med Decis Making* 1989; 9:142–149.
232. Hyder AA, Rotllant G, Morrow RH. Measuring the burden of disease. Healthy life years. *Am J Pub Health* 1998; 88:196–202.
233. Fine PEM. Herd immunity: History, theory, practice. *Epidemiol Rev* 1993; 15:265–302.
234. Müller-Wille S, Rheinberger HJ, eds. *Heredity Produced: At the Crossroads of Biology, Politics, and Culture, 1500–1870*. Cambridge, MA: The MIT Press, 2007.
235. Cobb M. Heredity before genetics: a history. *Nat Rev Genet* 2006; 7:953–958.
236. Canadian Task Force on the Periodic Health Examination. *The Canadian Guide to Clinical Preventive Health Care*. Ottawa: Canada Communication Group,1994.
237. U.S. Preventive Services Task Force. *Guide to Clinical Preventive Services 2006*. Baltimore, MD: Williams & Wilkins, 2006.

238. Hill AB. The environment and disease: association or causation. *Proc R Soc Med* 1965; 58:295–300.
239. Popper K. *The Logic of Scientific Discovery*. 11th ed. London: Hutchinson, 1983.
240. Gifford SM. The meaning of lumps: a case study of the ambiguities of risk. In: Janes CR, Stall R, Gifford SM, eds. *Anthropology and Epidemiology. Interdisciplinary Approaches to the Study of Health and Disease*. Dordrecht: Reidel, 1986. pp. 213–246.
241. Last JM. The iceberg. *Lancet* 1963; 2:28–31.
242. Heller RF, Dobson AJ, Attia J, Page J. Impact numbers: measures of risk factor impact on the whole population from case-control and cohort studies. *J Epidemiol Community Health* 2002; 56:606–610.
243. King RC, Stansfield WD, Mulligan PK. *A Dictionary of Genetics*. Oxford, UK: Oxford University Press, 2007.
244. Council for International Organizations of Medical Sciences. www.cioms.ch.
245. Relman AS. The Ingelfinger Rule. *N Engl J Med* 1981; 305:824–826.
246. Angell M, Kassirer JP. The Ingelfinger Rule revisited. *N Engl J Med* 1991; 325: 1371–1373.
247. Altman LK. The Ingelfinger rule, embargoes, and journal peer review. Part 1. *Lancet* 1996; 347:1382–1386. Part 2. *Lancet* 1996; 347:1459–1463.
248. Cavallis L, Feldman MW. Models for cultural inheritance.1: Group mean and within group variation. *Theoret Popul Biol* 1973; 4:42–55.
249. Cloninger CR, Rice J, Reich T. Multifactorial inheritance with cultural transmission and assortative mating. 2: General-model of combined polygenic and cultural inheritance. *Am J Hum Genet* 1979; 31:176–198.
250. McGue M, Rao DC, Iselius L, Russell JM. Resolution of genetic and cultural inheritance in twin families by path-analysis. application to HDL-cholesterol. *Am J Hum Genet* 1985; 37:998–1014.
251. Hamsten A, Defaire U, Iselius L, Blomback M. Genetic and cultural inheritance of plasma-fibrinogen concentration. *Lancet* 1987; 2:988–991.
252. Baker SP, O'Neill B, Ginsburg MJ, et al, eds. *The Injury Fact Book*. New York: Oxford University Press, 1992.
253. Hernán MA, Robins JM. Instruments for causal inference: an epidemiologist's dream? *Epidemiology* 2006; 17:360–372.
254. Porta M, Hernández-Aguado I, Lumbreras B, Crous-Bou M. "Omics" research, monetization of intellectual property and fragmentation of knowledge: can clinical epidemiology strengthen integrative research? *J Clin Epidemiol* 2007; 60:1220–1225.
255. Schwartz D, Lellouch J. Explanatory and pragmatic attitudes in therapeutic trials. *J Chronic Dis* 1967; 20:637–648.
256. Schwartz D, Flamant L, Lellouch J. *L'essai therapéutique chez l'homme*. 2nd ed. Paris: Flammarion, 1981.
257. Classification Committee of the World Organization of National Colleges, Academies, and Academic Associations of General Practitioners/Family Physicians (WONCA). *International Classification of Primary Care (ICPC-2)*. 2nd ed. Oxford, UK: Oxford University Press, 1998. www.globalfamilydoctor.com and www.woncaeurope.org.
258. Classification Committee of the World Organization of National Colleges, Academies, and Academic Associations of General Practitioners/Family Physicians (WONCA). *International Classification of Primary Care (ICPC-2-R)*. 2nd ed, rev. Oxford, UK: Oxford University Press, 2005.

259. Horton R. The rhetoric of research. *BMJ* 1995; 310:985–987.
260. Vandenbroucke JP. Medical journals and the shaping of medical knowledge. *Lancet* 1998; 352:2001–2006.
261. Rothenburg R, Ford ES, Vaitianen R. Ischemic heart disease: estimating the impact of interventions. *J Clin Epidemiol* 1992; 45:1:21–29.
262. Hernán MA, Robins JM. Estimating causal effects from epidemiological data. *J Epidemiol Community Health* 2006; 60:578–586.
263. Murphy EA. *The Logic of Medicine*. Baltimore: Johns Hopkins University Press, 1976. p. 16.
264. Jarman B. Identification of underprivileged areas. *Br Med J* 1983; 286:1705–1709.
265. Jellinek EM: The disease concept of alcoholism. New Haven, CT: College & University Press, 1960.
266. García AM, Checkoway H. A glossary for research in occupational health. *J Epidemiol Community Health* 2003; 57; 7–10.
267. Kaplan EL, Meier P. Non-parametric estimation for incomplete observations. *J Am Stat Assoc* 1958; 53:457–481.
268. Merz M. Knowledge construction. In: Restivo S, ed. *Science, Technology, and Society. An Encyclopedia*. Oxford, UK: Oxford University Press, 2005.
269. Carrat F, Valleron AJ. Epidemiologic mapping using the "Kriging" method: application to an influenza-like illness in France. *Am J Epidemiol* 1992; 135:1293–1300.
270. Ledermann S. *Alcool, Alcoolisme et Alcoolisation.* Paris: Presses Universitaires de France, 1956.
271. Holmes TH, Rahe RH. The social readjustment rating scale. *J Psychosom Res* 1967; 1:213–218.
272. Mantel N, Haenszel W. Statistical aspects of the analysis of data from retrospective studies of disease. *J Natl Cancer Inst* 1959; 22:719–748.
273. Robins JM, Hernán MA, Brumback B. Marginal structural models and causal inference in epidemiology. *Epidemiology* 2000; 11:550–560.
274. Hamer W. Epidemic disease in England. Lancet 1906; 1:733–739.
275. Fine PEM. Herd immunity: History, theory, practice. *Epidemiol Rev* 1993; 15:265–302.
276. Meade MS, Earickson RJ. *Medical Geography*. 2nd. ed. London: Guilford, 2005.
277. Learmonth ATA. *Disease Ecology. An Introduction*. Oxford: Blackwell, 1988.
278. Davey Smith G, Ebrahim S. "Mendelian randomization": can genetic epidemiology contribute to understanding environmental determinants of disease? *Int J Epidemiol* 2003; 32:1–22.
279. Dickerson K, Berlin JA. Meta-analysis: state of the science. *Epidemiol Rev* 1992; 14:154–176.
280. Petitti DB. *Meta-Analysis, Decision Analysis and Cost-Effectiveness Analysis: Methods for Quantitative Synthesis in Medicine*. 2nd ed. New York: Oxford University Press, 1999.
281. www.undp.org/mdg/basics.shtml.
282. McMichael AJ. "Molecular epidemiology": New pathway or new travelling companion? *Am J Epidemiol* 1994; 140:1–11.
283. Schulte PA, Perera FP. *Molecular Epidemiology. Principles and Practices*. Orlando, FL: Academic Press, 1993.
284. Carrington M, Hoelzel R. *Molecular Epidemiology*. New York: Oxford University Press, 2001.
285. Hunter DJ. The future of molecular epidemiology. *Int J Epidemiol* 1999; 28:S1012–S1014.

286. Stroup DF, Berlin JA, Morton SC, et al. Meta-analysis of observational studies in epidemiology (MOOSE) group. Meta-analysis of observational studies in epidemiology: a proposal for reporting. *JAMA* 2000; 283:2008–2012.
287. Diez-Roux A. Bringing context back into epidemiology: variables and fallacies in multilevel analysis. *Am J Public Health* 1998; 88:216–222.
288. Von Engelhardt D. Causality and conditionality in medicine around 1900. In: Delkeskamp-Hayes C, Cutter MAG, eds. *Science, Technology, and the Art of Medicine*. Dordrecht: Kluwer, 1993. pp. 75–104.
289. Snow J. *On the Mode of Communication of Cholera*. London; 1855.
290. Wright J, Williams R, Wilkinson JR. Development and importance of health needs assessment. *BMJ* 1998; 316:1310–1313.
291. Wacholder S, McLaughlin JK, Silverman DT, Mandel JS. Selection of controls in case-control studies. I. Principles. *Am J Epidemiol* 1992; 135:1019–1028. II. Types of controls. Am *J Epidemiol* 1992; 135:1029–1041. III. Design options. *Am J Epidemiol* 1992; 135:1042–1050.
292. Guyatt G, Sackett D, Taylor DW, et al. Determining optimal therapy: randomized trials in individual patients. *N Engl J Med* 1986; 314:889–892.
293. McLeod RS, Taylor DW, Cohen Z, Cullen JB. Single-patient randomised clinical trial. Use in determining optimum treatment for patient with inflammation of Kock continent ileostomy reservoir. *Lancet* 1986; 1:726–728.
294. Porta M. The search for more clinically meaningful research designs: single patient clinical trials [editorial]. *J Gen Intern Med* 1986; 1:418–419.
295. Shackelford RE, Kaufmann WK, Paules RS. Cell cycle control, checkpoint mechanisms, and genotoxic stress. *Environ Health Perspect* 1999; 107(Suppl 1):5–24.
296. Faber K. *Nosography in Modern Internal Medicine*. New York: Hoeber, 1923.
297. Laupacis A, Sackett DL, Roberts RS. An assessment of clinically useful measurements of the consequences of treatment. *N Engl J Med* 1988; 318:1728–1733.
298. Chatellier G, Zapletal E, Lemaitre D, et al. The number needed to treat: a clinically useful nomogram in its proper context. *BMJ* 1996; 312:426–429.
299. Checkoway H, Pearce N, Kriebel D. *Research Methods in Occupational Epidemiology*. 2nd ed. New York: Oxford University Press, 2004.
300. Monson RR. *Occupational Epidemiology*. 2nd ed. Boca Raton, FL: CRC Press, 1990.
301. Lowe EJ. *The Oxford Companion to Philosophy*. Oxford, UK: Oxford University Press, 2005.
302. Kuhn T. *The Structure of Scientific Revolutions*. Chicago: University of Chicago Press, 1962.
303. Strom BL, ed. *Pharmacoepidemiology*. 4th. ed. Chichester: Wiley, 2005.
304. Porta M, Carné X. Pharmacoepidemiology. In: Trichopoulos D, Olsen J, eds. *Teaching of Epidemiology*. Oxford, UK: Oxford University Press, 1992. pp. 285–304.
305. Pickles WN. *Epidemiology in Country Practice*. Bristol: John Wright, 1939.
306. Porta M, Alvarez-Dardet C. Epidemiology: bridges over (and across) roaring levels [editorial]. *J Epidemiol Community Health* 1998; 52:605.
307. Franco A, Álvarez-Dardet C, Ruiz MT. Effect of democracy on health: ecological study. *BMJ* 2004; 329:1421–1424.
308. Morgan LM. Political economy of health. In: Restivo S, ed. *Science, Technology, and Society. An Encyclopedia*. Oxford, UK: Oxford University Press, 2005.

309. Vineis P, Malats N, Lang M, et al, eds. *Metabolic Polymorphisms and Susceptibility to Cancer.* IARC Scientific Publications, no. 148. Lyon, France: International Agency for Research on Cancer, 1999.
310. MacMahon B, Pugh TF. *Epidemiology. Principles and Methods*. Boston: Little, Brown, 1970.
311. Cole P, MacMahon B. Attributable risk percent in case-control studies. *Br J Prev Soc Med* 1971; 25:242–244.
312. Young TK. *Population Health. Concepts and Methods*. New York: Oxford University Press, 1998.
313. Beaglehole R, Bonita R, Kjellström T. *Basic Epidemiology*. Geneva: WHO, 1993. pp. 85–88.
314. Bentzen N, ed. *WONCA Dictionary of General/Family Practice*. Copenhagen: Laegeforeningens Forlag, 2003.
315. Frank E. Osler was wrong: you are a preventionist. *Am J Prev Med* 1991; 7:128.
316. Hannaford PC, Smith BH, Elliott AM. Primary care epidemiology: its scope and purpose. *Family Practice* 2006; 23:1–7.
317. Starfield B. *Primary Care: Concept, Evaluation and Policy*. New York: Oxford University Press, 1992.
318. World Health Organization. *Glossary of Terms Used in the Health for All Series, No. 1–8*. Geneva: WHO, 1984.
319. Olsen J, Bréart G, Saracci R, et al., on behalf of the International Epidemiological Association—IEA European Epidemiology Group. Directive of the European Parliament and of the Council on the protection of individuals with regard to the processing of personal data and on the free movement of such data. *Int J Epidemiol* 1995; 24:462–463.
320. Weed LL. Medical records that guide and teach. *N Engl J Med* 1968; 278:593–600, 652–657.
321. Feinstein AR. *Clinical Epidemiology. The Architecture of Clinical Research*. Philadelphia: Saunders, 1985.
322. Feinstein AR. Clinical biostatistics: LVII. A glossary of neologisms in quantitative clinical science. *Clin Pharmacol Ther* 1981; 30:564–577.
323. D'Agostino RB Jr. Propensity score methods for bias reduction in the comparison of a treatment to a non-randomized control group. *Stat Med* 1998; 17:2265–2281.
324. *Public Health in England: The Report of the Committee of Inquiry into the Future Development of the Public Health Function*. Cmnd 289. London: HMSO, 1988.
325. *Higher Education for Public Health: A Report of the Milbank Memorial Fund Commission*. New York: Milbank Memorial Fund, 1976.
326. European Observatory on Health Systems and Policies. Research topics: Health impact assessment. www.euro.who.int/observatory.
327. Whiting P, Rutjes AW, Reitsma JB, et al. The development of QUADAS: a tool for the quality assessment of studies of diagnostic accuracy included in systematic reviews. *BMC Med Res Methodol* 2003; 3:25.
328. Schwandt TA. *Qualitative Inquiry: A Dictionary of Terms*. Thousand Oaks, CA: Sage Publications, 1997.
329. Donabedian A. A. *Guide to Medical Care Administration*. Vol 2. New York: American Public Health Association, 1969.
330. Moher D, Cook DJ, Eastwood S, et al. Improving the quality of reports of meta-analyses of randomised controlled trials: the QUOROM statement. *Lancet* 1999; 354:1896–1900.

331. *A Dictionary of Biology*. Oxford, UK: Oxford University Press, 2004.
332. Omi M, Winant H. On the theoretical status of the concept of race. In: McCarthy C, Crichlow W, eds. *Race, Identity and Representation*. New York: Routledge, 1993:1–9.
333. Rapid epidemiological assessment. *Int J Epidemiol* 1989; 18 (Suppl 2):S1-S67.
334. *Newcombe HB. Handbook of Record Linkage*. Oxford, UK: Oxford Medical Publications, 1988.
335. Dunn HL. Record linkage. *Am J Public Health* 1946; 36:1412.
336. Lambert ML, Hasker, E, Van Deun A, Roberfroid D, Boelaert M, Van der Stuyft P. Recurrence in tuberculosis: relapse or reinfection? *Lancet Inf Dis* 2003; 3:282–287.
337. Wilcox AJ. The analysis of recurrence risk as an epidemiological tool. *Paediatr Perinat Epidemiol* 2007; 21(Suppl 1):4–7.
338. World Health Organization. International Union against Tuberculosis and Lung Disease, Royal Netherlands Tuberculosis Association. Revised international definitions in tuberculosis control. *Int J Tuberc Lung Dis* 2001; 5:213–215.
339. Vickers GR. What sets the goals of public health? *Lancet* 1958; 1:599–604.
340. Fox JP, Elveback L, Scott, W, et al. Herd immunity: Basic concept and relevance to public health immunization practices. *Am J Epidemiol* 1971; 94:179–189.
341. Goldberg J, Gelfand HM, Levy PS. Registry evaluation methods. *Epidemiol Rev* 1980; 2:210–220.
342. World Health Organization, International Union against Tuberculosis and lung disease, Royal Netherlands Tuberculosis Association. Revised international definitions in tuberculosis control. *Int J Tuberc Lung Dis* 2001; 5:213–215.
343. Verver S, Warren RM, Beyers N, et al. Rate of reinfection tuberculosis alter successful treatment is higer than rate of new tuberculosis. *Am J Resp Crit Med Care Med* 2005; 17:1430–1435.
344. Suissa S. Relative excess risk: an alternative measure of comparative risk. *Am J Epidemiol* 1999; 150:279–282.
345. Patrick DL, Erickson P. *Health Status and Health Policy: Allocating Resources to Health Care.* New York: Oxford University Press, 1993.
346. Dawber TR, Kannel WB, Revotskie N, et al. Some factors associated with the development of coronary heart disease: six years' follow-up experience in the Framingham study. *Am J Public Health* 1959; 49:1349–56.
347. Bailey JE. Lessons from metabolic engineering for functional genomics and drug discovery. *Nature Biotechnol* 1999; 17:616–618.
348. Feinstein AR. The Santayana syndrome. I: Errors in getting and interpreting evidence. *Perspect Biol Med* 1997; 41:45–57.
349. Feinstein AR. The Santayana syndrome. II: Problems in reasoning and learning about error. *Perspect Biol Med* 1997; 41:73–85.
350. Santayana G. Reason in common sense. In: *The Life of Reason*. Vol. 1. New York: Scribner's, 1905 (Amherst, NY: Prometheus Books, 1998).
351. Sartwell PE. The incubation period of infectious diseases. *Am J Hygiene* 1950; 51:310–318.
352. Brouwer JJ, Schreuder RF. *Scenarios and Other Methods to Support Long Term Health Planning.* Utrecht: Jan van Arkel, 1988.
353. Medawar P. *Pluto's Republic. The Art of the Soluble. Induction and Intuition in Scientific Thought.* Oxford, UK: Oxford University Press, 1984.
354. Wilson JMG, Jungner G. *The Principles and Practice of Screening for Disease*. Geneva: WHO, 1968.

355. Raffle AE, Gray M. *Screening. Evidence and Practice*. Oxford, UK: Oxford University Press, 2007.
356. Hernán MA, Hernández-Díaz S, Robins JM. A structural approach to selection bias. *Epidemiology* 2004; 15:615–625.
357. Olson SH, Voigt LF, Begg CB, Weiss NS. Reporting participation in case-control studies. *Epidemiology* 2002; 13:123–126.
358. Kunzli N, Tager IB. The semi-individual study in air pollution epidemiology: a valid design as compared to ecologic studies. *Environ Health Perspect* 1997; 105:1078–1083.
359. Colman AM. *A Dictionary of Psychology*. Oxford, UK: Oxford University Press, 2006.
360. Schneeweiss S. Sensitivity analysis and external adjustment for unmeasured confounders in epidemiologic database studies of therapeutics. *Pharmacoepidemiol Drug Safety* 2006; 15:291–303.
361. Rothman KJ. A pictorial representation of confounding in epidemiologic studies. *J Chronic Dis* 1975; 28:101–108.
362. Reintjes R et al. Simpson's paradox: an example from hospital epidemiology. *Epidemiology* 2000; 11:1–3.
363. Berkman LF, Kawachi I. *Social Epidemiology*. New York: Oxford University Press, 2000.
364. Marmot M, Wilkinson RG. *Social Determinants of Health*. 2nd ed. New York: Oxford University Press, 2005.
365. Krieger N. Sticky webs, hungry spiders, buzzing flies, and fractal metaphors: on the misleading juxtaposition of "risk factor" versus "social" epidemiology. *J Epidemiol Community Health* 1999; 53:678–680.
366. Berkman LF, Breslow L. *Health and Ways of Living: The Alameda County Study*. New York: Oxford University Press, 1983.
367. Galobardes B, Lynch J, Davey-Smith G. Measuring socioeconomic position in health research. *Br Med Bull* 2007; 81–82:21–37.
368. Alexander F. Estimation of sojourn time distributions and false negative rates in screening programmes which use two modalities. *Stat Med* 1989; 8:743–755.
369. Ransohoff DF, Feinstein AR. Problems of spectrum and bias in evaluating the efficacy of diagnostic tests. *N Engl J Med* 1978; 299:926–930.
370. Mulherin SA, Miller WC. Spectrum bias or spectrum effect? Subgroup variation in diagnostic test evaluation. *Ann Intern Med* 2002; 137:598–602.
371. Bossuyt PM, Reitsma JB, Bruns DE, et al. Towards complete and accurate reporting of studies of diagnostic accuracy: the STARD initiative. *BMJ* 2003; 326:41–44.
372. Leeflang M, Reitsma J, Scholten R, et al. Impact of adjustment for quality on results of metaanalyses of diagnostic accuracy. *Clin Chem* 2007; 53:164–172.
373. Von Elm E, Altman D, Egger M, et al. Strengthening the reporting of observational studies in epidemiology: the STROBE statement. *Prev Med* 2007;45:247–251.
374. Centers for Disease Control. *Comprehensive Plan for Epidemiologic Surveillance*. Atlanta, GA: CDC, 1996.
375. Estève J, Benhamou E, Croasdale M, Raymond L. Relative survival and the estimation of net survival: elements for further discussion. *Stat Med* 1990; 9:529–538.
376. Vineis P. Individual susceptibility to carcinogens. *Oncogene* 2004; 23:6477–6483.
377. Hirschhorn JN, Lohmueller K, Byrne E, Hirschhorn K. A comprehensive review of genetic association studies. *Genet Med* 2002; 4:45–61.
378. Zolg W. The proteomic search for diagnostic biomarkers: lost in translation? *Mol Cell Proteomics* 2006; 5:1720–1726.

379. Torrance GW. The measurement of health status utilities for economic appraisal. A review. *J Health Economics* 1986; 5:1–30.
380. Townsend P, Phillimore P, Beattie A. *Health and Deprivation: Inequality and the North*. London: Croom Helm, 1988.
381. Kessner DM, Snow CK, Singer J. *Assessment of Medical Care for Children*. Washington DC: National Academy of Sciences, Institute of Medicine, 1974.
382. Transdisciplinarity. Stimulating Synergies, Integrating Knowledge. Paris: UNESCO, 1998. http://unesdoc.unesco.org/images/0011/001146/114694eo.pdf
383. Des Jarlais DC, Lyles C, Crepaz N. TREND Group. Improving the reporting quality of nonrandomized evaluations of behavioral and public health interventions: the TREND statement. *Am J Public Health* 2004; 94:361–366.
384. http://www.who.int/mediacentre/factsheets/fs104/en.
385. Porter JDH, McAdam KPWJ. The re-emergence of tuberculosis. *Annu Rev Public Health* 1994; 15:303–323.
386. Webb EJ, Campbell DT, Schwartz RD, Sechrest L. *Unobtrusive Measures*. Chicago: Rand McNally, 1966.
387. Khoury MJ. *Human Genome Epidemiology. A Scientific Foundation for Using Genetic Information to Improve Health and Prevent Disease*. New York: Oxford University Press, 2003.
388. Chandramohan D, Maude GH, Rodriques LC, Hayes RJ. Verbal autopsies for adult deaths: Issues in their development and validation. *Int J Epidemiol* 1994; 23:213–230.
389. Von Neumann J, Morgenstern O. *Theory of Games and Economic Behavior*. Princeton, NJ: Princeton University Press, 1944.
390. Dawber TR, Kannel WB, Revotskie N, et al. Some factors associated with the development of coronary heart disease: six years' follow-up experience in the Framingham study. *Am J Public Health* 1959; 49:1349–1356.
391. MacMahon B, Pugh TF, Ipsen J. *Epidemiologic Methods*. Boston: Little, Brown, 1960.
392. Zelen M. The randomization and stratification of patients to clinical trials. *J Chronic Dis* 1974; 27:365–373.
393. Robins JM. The Analysis of randomized and non-randomized AIDS treatment trials using a new approach to causal inference in longitudinal studies. Health Service Research Methodology: A Focus on AIDS. In: Sechrest L, Freeman H, Mulley A, eds. Washington, DC: U.S. Public Health Service, National Center for Health Services Research, 1989; 113–159.
394. Robins JM, Hernán MA. Estimation of the causal effects of time-varying exposures. In: Fitzmaurice G, Davidian M, Verbeke G, Molenberghs G, eds. Advances in Longitudinal Data Analysis. New York: Chapman and Hall/CRC Press, 2008.
395. Norman G, Description and prescription in dictionaries of scientific terms. Int J Lexicography 2002; 15:259–276.